Atlas of Diagnostic Cytopathology

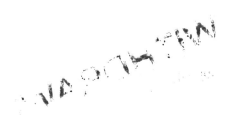

For Churchill Livingstone

Commissioning Editor: Gavin Smith
Copy Editor: Liz Graham
Project Controller: Sarah Lowe
Cover Design: Jeanette Jacobs
Indexer: Monica Trigg

Atlas of Diagnostic Cytopathology

Gabrijela Kocjan

Consultant Cytopathologist, University College Hospital, London

SECOND EDITION

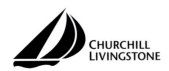

CHURCHILL
LIVINGSTONE

NEW YORK EDINBURGH LONDON MADRID MELBOURNE SAN FRANCISCO TOKYO 1997

CHURCHILL LIVINGSTONE
Medical Division of Pearson Professional Limited

Distributed in the United States of America by
Churchill Livingstone Inc., 650 Avenue of the Americas, New York,
N.Y. 10011, and by associated companies, branches and
representatives throughout the world.

First published 1988
Second Edition 1997

ISBN 0 443 05174 7

British Library Cataloguing in Publication Data
A catalogue record for this book is available from the British Library.

Library of Congress Cataloging in Publication Data
A catalog record for this book is available from the Library of Congress.

The
publisher's
policy is to use
**paper manufactured
from sustainable forests**

Produced by Longman Asia Ltd, Hong Kong
WW/01

Contents

Preface to the First Edition   vi

Preface to the Second Edition   vii

1. Female reproductive system   1

2. Breast   52

3. Respiratory tract   83

4. Serous effusions   130

5. Cerebrospinal fluid   165

6. Oesophagogastrointestinal tract   173

7. Pancreas, liver and extrahepatic bile ducts   184

8. Urinary system   207

9. Male genital system   218

10. Lymph nodes and thymus   225

11. Cytology of salivary glands   236

12. Skin and subcutaneous lesions   250

13. Thyroid   257

14. Bone and soft tissue   272

15. Cellular changes due to treatment   297

Index   305

Preface to the first edition

Recent years have seen a virtually explosive increase in the demand for cytopathology services. The reasons are simple. Cytopathology can be applied to spontaneously desquamated cells in a large proportion of cases. Its scope has been greatly extended by technical advances in fibre-optic endoscopy and interventional radiology. The morbidity associated with invasive methods required to obtain cytological specimens is significantly lower than with methods employed to obtain a formal biopsy. Furthermore, cytology is rapid and cost-effective.

The demand is expected to be met by increasing numbers of trainee histopathologists whose curriculum now includes cytopathology, medical laboratory scientists whose traditional role as cytoscreeners of cervical smears is widened to include newer techniques, and pathologists whose interests were formerly confined to histopathology.

The provision of an expert cytopathology service rests on correct interpretation of cytological artefacts; this in turn, rests on study and experience. This book is intended to help towards that study. It has been designed as a text atlas in which the relatively new brush and aspiration techniques are included with exfoliative cytology in the consideration of organ systems. The specially prepared illustrations are of specimens submitted to a diagnostic and teaching laboratory and represent its day to day work. The two staining procedures favoured by most cytology laboratories and routinely used in the author's department are the Papanicolaou and the Romanowsky methods; both are represented in the book. Special staining methods, including immunocytochemical procedures, have been included where appropriate. The text has been designed to provide background information and teaching discussion in addition to descriptive legends. In some instances, selected cases have been included to reinforce a clinical or diagnostic point.

Guidelines to the cytodiagnostic approach to malignancy, applicable to all types of tumours and all tissue systems, have been placed in a separate introductory chapter.

Moraira, Spain   Chandra Grubb
1988

Preface to the second edition

It is with great enthusiasm that I have taken up the challenge of preparing the second edition of this popular cytology atlas, which already has a firmly established place on our laboratory benches. My task was to fill in on some of the areas where progress in diagnostic techniques has been made in recent years, e.g. fine needle aspiration (FNA) and immunocytochemistry; to introduce some of the newly recognized pathological conditions, particularly those associated with the HIV-AIDS spectrum of conditions; and to update some of the diagnostic concepts, particularly in cervical cytology, which are constantly under review after the introduction of population-based cervical screening in Britain.

Following on from the above, the second edition contains a greatly expanded number of illustrations mainly associated with new chapters on pancreas and liver, salivary gland, thyroid, and soft tissue cytology. It also contains many new illustrations within the existing chapters, in particular within the chapters on fluid, lymph node, breast and cervical cytology, incorporating newly described entities and immunocytochemistry. The revised and updated text takes account of current scientific concepts while maintaining the practical approach aimed at the diagnostic cytopathologist. The atlas as a whole attempts to cover the main areas likely to be encountered in the daily work, with common pathologies featuring prominently, whilst showing examples of some of the rarer conditions and diagnostic pitfalls.

My thanks go to all the clinicians who provided the samples illustrated in this edition, in particular Mr A. C. Silverstone, Dr R. F. Miller, Dr M. F. Spittle, Mr T. Davidson, Dr A. Schneidau and other members of the University College London Hospitals. I am also grateful to all those cytopathologists who contributed illustrations of rare cases. This edition would not have been possible without the support of the technical staff and my colleagues in the department, in particular Dr A. Nisbet Smith. My gratitude is also for my teachers and mentors, Dr Z. Znidarcic-Bauer of the University of Zagreb, Croatia and Dr O. A. N. Husain of Charing Cross Hospital, London, who have inspired my love of cells. Finally, my task would not have been such a pleasure without the support and encouragement of my family for which I am deeply grateful.

Gabrijela Kocjan
London, 1995

1. Female reproductive system

The female reproductive system consists of the ovaries, the genital tract and the breasts. The genital tract comprises the two oviducts or fallopian tubes, the uterus, the vagina and the vulva. The fimbrial ends of the fallopian tubes are open to the peritoneal cavity close to the ovaries. The uterus is divided into the body or corpus uteri and a neck—the cervix uteri—part of which protrudes into the vagina (pars vaginalis). The fallopian tubes and the uterine corpus constitute the upper genital tract; the cervix, vagina and vulva form the lower genital tract.

The entire tract has an outer wall of smooth muscle, an internal mucosal lining and an intervening layer of loose connective tissue. The muscle coat is thickest in the uterine corpus. The connective tissue of the cervix is rich in collagen fibres which interlace with the fibres of its muscle coat. The mucosa lining varies greatly in morphology and function in the different parts of the tract.

The vagina and the vaginal aspect of the cervix are lined by an identical protective, non-keratinized, stratified, squamous epithelium. The endocervical canal is lined by a simple mucus-secreting columnar epithelium which invaginates the mucocollagenous substance of the cervix to form deep branching crypts. The junction between the ectocervical squamous epithelium and the endocervical columnar epithelium (squamocolumnar junction) is an abrupt one and usually coincides with the external os, the opening of the endocervical canal into the vagina. At the internal os at the upper end of the canal, the endocervical mucosa merges into the endometrium, the mucosal lining of the body of the uterus. The fallopian tubes are lined by ciliated and non-ciliated columnar cells.

THE OVARIAN CYCLE

From puberty to menopause, the reproductive system is subject to repeated hormonal cycles programmed to produce mature ova and to prepare a suitable environment in the endometrium for the implantation of a fertilized ovum. If pregnancy occurs, the cycle is suspended at this stage.

The ovary, at birth, contains numerous primordial follicles, each composed of a germ cell surrounded by a single row of flattened granulosa or follicular cells. The ovarian cycle is initiated after sexual maturity is reached. Under the influence of the follicle-stimulating hormone (FSH) of the anterior pituitary, several primordial follicles begin to mature. The granulosa cells multiply and the surrounding stromal cells are organized into a theca interna and a theca externa. Rising levels of circulating oestrogen secreted by the cells of the theca interna induce proliferation of the endometrium, inhibit FSH and initiate release of the luteinizing hormone (LH) by the anterior pituitary. As a rule only one follicle matures into a Graafian follicle; the rest undergo atresia and plasma oestrogen levels drop.

The mature Graafian follicle ruptures to release an ovum and under the influence of LH is converted into a corpus luteum. The luteinized theca interna cells continue to secrete oestrogen, the granulosa cells enlarge into granulosa lutein cells and begin secretion of progesterone which promotes secretory activity in the endometrium. A feedback mechanism operates via the hypothalamus whereby rising levels of progesterone inhibit the continued secretion of LH. The corpus luteum regresses into an inactive corpus albicans, production of oestrogen and progesterone ceases, the endometrium is shed in the menstrual flow and a new cycle commences.

The menstrual cycle is of variable duration but usually takes 28 days and is divided into the menstrual phase (days 1–4), the preovulatory proliferative phase (days 5–14) and the postovulatory secretory phase (days 15–28). Ovulation usually occurs at or immediately prior to day 15 of a 28-day cycle. Although the histological and functional cyclical changes are most marked in the endometrium, subtler changes occur in parallel in the vaginal and cervical epithelia.

The specimens illustrated in this section are cervical scrape smears except where otherwise stated.

Squamous epithelium

The vaginal and ectocervical squamous epithelium of a woman in the child-bearing years may be divided into four strata:

1. Stratum germinativum or the basal layer consists of a single row of vertically oriented cuboidal cells.
2. Stratum spinosum profundum or the parabasal zone has several layers of larger polygonal cells.
3. Stratum spinosum superficiale or the intermediate zone is subdivided into an inner zone of ovoid cells and an outer zone of large polyhedral cells.
4. Stratum superficiale or the superficial layer is made up of large flat polyhedral cells with pyknotic nuclei.

Cell division occurs in the basal germinal layer. Thereafter, the postmitotic cells do not divide further but mature and move towards the surface. In the course of maturation, they undergo morphological and functional differentiation through the parabasal and intermediate stages into superficial cells which are continuously exfoliated. In a vital process the changes are gradual and cells will be met which appear to be transitional between arbitrarily separated strata.

The extent of maturation, the thickness of the different strata and the cohesiveness of the cells vary with the stage of the menstrual cycle. The date of ovulation preferred in some countries as day 1 of the menstrual cycle is a convenient and customary starting point for the study of changing cell patterns in smears. The cells seen, whether desquamated or scraped, come from the upper few layers; deeper layer cells are not normally recovered from an intact mature squamous epithelium.

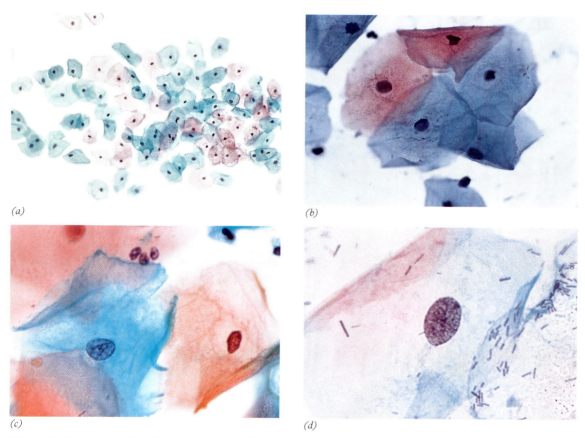

(a)   (b)   (c)   (d)

Fig. 1.1 Superficial and outer intermediate squamous cells

(a) Papanicolaou ×840 (b) ×1260 (c) ×2100 (d) ×2100

The superficial and outer intermediate cells are the end-point in the differentiation of the oestrogen-responsive squamous epithelium of the vagina and ectocervix. They are large flat polyhedral cells, approximately 60 mm in diameter, generally eosinophilic (a) and occasionally cyanophilic (b, c). Distanced from its submucosal source of nourishment, superficial cell is characterized by a pyknotic nucleus of 5 mm or less (a–c) whilst intermediate cell has a larger, round, open, viable nucleus (c, d).

The proportion of superficial cells, low at the commencement of a menstrual cycle, increases progressively during the proliferative phase and peaks at 60–80% of cell population at the time of ovulation. The fully oestrogenized mid-cycle smear is typically sparse and the background is clear apart from the normal bacterial flora (d). The cells are mainly dissociated and flat, eosinophilic, superficial cells dominate the picture.

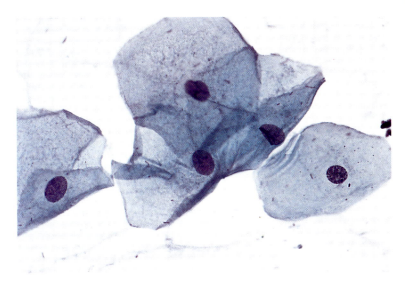

Fig. 1.2 Navicular cells

Papanicolaou ×1740: mid-secretory vaginal smear

In the postovulatory luteal phase, the proportion of superficial and intermediate squamous cells is reversed. As progesterone levels rise and the secretory phase progresses, the smear becomes more cellular and consists mainly of sheets of closely adherent, inner intermediate cells, referred to as navicular cells on account of their boat-like shape. The individual navicular cell is smaller than the outer intermediate cell and has a thick rolled edge and a thinner centre. This appearance is due to an abundance of glycogen which is aggregated in the central part of the cell around or near the usually eccentric nucleus. The glycogen sometimes imparts a yellow-brown tinge to the Papanicolaou-stained cytoplasm (possibly due to the counterstain Bismarck brown). Navicular cells are most abundant in the mid secretory phase and in the early weeks of pregnancy.

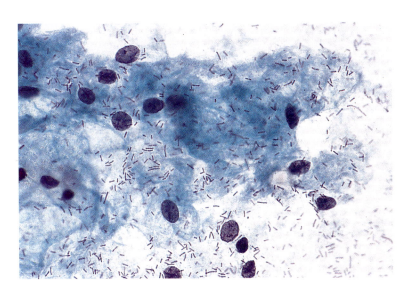

Fig. 1.3 Cytolytic pattern. Döderlein bacilli

Papanicolaou ×1740: premenstrual vaginal smear

In the last few days of the secretory phase which correspond with the formation of the inert corpus albicans, and the imminent dissolution of the endometrium, the intermediate squamous cells disintegrate and the smear is covered with fragments of cytoplasm and stripped nuclei. Slender commensal bacilli, present throughout the cycle, become more conspicuous amongst the cell debris. These bacilli, known as Döderlein's bacilli, form lactic acid by anaerobic metabolism of the epithelial glycogen and thereby produce and maintain the acid pH of a healthy vagina.

Endocervical columnar cells

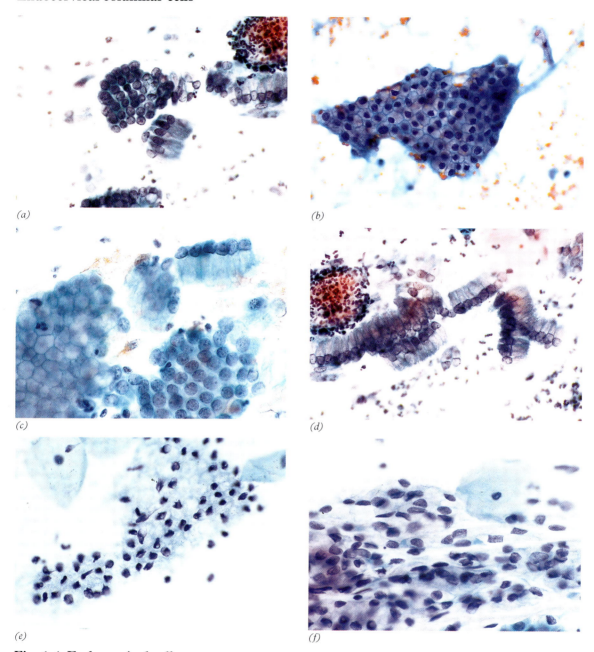

(a)   (b)

(c)   (d)

(e)   (f)

Fig. 1.4 Endocervical cells

(a) Papanicolaou ×840 (b) ×1260 (c) ×1260 (d) ×840 (e) ×840 (f) ×1260

A smear taken from the squamocolumnar junction contains endocervical, mucus-secreting columnar cells in addition to ectocervical squamous cells. The columnar cells are tall, slender and cylindrical (a). They appear singly or, more commonly, in sheets (b). Viewed in profile, they appear in a palisade with basally located nuclei (c); in cross-section they are arranged in a characteristic honeycomb pattern (b, d). Some alteration occurs in the height and distension of the columnar cells during the menstrual cycle but is not of particular note; cyclical changes in the quality of their secretion are of greater significance. The mucus secreted is alkaline. During the proliferative phase, it is quite thin. At the time of ovulation, it becomes thinner still to facilitate the entry of the spermatozoa into the uterine cavity, and may flow into the vagina as a mid-cycle 'discharge'. In response to postovulatory progesterone, the mucus becomes viscid, plugs the external os and provides a protective barrier against invasion of the uterine cavity by infective organisms. In addition, the cervical mucus lubricates the vaginal epithelium and obviates the need for further squamous differentiation to the level of keratin formation. Due to the presence of mucus, cytoplasmic outline is sometimes vague and nucleus pushed to the periphery of the cell (e). Smears taken with cytobrush often contain distorted endocervical cells (f).

NORMAL POSTMENOPAUSAL AND POSTNATAL PATTERNS

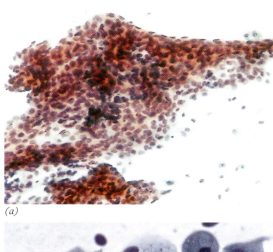

(a)

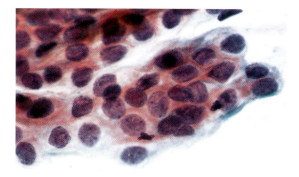

(b)

Fig. 1.5 Atrophic squamous cells

Papanicolaou (a) ×133 (b) ×525 (c) ×1260

Atrophic smears are those obtained from peri- or postmenopausal women, postnatal or breast-feeding women and women with low oestrogen or progestogen levels. These smears are often scanty and air-dried. 'Normal' atrophic smears contain: cells forming a 'crazy paving' or pavement-like pattern due to air-drying; cells with a high nuclear-cytoplasmic ratio; cells with dense orangeophilic cytoplasm with smaller cells looking as though they have denser cytoplasm and nuclei than larger ones; a variation in cytoplasmic staining, often of an orange-yellow hue; nuclear pyknosis and karyorrhexis.

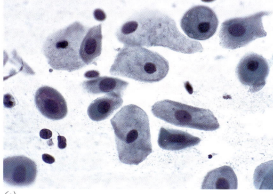

(c)

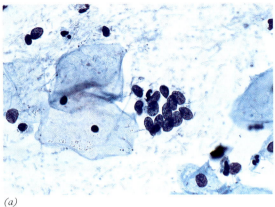

(a)   (b)

Fig. 1.6 Reserve cells

(a) Papanicolaou ×1260 (b) ×1260

Reserve cells represent a basal layer of epithelium which is rarely seen in smears. Cells are small, oval, have no discernible cytoplasm (a), often in loose aggregates showing branching. Their chromatin is uniformly dense and, although occasionally hyperchromatic, they are very uniform in appearance. They are most commonly seen in atrophic smears but may be seen in mature cell smears as a reflection of reserve cell hyperplasia (a).

SQUAMOUS METAPLASIA

In addition to the effect on the mucosal lining of the genital tract, the female sex hormones, particularly oestrogen, induce expansion of the collagen-rich cervical stroma, thereby increasing its bulk. The cervix becomes everted at the external os and the lower end of the endocervical mucosa is exposed to the vagina. The subepithelial vasculature, visible through the simple columnar epithelium, imparts a red colour to the area around the os. This appearance, the result of anatomical cervical ectropion, is referred to in common clinical practice as cervical erosion—a misleading term as the cervical mucosa is in no way eroded.

The normal pH of the endocervical canal is alkaline. Exposure of the endocervical mucosa to the acid environment of the vagina stimulates the formation of a protective squamous epithelium. The process begins peripherally at the squamocolumnar junction and extends inwards until the exposed columnar epithelium is replaced by a newly formed metaplastic squamous epithelium. The cervix now has two epithelial junctions: a distal one between the native and metaplastic squamous epithelia and a proximal junction between the metaplastic squamous epithelium and columnar epithelium.

The formation of the metaplastic epithelium begins initially below an intact columnar cell layer. Opinions vary as to the origin of the progenitor cell. One theory is that of a bipotential, subcylindrical reserve cell which normally replenishes the columnar cell layer, but is capable of squamous differentiation if suitably stimulated. Another theory, advanced more recently, is that of a migrant stromal cell which crosses the basement membrane and comes to lie below the mucous layer.

Cervical ectopy occurs to some extent in each menstrual cycle, but is most marked at puberty, pregnancy, postpartum and with some steroid oral contraceptives. The maternal hormones may exert a similar effect on a female neonate (erosion of the newborn). Squamous metaplasia will be seen to be a normal physiological response to environmental changes. It is, however, less stable than native squamous epithelium, and may become the site of neoplasia. Cervical ectropion covered with columnar and metaplastic squamous epithelium is referred to as the transformation zone.

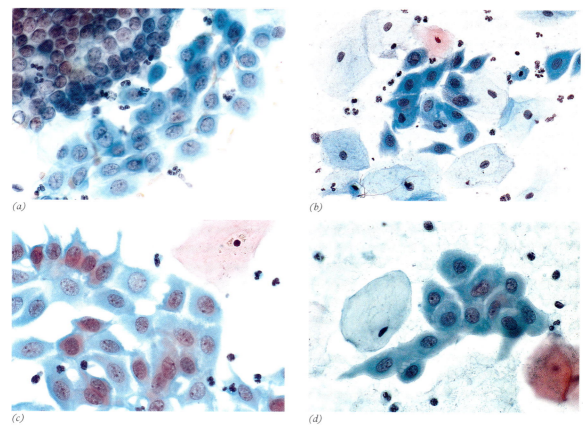

(a) *(b)* *(c)* *(d)*

Fig. 1.7 Squamous metaplasia

(a) Papanicolaou ×1260 (b) ×840 (c) ×1260 (d) ×1260

Cells from squamous metaplasia are polygonal or oval with a centrally placed oval nucleus. Nuclear characteristics are very similar to endocervical columnar cells (a) in that they are oval rather than round and have a discrete nucleolus. Cytoplasm is more or less plentiful depending on the maturity of the metaplastic epithelium and is usually densely cyanophilic compared to 'native' squamous cells (b). Nuclear–cytoplasmic ratio is higher than in mature squamous epithelium (b, d). Metaplastic cells form flat sheets with 'pulled-out' edges (c). Cells at the edges resemble kites, the pointed ends corresponding to intercellular bridges (c, d).

ENDOMETRIAL CELLS

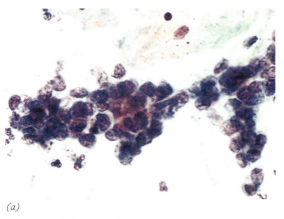

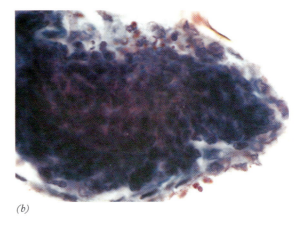

(a)   *(b)*

Fig. 1.8 Menstrual smear

Papanicolaou ×525: vaginal smear (a) endometrial glandular cells (b) endometrial stromal cells

The menstrual smear contains blood, macrophages and two types of endometrial cells. The exfoliated glandular cell is two to three times the size of a neutrophil, and is usually round with a narrow rim of cytoplasm virtually filled with a hyperchromatic granular nucleus (a). Degenerative changes are common and some nuclei may be pyknotic. The stromal cells are slender and elongated and have fusiform nuclei. Both types appear in a menstrual smear in substantial-sized clusters and the stromal cells are often seen on the periphery of a cone-shaped aggregate of cells, surrounding centrally positioned glandular cells (b).

Menstruation is preceded by ischaemic necrosis of the endometrium and endometrial cells are almost always present in a smear a day or two before the onset of overt bleeding. They are most abundant during the 3–5 days of the menstrual flow, but a few may persist to the 10th day of a normal cycle. They may be seen at mid-cycle on the rare occasion when rupture of the Graafian follicle is associated with a transient bleed. Desquamation of endometrial cells at times other than these is abnormal and may be caused by hormonal disturbances, underlying pathology or a local irritant such as an intrauterine contraceptive device (IUCD). The end of menstruation is marked by an outpouring of histiocytes; this appearance is known as the exodus.

Histiocytes

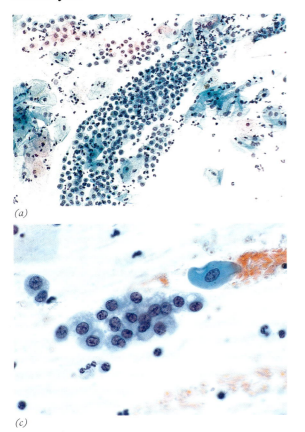

(a)

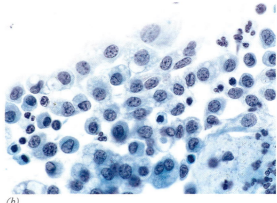

(b)

Fig. 1.9

(a) Papanicolaou ×420 (b) ×1260 (c) ×1260

Histiocytes may be found in menstrual smears, postcoital smears and a variety of inflammatory conditions. They often appear in streaks of single cells admixed with other inflammatory cells (a). High-power view reveals a single-cell population of cells with eccentrically placed nuclei and finely vacuolated cytoplasm (b). Nuclei are indented, kidney-shaped and vary in size. Their chromatin is clumped. Histiocytes can be mistaken for metaplastic cells although both nuclear and cytoplasmic features are different (c). Occasionally it is difficult to distinguish them from a hypochromatic metaplastic type of cervical intraepithelial neoplasia type 3 (CIN 3) cells (see Fig. 1.27a–c).

(c)

INFLAMMATORY SMEARS, EPITHELIAL REPAIR AND BORDERLINE NUCLEAR CHANGES

The presence of neutrophils in cervical smears does not necessarily denote inflammation. They can be present during various stages of the menstrual cycle, pregnancy and in postcoital smears. Similarly, the presence of bacteria, e.g. *Gardnerella vaginalis*, does not necessarily result in inflammatory cell changes.

Inflammatory cell changes include a spectrum of minor changes affecting both nucleus and cytoplasm. These reflect both increased cell activity and degeneration. Nuclei show mild enlargement, bi- and multinucleation, chromatin clumping, karyopyknosis and karyorrhexis. Cytoplasm may show perinuclear halo, polychromasia and vacuolation.

Epithelial repair is a term applied to regenerating, usually metaplastic epithelium of the transformation zone in which the cells show nuclei 1–2.5 times larger than intermediate cells. The nucleoli are very prominent and these cells can be mistaken for neoplasia. The key to their benign nature is the uniformly granular chromatin pattern, preserved nuclear-cytoplasmic ratio, their arrangement in flat sheets with evidence of cytoplasmic differentiation and 'pulled-out' edges. Polymorphs may be admixed to the epithelial cells and the clinical impression is usually that of erosion. It is our experience that these changes are most pronounced in very young patients, usually under the age of 20, but can occur at any age, usually following recent therapy, e.g. radiation, cauterization or biopsy.

The term *borderline* abnormality is used in cases where there is doubt as to whether cell changes are inflammatory or neoplastic. It is, so far, a management category rather than a diagnosis. Borderline nuclear changes are most frequently reported in the presence of human papillomavirus (HPV) infection, inflammatory smear, in the presence of an IUCD or cervical polyp (where they may include equivocal changes in endocervical epithelium and should not be categorized as ? glandular neoplasia) and in atrophic smears. The smear with even a few dyskaryotic cells should not be reported as borderline but classified appropriately.

Fig. 1.10 Inflammatory smear

(a) Papanicolaou ×1260 (b) Papanicolaou ×840: inflammatory smear (c) ×1260: epithelial repair (d) ×1260: same case

Inflammatory smears have the following features which can be reported as negative or normal: a minor variation in nuclear shape but with smooth nuclear membranes (a); nuclear pyknosis or karyorrhexis; presence of nucleoli which do not have an irregular outline; the condensation of chromatin under nuclear membrane; bi- or multinucleation; intracytoplasmic polymorphs; increased density of cytoplasmic staining (b); metachromatic cytoplasmic staining; pulled-out strands of cytoplasm; so-called spider cells.

Epithelial repair has been discussed in the introduction. Cells are metaplastic with extreme nuclear and cytoplasmic enlargement and very prominent nucleoli (c, d). The key to the benign nature is their relative architectural regularity and preserved nuclear-cytoplasmic ratio as well as their almost invariable arrangement in sheets and aggregates, rather than singly, often admixed with polymorphs. Their bizarre, worrisome appearances are best resolved by analysing the cells at the edge of the sheet: this should reveal some of the characteristics mentioned above. No premalignant condition of the cervix has quite so pleomorphic appearances. Differential diagnosis includes invasive squamous cell carcinoma and adenocarcinoma.

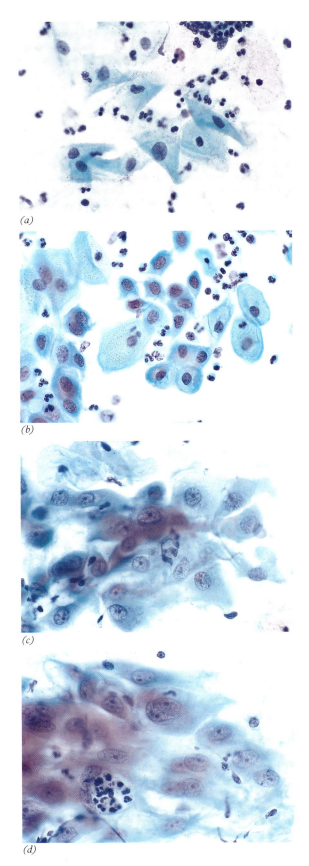

(a)

(b)

(c)

(d)

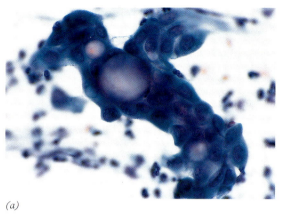

(a)

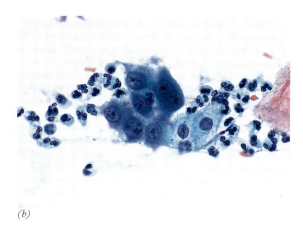

(b)

Fig. 1.11 Endocervicitis

(a) Papanicolaou ×1260 (b) ×1260

Inflammatory changes of endocervical epithelium which can be reported as negative or normal include: substantial variation in nuclear size but with maintenance of normal nuclear-cytoplasmic ratio; rounded or ballooned nuclei (a) with minimal or no irregularity of contour; even, clearly defined nuclear membrane with condensation of the nuclear chromatin at the nuclear margin; prominent, often multiple nucleoli but not irregularly shaped or disproportionately enlarged nucleoli (b); mitoses of normal form; pulled-out strands of cytoplasm; pink cytoplasm with a hazy pink overlay on the cells; cytoplasmic vacuolation.

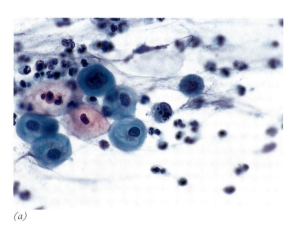

(a)

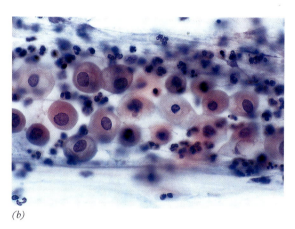

(b)

Fig. 1.12 Atrophic vaginitis

(a) Papanicolaou ×1260 (b) ×1260

Postmenopausal atrophy of the squamous epithelium may lead to atrophic vaginitis. The condition is caused by insufficiency of hormonal support to the epithelium and responds to oestrogen therapy; it is rarely due to a specific pathogen. The cells tend to dissociation, appear attenuated and the majority are somewhat amphophilic (a). A common feature of atrophic vaginitis is the presence of eosinophilic parabasal cells which vary from occasional to half or more of the cell population. In a Papanicolaou-stained smear, degenerate cytoplasm often displays an anomalous staining reaction and eosinophilia of parabasal cells in atrophic vaginitis should not be misinterpreted as pathological dyskeratosis. The nuclei are generally degenerate. The condensed chromatin of a pyknotic or fragmented nucleus may be pulled out in long threads, which mimic condensed mucus threads. When karyolysis occurs, the cell appears as a blue blob, the ghost nucleus being represented by a central circumscribed zone of pallor.

Another common finding in extreme senile atrophy and vaginitis is the presence of variable-sized multinucleated cells which resemble giant histiocytes. The similarity between their nuclei and the nuclei of parabasal cells suggests an epithelial syncytium rather than a phagocytic macrophage.

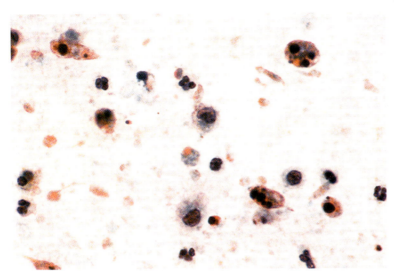

Fig. 1.13 Apoptosis

Papanicolaou ×720

A form of cell death, not related to injury and necrosis but considered to form part of a cell population regulatory process, has been termed apoptosis. Fragments of cytoplasm, which vary in size from the dot-like to small cuboidal cell size, are seen concentrated in one or two microscopic fields or even part of one field. The staining reaction is also variable. Several fragments are devoid of nuclear material; others contain highly condensed pinpoint granules of chromatin, while yet others resemble small cells undergoing karyorrhexis. The appearance has been noted by the author in postcoital smears, in cases of endometrial carcinoma and in atrophic vaginitis

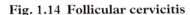

Fig. 1.14 Follicular cervicitis

Papanicolaou (a) ×183 (b) ×720

In chronic cervicitis, the cervix may contain lymph follicles with germinal centres. Chance scraping of a follicle produces a characteristic cytological picture. Numerous small discrete cells are seen streaked across two or three contiguous low-power fields (a). High-power examination shows an admixture of lymphoid cells (b): small mature lymphocytes with condensed hyperchromatic nuclei, larger prolymphocytes with small nucleoli, large lymphoblasts with more open pale nuclei and one or several nucleoli, and an occasional histiocyte with a reniform nucleus and phagocytosed intracytoplasmic debris. Mitotic figures occur in reactive lymphoid hyperplasia; one is seen near the centre of the field (b).

(a)

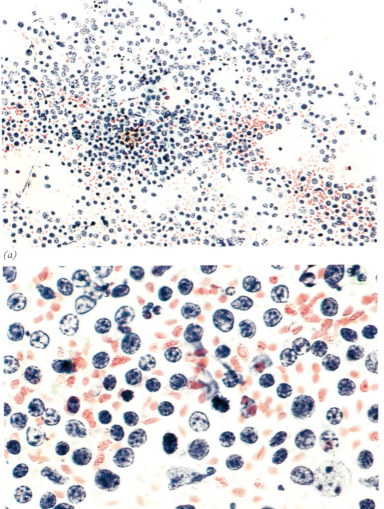

(b)

Flora and fauna

A number of pathogens that invade the genital tract may be recognized in smears. Several are sexually transmitted and some of these have a probable role as aetiological agents in the causation of cervical squamous neoplasia.

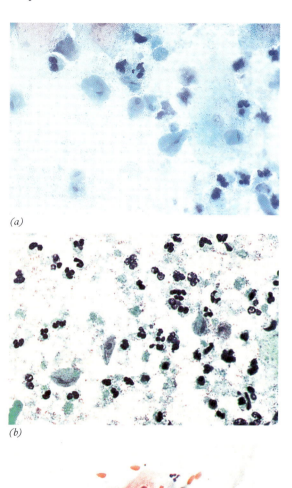

(a)

(b)

(c)

Fig. 1.15 *Trichomonas vaginalis* (TV)

(a) Papanicolaou ×525: flagellated forms (b) ×525: acute TV cervicitis (c) ×333: chronic TV cervicitis

One of the commonest pathogens is *Trichomonas vaginalis*, a flagellated unicellular protozoon with a size range of 10–30 μm. The flagellae illustrated in (a) are rarely evident in an alcohol-fixed smear and are not required for correct identification. The parasite usually appears as a greyish-blue, pear-shaped body with a single ovoid or crescentic nucleus (b). Some may contain a dusting of fine intracytoplasmic granules (a). Visualization of the nucleus is essential to discriminate between the parasite, fragments of cytoplasm and degenerate karyolytic parabasal squamous cells, which are particularly common in atrophic smears. *Trichomonas vaginalis* is usually, but not invariably sexually transmitted and causes an initial acute vaginitis and cervicitis associated with a frothy discharge. The smear at this stage shows many parasitic forms, large numbers of neutrophils and much proteinaceous debris (b). A chronic phase may follow, and in persistent or recurrent infestation, the epithelium shows degenerative changes which consist of pseudoeosinophilia of intermediate squamous cells which often contain small perinuclear haloes (c). Although this appearance is commonly associated with trichomonal infestation, it is not specific. The parasites may be few in number at this stage and a diligent search may be necessary for the identification of the organism and firm diagnosis. Trichomonads are more easily identified by their motility in a wet preparation of a fresh vaginal discharge.

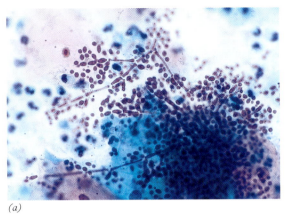

(a)

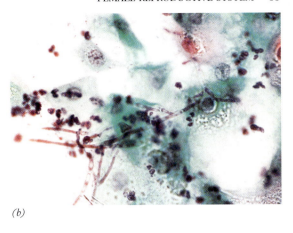

(b)

Fig. 1.16 *Candida albicans*

Papanicolaou (a) ×1260 (b) ×525

The widely prevalent yeast *Candida albicans* is one of the normal flora of the body, and dormant spore forms may be present in a routine smear from an asymptomatic woman. The vegetative stage, developed when spores bud into blastospores (a), pseudohyphae and branching septate hyphae (b), is a common cause of vulvovaginitis, which presents with intense itching and a thick, curd-like discharge. Vegetative forms of *Candida albicans* are particularly common in smears of some women on steroid oral contraceptives and in pregnancy. Although not one of the usual venereally transmitted pathogens, it may on occasion be conveyed to the male partner and cause penile irritation.

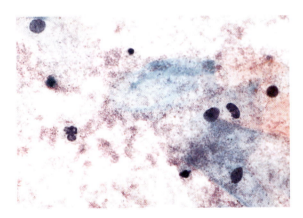

Fig. 1.17 *Gardnerella vaginalis*

Papanicolaou ×525

Gardnerella vaginalis, a sexually transmitted coccobacillus, is associated with a thin, foul-smelling discharge and a characteristic smear pattern. The smear contains myriads of coccobacilli and the cell population consists almost exclusively of intermediate squamous cells covered with bacteria; leukocytes are conspicuous by their absence. Although the cells overlaid with the coccobacilli have been designated 'clue' cells, the appearance is suggestive, but not pathognomonic, of *Gardnerella* infection which should be proved by appropriate bacteriological studies.

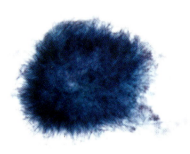

(a)

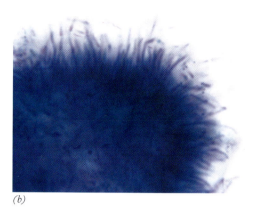

(b)

Fig. 1.18 *Actinomyces* spp.

Papanicolaou (a) ×1260 (b) ×2100

An opportunistic infection of the uterine cavity may be caused in a woman fitted with an inert IUCD by *Actinomyces israelii*, a filamentous bacterium which branches freely and resembles fungal hyphae. The bacterial filament is 1 μm in width and is studded with numerous punctate coccal forms. The characteristic morphology of *Actinomycetes* species seen in a smear is non-specific as to type. The only pathogenic member, *A. israelii*, is difficult to culture in the laboratory but may be correctly identified by immunofluorescent demonstration of specific antigen-antibody reaction. The bacterium may occur in smears of asymptomatic subjects; in others, it may cause pelvic inflammatory disease. An *Actinomycetes*-encrusted IUCD has been known to rupture through the uterine wall into the abdominal cavity, producing an actinomycetoma.

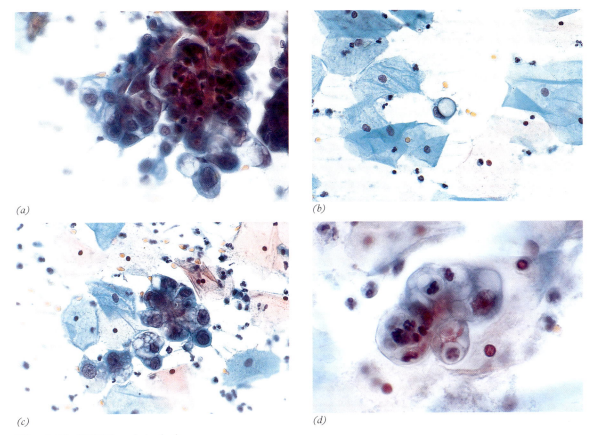

(a)

(b)

(c)

(d)

Fig. 1.19 IUCD-related change

(a) Papanicolaou ×1180 (b) ×840 (c) ×840 (d) ×2100

An intrauterine contraceptive device may provoke an inflammatory reaction. This is sometimes reflected in the atypical changes of endocervical and/or endometrial epithelium which may appear in papillary clusters of slightly hypertrophic vacuolated cells (bubblegum cells) (a–c) or as discrete hypertrophic "brown cells". Engulfing of polymorphs, variation in nuclear size and shape as well as hyperchromasia may be seen (d, e). *Actinomycetes* organisms are a frequent concomitant finding (Fig. 1.18). The importance of recognizing the IUCD effect is in distinguishing it from glandular neoplasia.

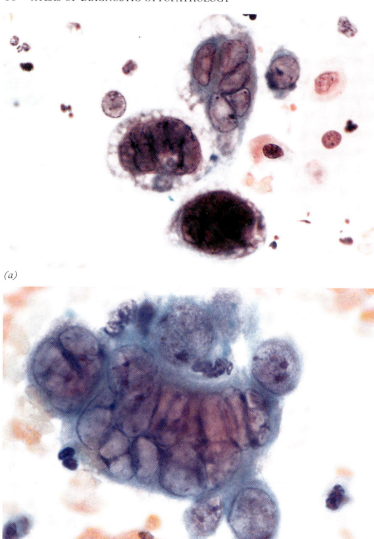

(a)

(b)

Fig. 1.20 Herpes simplex virus (HSV)-associated cell change

(a) ×720 (b) ×1740

Infection of the lower genital tract by HSV may be due to HSV type 1, but is more often caused by the sexually transmitted type 2, referred to as herpes genitalis. Characteristic cytopathic effects are seen in both squamous and endocervical columnar cells. The infected cell may be mononuclear, but more often contains several nuclei which mould one another (a). The nucleus has a ground-glass appearance due to accumulation of intranuclear viral particles; the chromatin, pushed to the periphery, sharply demarcates the nuclear margin. One or two clumps of chromatin may be seen attached to the inner surface of the nuclear membrane, in simulation of a Barr body (a). The large dense intranuclear inclusions illustrated in (b) are considered to appear in a recurrent infection or in a reactivated phase of a latent infection. The pathognomonic cytopathic appearance is obtained from the fluid and the base of an intact herpetic vesicle, and is quickly lost once the vesicle has ruptured and become secondarily infected.

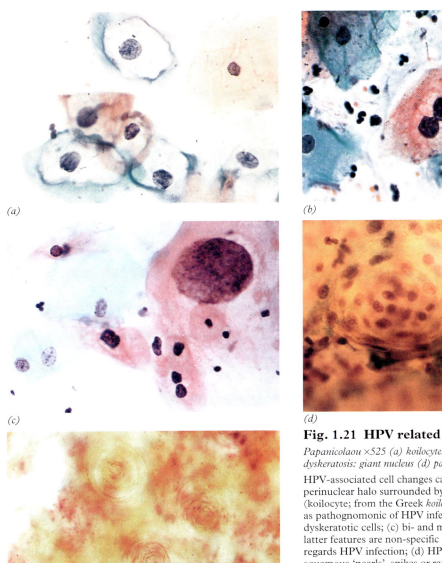

(a)

(b)

(c)

(d)

(e)

Fig. 1.21 HPV related cell change

Papanicolaou ×525 (a) koilocytes (b) binucleate koilocyte (c) dyskeratosis: giant nucleus (d) parakeratosis (e) hyperkeratosis

HPV-associated cell changes can be manifold: (a) a sharp perinuclear halo surrounded by a dense rim of cytoplasm (koilocyte; from the Greek *koilos*, hole). These are regarded as pathognomonic of HPV infection; (b) single or groups of dyskeratotic cells; (c) bi- and multinucleation—the two latter features are non-specific but are very sensitive as regards HPV infection; (d) HPV-affected smears often show squamous 'pearls', spikes or rafts depending on the direction of the nuclei in these aggregates. Although these sheets may overlie a more serious abnormality and should be screened carefully, in the absence of dyskaryotic, disorderly, enlarged nuclei, they can be reported as negative; (e) anucleate squamous cells can be also a reflection of HPV infection (hyperkeratosis) but can also be found in prolapse.

Smears showing signs of HPV infection are reported as showing borderline nuclear changes and followed up with repeat smears provided that nuclear change in koilocytes is less than mild dyskaryosis; and that there are small dyskeratotic cells in groups with variable nuclear enlargement, increased nuclear-cytoplasmic ratio and condensed nuclear chromatin. Persistent abnormality is being clinically assessed and biopsied. Smears with dyskaryotic nuclei alongside HPV infection are being reported according to the degree of dyskaryosis.

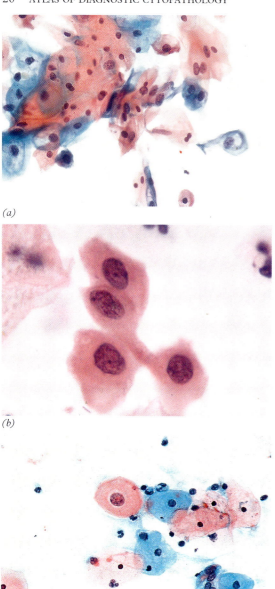

(a)

(b)

(c)

Fig. 1.22 Borderline nuclear changes

(a) ×840 (b) ×1260 (c) ×840 (after oestrogens)

The term *borderline nuclear abnormality* was introduced in 1986 by the British Society of Clinical Cytology in its recommendations on the terminology of cervical smears. It is to be used in cases where there is doubt whether nuclear changes are reactive or neoplastic.

There are two broad situations in which the term 'borderline' is used. The commonest is in the presence of HPV infection where distinction between borderline nuclear changes and mild dyskaryosis may be difficult. The second situation covers a variety of conditions in which it may be difficult to distinguish benign, reactive changes from higher degrees of dyskaryosis or occasionally even invasive cancer.

Borderline nuclear changes should be reported in *cells with HPV-related change* only when koilocytes show milder nuclear changes than those required for mild dyskaryosis (a), and when there are small dyskeratotic cells, often arranged in groups which have variable nuclear enlargement with increased nuclear-cytoplasmic ratios and condensed nuclear chromatin.

Metaplastic cells show borderline changes (b) when there is an increase in the nuclear-cytoplasmic ratio in the absence of cell degeneration or overt dyskaryosis; mild hyperchromasia occurs in enlarged nuclei and the chromatin pattern is slightly coarsened.

Atrophic smears can occasionally show borderline changes. Cells show increased nuclear-cytoplasmic ratios and degenerate but irregular nuclei. If dyskaryosis cannot be confidently excluded, a repeat after a course of local oestrogen is recommended (c).

CERVICAL INTRAEPITHELIAL NEOPLASIA (CIN)

CIN classification refers to a spectrum of preneoplastic changes of cervical epithelium and corresponds to dysplasia and carcinoma-*in-situ* terms used in the older classifications. CIN is histologically graded according to the proportion of the epithelium replaced by dyskaryotic cells.

Cytological grading of CIN lesions relies on the cell morphology alone, assuming that the sample from the surface reflects the changes that have occurred throughout the epithelium. Dyskaryosis is a term generally used to describe nuclear abnormalities greater than those associated with inflammation. Dyskaryosis means 'abnormal nucleus'. It is appropriate to use it to mark both squamous and endocervical cell abnormalities. The term is now seldom used outside the UK, where description of cell changes is avoided and terminology is related to histological changes believed to be present: The term dysplasia is frequently used instead of dyskaryosis. The most important change in nuclear appearance is the irregularity of its chromatin pattern. It can be accompanied by irregularity of form or outline, hyper- or hypochromasia and further nuclear enlargement. Dyskaryotic cells are classified into mild, moderate and severe, according to the diversity of abnormal nuclear characteristics and the degree of morphological abnormality, and the cytoplasmic characteristics which include quantity, density, shape and staining quality. When classifying dyskaryotic cells, attention must be given to the three main types of CIN lesions: large cell non-keratinising, keratinising and small cell lesions and their various characteristics as described below.

There are currently other classifications, e.g. the Bethesda classification used in the USA, which propose to classify squamous intraepithelial lesions (SIL) into low and high grade. Low-grade SIL encompasses borderline and mildly dyskaryotic cells (CIN 1) and high-grade SIL includes moderately and severely dyskaryotic cells (i.e. CIN 2 and CIN 3). Diagnostic categories of the Bethesda classification mirror the management policies associated with CIN classification whereupon mild dyskaryosis (CIN 1) is initially followed up cytologically, whilst moderate and severe dyskaryosis (CIN 2 and CIN 3) are biopsied and treated early.

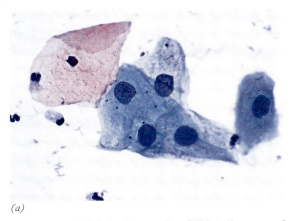
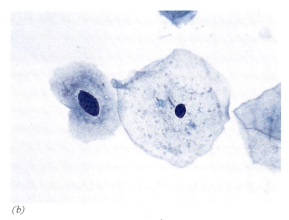

(a)   *(b)*

Fig. 1.23 Mild dyskaryosis: CIN 1 (low-grade SIL)

(a) Papanicolaou ×1260 (b) ×1260

Mildly dyskaryotic cells correspond to the CIN 1 lesion. They have an enlarged nucleus which occupies less than half of the total cell surface (a, b), with irregular nuclear outline, abnormal chromatin pattern and hyperchromasia (not invariably). The cytoplasm is that of mature squamous cells reflecting relatively normal cell maturation to superficial cells. Mild dyskaryosis may, however, involve immature squamous metaplasia or atrophic epithelium. In these instances the degree of dyskaryosis should be assessed in relative proportion to the nuclear:cytoplasmic ratio normal for that cell which is likely to be higher.

Smears showing mild dyskaryosis should be followed up in the first instance and referred to colposcopy and biopsy if abnormality persists on subsequent smears. Following colposcopy, mild dyskaryosis should be managed at the discretion of the cytopathologist in consultation with the gynaecologist.

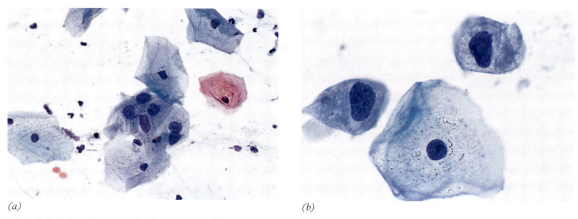

(a)   *(b)*

Fig. 1.24 Moderate dyskaryosis: CIN 2 (high-grade SIL)

(a) Papanicolaou ×1260 (b) ×1260

Nuclear enlargement of moderately dyskaryotic cells is such that it occupies one-half to two-thirds of the cell diameter (a, b). Moderately dyskaryotic cells usually do not show cytoplasmic maturation beyond intermediate cells. Cytoplasm may resemble that of intermediate, parabasal or metaplastic cells. Nuclear changes are variable but tend to be less than in severe dyskaryosis.

Dyskaryotic cells which are difficult to grade, usually because of their scarcity in the smear, should be coded and managed as for moderate dyskaryosis. This applies particularly to follow-up smears of previous severe dyskaryosis where there may be few abnormal cells in the smear.

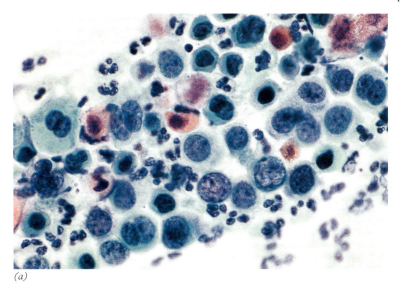

(a)

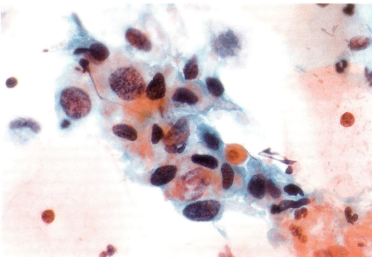

(b)

Fig. 1.25 Severe dyskaryosis: CIN 3 (high-grade SIL)

(a) Papanicolaou ×720 (b) ×1160

Severely dyskaryotic cells have nuclei occupying more than two-thirds of the cell diameter with only a thin rim of cytoplasm remaining (high nucleo:cytoplasmic ratio) reflecting abnormal cytoplasmic maturation. Nuclei are irregularly shaped, chromatin is clumped and they are usually hyperchromatic (a, b). Severe dyskaryosis may, however, occur in cells with intracytoplasmic keratinization which should not be mistaken for HPV change.

Morphologically there are three main patterns of CIN 3 lesions depending on the presence and type of cytoplasmic differentiation and dyskaryosis: large cell non-keratinizing, keratinizing and small cell/undifferentiated type.

Potential pitfalls (*false negatives*) in diagnosis of severe dyskaryosis include: small cell severe dyskaryosis (Fig 1.29), pale dyskaryosis (Fig 1.27), CIN 3 micro-biopsies, small keratinized cells, CIN 3 involving endocervical glands, and sparse dyskaryotic cells.

Potential *false positives* include endometrial cells/tuboendometrioid metaplasia (Figs 1.36, 1.37), histiocytes (Figs 1.9, 1.27 d, e) and follicular cervicitis (Fig 1.14).

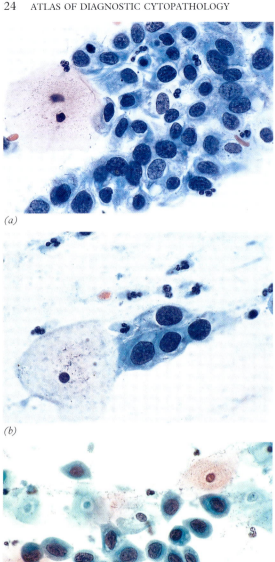

(a)

(b)

(c)

Fig. 1.26 Large cell non-keratinizing type of CIN

(a) Papanicolaou ×1260 (b) ×1260 (c) ×1260

This is the most common appearance of CIN 3 lesion in cervical smears, reflecting the fact that the majority of the lesions originate in the transformation zone. Cells with dyskaryotic nuclei are round, oval or polygonal, usually 4–6 times the size of neutrophils, and abnormal nuclei easily fulfil criteria of increased nuclear-cytoplasmic ratio, with the nucleus occupying more than two-thirds of the total cell area (a–c). Cells are usually lying singly, often in characteristic streaks or chains, sometimes admixed with inflammatory exudate. Nuclei are usually hyperchromatic (but may be hypochromatic), have abnormal chromatin pattern and have an irregular outline. Anisonucleosis and irregular nuclear outline are often clues to differentiating these cells from immature squamous metaplasia and macrophages. Cytoplasmic keratinization may be seen but is rare.

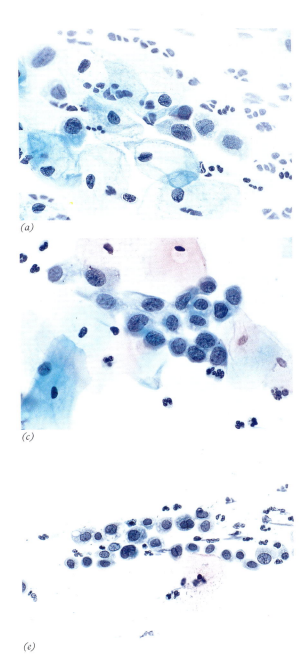

(a)

(b)

(c)

(d)

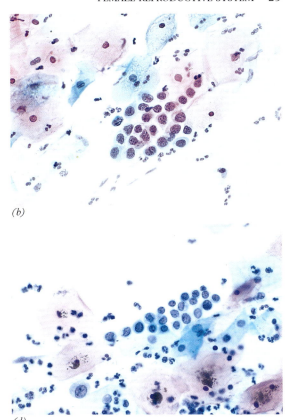

(e)

Fig. 1.27 CIN 3: pale dyskaryosis vs macrophages

(a) Papanicolaou ×1260: CIN 3 (b) ×840: CIN 3 (c) ×840: CIN 3 (d) ×840: macrophages (e) ×840: macrophages

Cells with pale dyskaryosis may be shed from various degrees of CIN, including CIN 3. They have high nuclear-cytoplasmic ratios (a–c), nuclei which are paler than the surrounding polymorphs (a), do not have any chromatin condensation at the nuclear membrane (a), have an irregularly distributed, although pale, chromatin pattern which may vary from cell to cell (this irregularity may be minimal) and they can occur without more typical dyskaryosis. The cell arrangement (mainly single cells), admixture of inflammatory exudate and hypochromasia may make distinction between the hypochromatic type of CIN and macrophages difficult.

Macrophages illustrated in (d) and (e) have on medium-power view a similar pattern of spread and lie singly. High-power assessment of nuclear detail, with particular reference to grooved nuclei, foamy cytoplasm and low nuclear-cytoplasmic ratios of histiocytes, versus high nuclear-cytoplasmic ratio, anisonucleosis and irregularities of chromatin in CIN, should help to distinguish the two in most cases. On occasions, histiocytes may have granular chromatin which may mimic 'small cell' CIN 3 but other features including grooved nuclei and absence of cytoplasmic keratinisation should help distinguish the two.

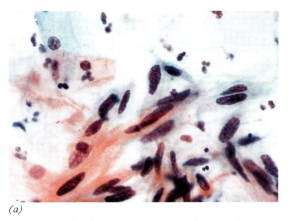

(a)

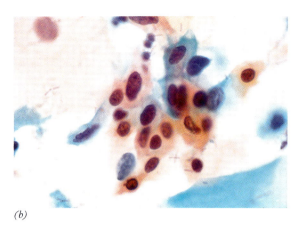

(b)

Fig. 1.28 CIN 3: keratinizing dysplasia

(a) Papanicolaou ×525 (b) ×2100

This is the most 'colourful' of dysplasias, its origin entirely from the ectocervix, with adundant keratinized cells, many showing bizarre features including fibre and tadpole cells. Nuclei are usually hyperchromatic and severely dyskaryotic (a, b), they occupy less than 2/3 of the cytoplasmic area.

Sometimes, small keratinized cells may be difficult to recognize, particularly in atrophic smear when associated with inflammation. An early repeat smear after the course of local oestrogen should elucidate the problem.

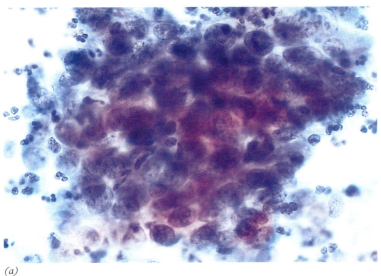

(a)

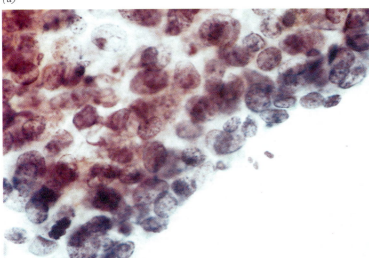

(b)

Fig. 1.29 Small cell type non-keratinizing of CIN 3

(a) Papanicolaou ×1740 (b) ×720

This lesion usually involves endocervical canal. Smears contain sheets of monotonous, hyperchromatic cells with oval, round or irregular nuclei, scanty poorly defined cytoplasm and coarse granular chromatin with occasional mitoses (a). Sheets of these cells are best analysed at the edges (b) because the extreme crowding of nuclei often prevents their assessment in the middle of the cell aggregate. The cells from this type of CIN 3 can be mistaken for endometrial cells, reactive endocervical cells, reserve cell hyperplasia or glandular neoplasia. They can be scanty or very scanty and may be obscured by inflammatory cells.

The latter may particularly be true of *CIN 3 lesions involving endocervical glands*. These lesions may have severely dyskaryotic squamous cells intimately associated with slightly enlarged endocervical cells, in such a way that a whole group may be considered glandular. The characteristic features of glandular neoplasia are not seen in these cell groups. Helpful distinguishing features are: CIN 3 clusters are usually well rounded with a well defined rim of cytoplasm, peripheral flattening of the nuclei, mild anisonucleosis, uneven chromatin pattern within the group and central whorling of nuclei within the group.

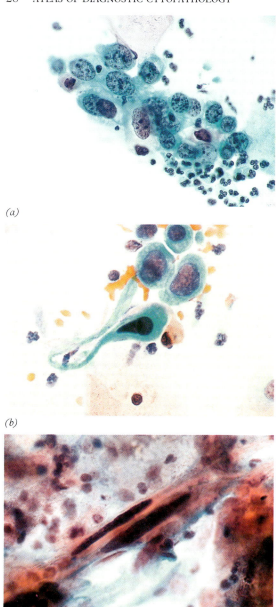

(a)

(b)

(c)

Fig. 1.30 Microinvasive squamous cell carcinoma

(a) Papanicolaou ×1260 (b) ×525 (c) ×525

It is generally agreed that the treatment of microinvasive carcinoma need not be different from that of CIN 3. The precise definition of what constitutes a microinvasive carcinoma as distinct from an invasive carcinoma continues to be the subject of debate and has been revised more than once. The term is provisionally accepted to describe lesions in which the penetration of the basement membrane by a single or multiple non-confluent tongues of neoplastic cells is no greater than 3 mm deep from the base of the epithelium. A definitive diagnosis of microinvasion requires histological examination of a biopsy of adequate size and depth, and is facilitated by the well-established observation that the invading cells are usually better differentiated than the overlying CIN from which they are derived. The cytological presentation may be indistinguishable from CIN 3. In some cases of microinvasive carcinoma, foci of better differentiated cells, similar to the invading cells, are present within the CIN, some of them close enough to the surface to be recoverable in a smear. The CIN may appear exceptionally pleomorphic or it may contain dyskeratotic cells which are arranged in whorls and form incipient or actual squamous pearls. The neoplastic epithelium acquires an appearance which has been described as restless. The smear pattern may be similar to that seen in an invasive carcinoma.

In about 50% of cases, a different picture is seen, and a cytodiagnosis of probable microinvasive carcinoma is feasible.

The overall appearance of the smear is compatible with CIN 3, but a small number of malignant cells inconsistent with a typical intraepithelial lesion are present in addition. Variants of the suggestive picture are illustrated by three cases in which a cytological diagnosis of a probable microcarcinoma was confirmed by cone biopsy histology. None of the smears showed a cancer diathesis. All contained poorly differentiated dyskaryotic squamous cells: these are shown from one case in (a). In the second case shown, the CIN 3 cells were accompanied by a few better differentiated malignant squamous cells and an occasional bizarre caudate cell (b). In the third case, the cells that do not fit a CIN 3 are large and keratinized and contain grossly abnormal spindle-shaped nuclei (c).

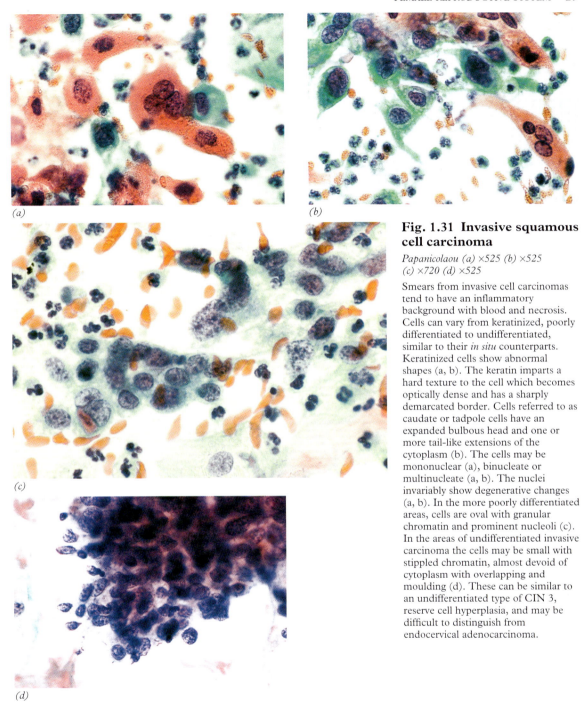

(a)

(b)

(c)

(d)

Fig. 1.31 Invasive squamous cell carcinoma

Papanicolaou (a) ×525 (b) ×525 (c) ×720 (d) ×525

Smears from invasive cell carcinomas tend to have an inflammatory background with blood and necrosis. Cells can vary from keratinized, poorly differentiated to undifferentiated, similar to their *in situ* counterparts. Keratinized cells show abnormal shapes (a, b). The keratin imparts a hard texture to the cell which becomes optically dense and has a sharply demarcated border. Cells referred to as caudate or tadpole cells have an expanded bulbous head and one or more tail-like extensions of the cytoplasm (b). The cells may be mononuclear (a), binucleate or multinucleate (a, b). The nuclei invariably show degenerative changes (a, b). In the more poorly differentiated areas, cells are oval with granular chromatin and prominent nucleoli (c). In the areas of undifferentiated invasive carcinoma the cells may be small with stippled chromatin, almost devoid of cytoplasm with overlapping and moulding (d). These can be similar to an undifferentiated type of CIN 3, reserve cell hyperplasia, and may be difficult to distinguish from endocervical adenocarcinoma.

CERVICAL INTRAEPITHELIAL GLANDULAR NEOPLASIA (CIGN)

High grade cervical intraepithelial glandular neoplasia (CIGN) or adenocarcinoma-*in-situ* (AIS) and its possible antecedent, glandular atypia or low grade CIGN, have been identified histologically and cytologically since 1952 and 1970 respectively. It is relatively uncommon (0.1% of predictions in UK screening programme) but with increased awareness the expected proportions, glandular to squamous, on cone biopsy and hysterectomy specimens performed for cytological reasons, has increased 10 fold from 1979 to 1988.

Cervical smear is not as efficient in diagnosing these precursors of adenocarcinoma as it is in detecting those of squamous carcinoma, sensitivity being between 74% and 88%. The problem is partly due to sampling, partly to interpretation; these lesions usually occur in the endocervical canal, their distribution within the canal is uncertain, they are colposcopically non specific and may not be present on smears deemed adequate on standard criteria, i.e. squamous and metaplastic epithelium.

Cytological appearances of a well-differentiated and *in situ* endocervical adenocarcinoma may mimic benign conditions, such as reactive endocervical cells, tuboendometrioid metaplasia (TEM), cervical endometriosis, lower uterine segment cells, large stromal fragments and IUCD effect, particularly in the smears taken by cervical brush which tend to yield larger amounts of endocervical epithelium than is normally experienced by a routine screener. Screening for squamous lesions involves search for individual abnormal cells whereas identification of preinvasive glandular lesions involves often recognition of architectural features as well as individual cell characteristics.

Smears from AIS show characteristic architectural features: rosettes, pseudostratification, feathering (frayed) edges, and wispy cytoplasmic tags.

They also include palisading, monolayer sheets of cells and gland openings. Increased degree of nuclear crowding implies increasing severity of the lesion. Notable general features of AIS include : clean background, nuclear size: even within group, vary from 8–20 µm diameter; chromasia: even within each group, may be hypo to hyperchromatic.

Individual cell features include round to oval nuclei with smooth nuclear outline, mitoses are uncommon, nucleoli are not a constant feature. Chromatin is evenly dispersed with coarse granules (salt and pepper), cytoplasm is delicate, usually scanty, finely vacuolated or granular, fading towards periphery.

Distinction between in situ and microinvasive AIS may not be possible on cervical smears. Smears from *microinvasive endocervical adenocarcinoma* show supercrowded sheets, abundant mitoses, enlarged, round and irregularly shaped nuclei with variable chromasia and loss of architecture. Signs of squamoid differentiation may be seen. Smears from *frankly invasive endocervical adenocarcinoma* show nuclear pleomorphism, mitotic figures, irregular chromatin, prominent/abnormal nucleoli, increased N/C ratio, crowding or loss of cohesion and tumour diathesis (Wadell, personal communication). Both *in situ* and invasive endocervical adenocarcinoma appear to originate from reserve cells. However, due to the presence of poorly differentiated forms of AIS and well-differentiated invasive adenocarcinoma, cellular features alone, including nuclear size and macronucleoli, previously mentioned, may not be helpful. Similarly, blood and inflammatory background, thought to be associated with invasive tumours, may also be found in AIS.

CIGN may be subtyped into CIGN 1 (endocervical adenocarcinoma, well differentiated) and CIGN 2 (endometrioid, intestinal and very uncommon adenosquamous carcinoma in situ and clear cell adenocarcinoma in situ).

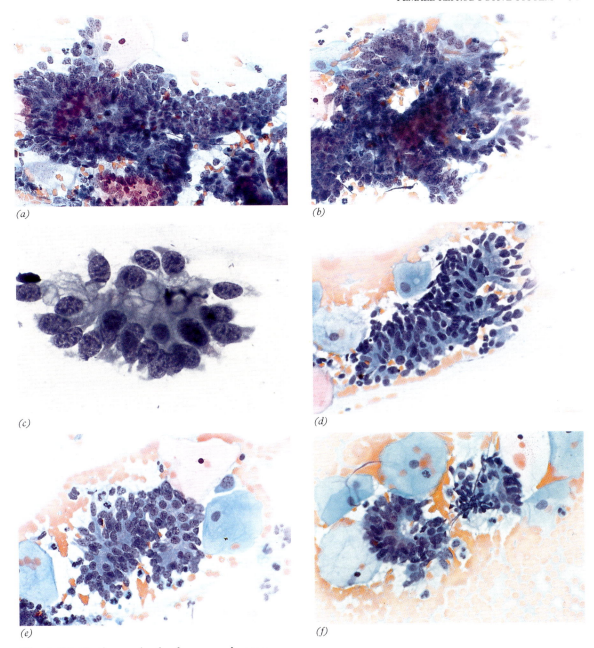

Fig. 1.32 Endocervical adenocarcinoma

(a) Papanicolaou ×840 (b) ×840 (c) ×1260 (d) ×840 (e) ×840 (f) ×840

Architectural features commonly encountered in smears from endocervical adenocarcinoma, as described above, are: polarization of long axes of nuclei with rosettes, pseudostratification, crowding of cells, feathering, wispy cytoplasmic tags, palisading and gland openings.

Illustrations show large clusters of hyperchromatic, crowded cells with oval, regular, even-sized nuclei, slightly larger than those of normal endocervical cells, with evenly dispersed slightly coarse chromatin (a, c). 'Feathering' refers to nuclear protrusions around the edges of the cell clusters with no discernible luminal border (a); cells often form rosettes with gland-like lumina (b, f). Clusters are often numerous and branching; strips of endocervical epithelium show pseudopalisading (d): nuclei are crowded and polarized towards one edge (c, e). Cells retain the delicate cytoplasmic appearance of glandular epithelium with wispy tags (c, d). Evenly dispersed granular chromatin and nuclear size regularity suggest *in situ* rather than invasive adenocarcinoma; increasing degree of nuclear crowding implies increased severity of the lesion, although the distinction on cervical smears may not be possible other than in advanced cases.

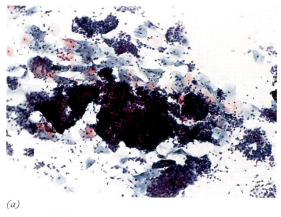

(a)

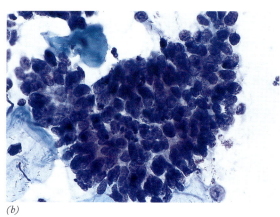

(b)

Fig. 1.33 CIGN 2: Endocervical adenocarcinoma

(a) Papanicolaou ×210 (b) ×1260 (c) ×1260

The smear from this CIGN 2 type lesion shows numerous clusters, strips and single glandular cells (a). High power (b, c) reveals glandular-type neoplasia with unevenly sized oval-shaped nuclei and a coarse chromatin pattern and variable chromasia within the group. In this case it is more difficult to distinguish this lesion from an undifferentiated CIN 3, particularly since they are both thought to arise from reserve cells. Helpful features in diagnosing CIN (squamous) with crypt involvement are: round or oval cell clusters with well defined cytoplasmic rim, peripheral flattening of nuclei, central whorling of nuclei, mild anisonucleosis and uneven chromasia within the group.

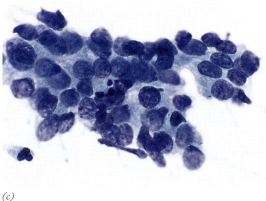

(c)

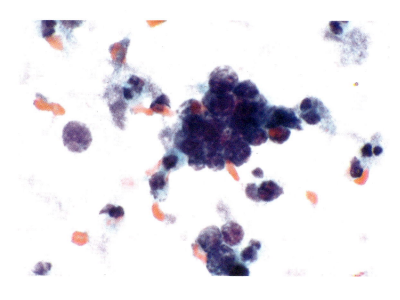

Fig. 1.34 Small-cell anaplastic-cell carcinoma of the cervix

Papanicolaou ×2900

This is a very rare tumour similar to others of its kind thought to be originating from the neuroendocrine type cells in other parts of the body, namely lung. Cells are very small, hyperchromatic and arranged in clusters. They have coarse chromatin, no discernible cytoplasm and show nuclear moulding. Immunocytochemistry shows positivity for neuroendocrine markers. They have to be distinguished from lymphocytes and reserve cells. The former are usually in flat sheets rather than three-dimensional clusters. Biological behaviour is aggressive; they metastasize widely. The case illustrated was diagnosed from the fine-needle aspiration of the breast which showed small cells with positivity for neuroendocrine markers. Review of previous cervical resection and preceding cervical smear revealed the same tumour.

BENIGN CONDITIONS MIMICKING CERVICAL INTRAEPITHELIAL GLANDULAR NEOPLASIA (CIGN)

Greater awareness of endocervical adenocarcinoma has resulted in better interpretation of abnormal smears but has also caused overdiagnosis in cases where 'atypical glandular cells' are reported. We show examples of microglandular hyperplasia, tuboendometrioid metaplasia and cervical endometriosis, all of which may be mistaken for glandular or squamous neoplasia of the cervix.

Other benign conditions that may be mistaken for CIGN include: reactive endocervical cells, overstaining of normal endocervical cells, tissue repair, follicular cervicitis, herpetic cervicitis and prolapsed fallopian tube (in vault smears).

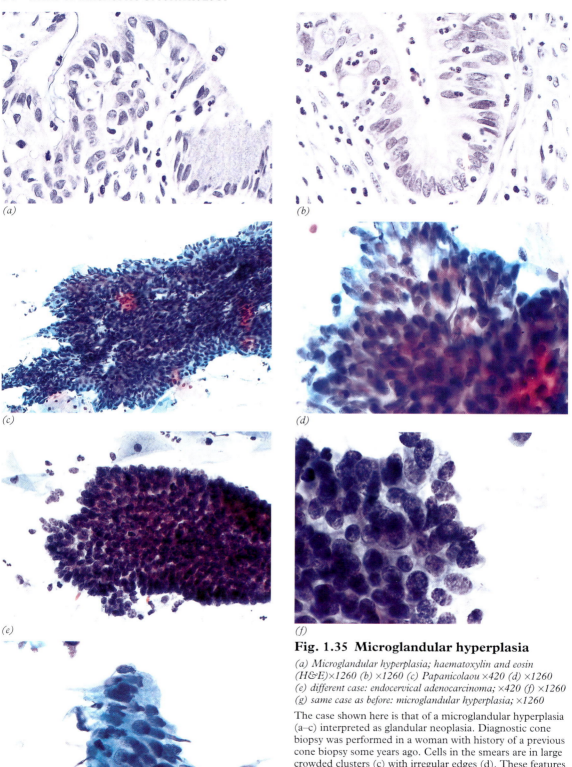

Fig. 1.35 Microglandular hyperplasia

(a) Microglandular hyperplasia; haematoxylin and eosin (H&E)×1260 (b) ×1260 (c) Papanicolaou ×420 (d) ×1260 (e) different case: endocervical adenocarcinoma; ×420 (f) ×1260 (g) same case as before: microglandular hyperplasia; ×1260

The case shown here is that of a microglandular hyperplasia (a–c) interpreted as glandular neoplasia. Diagnostic cone biopsy was performed in a woman with history of a previous cone biopsy some years ago. Cells in the smears are in large crowded clusters (c) with irregular edges (d). These features are similar to hypercrowding (e) and feathering (f) seen in endocervical adenocarcinoma. Strips of epithelium show pseudostratification (b, g) and may show mitoses.

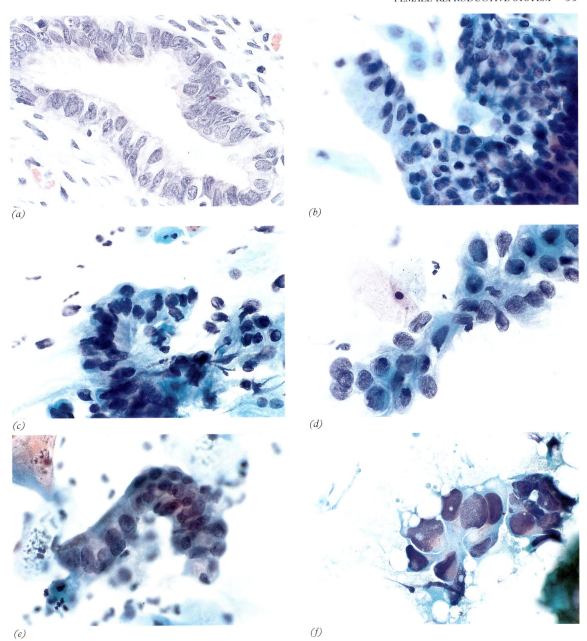

(a) (b) (c) (d) (e) (f)

Fig. 1.36 Tuboendometrioid metaplasia (TEM)

(a) H&E ×840 (b-f) Papanicolaou ×1260

This figure illustrates a case of tuboendometrioid metaplasia erroneously interpreted as residual endocervical adenocarcinoma. Tubal metaplasia is one of the known consequences of cone biopsies and as such is not rare. Apart from ciliated and secretory cell type, tubal epithelium has also intercalated cell. Histological section (a) shows a gland with large atypical nuclei showing pseudopalisading. Note the ciliated luminal border which gives the clue to the diagnosis. Smears from the same case show sheets of crowded glandular cells (b), attempting to form acini and showing anisonucleosis (c). Cytoplasm is distinct, denser than in endocervical cells. Cytoplasmic margins are blunted and may have terminal bars or cilia (d, e). Chromatin pattern is "smokey", pseudostratification and rosettes are seen (f).

Pseudostratification is usually a feature and a higher nucleo-cytoplasmic ratio than in normal endocervical cells is usually seen. Nucleoli may be prominent.

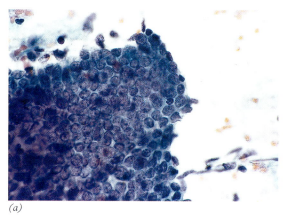

(a)

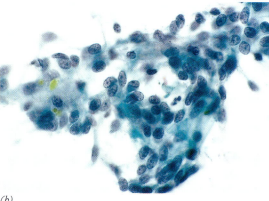

(b)

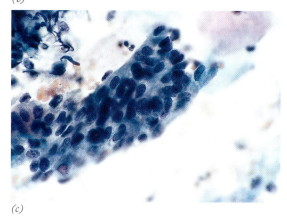

(c)

Fig. 1.37 Endometriosis

(a–c) Papanicolaou ×1260

Endometriosis of the cervix is not uncommon in patients with history of cone biopsy. At the same time these patients are usually under close scrutiny for possible residual/recurrent disease. This case illustrates architectural chaos in ragged, three dimensional, untidy sheets of small hyperchromatic cells (a) which showed overlapping of nuclei and no distinct cell borders (b). Hyperchromatic nuclei in apparent 'microbiopsy' fragments were erroneously interpreted as recurrent undifferentiated CIN 3 lesion (c) (compare Fig. 1.29a and b). Cone biopsy revealed cervical endometriosis.

ENDOMETRIAL ADENOCARCINOMA

Cervical smears may be a means of detecting endometrial adenocarcinoma. These tumours are most frequent in postmenopausal years and abnormal bleeding is a common and a relatively early symptom. Malignant endometrial cells are more likely to be recovered from a posterior vaginal fornix pool smear if the bleeding is heavy or recent; when this is not the case, the cells may be arrested in the cervical mucus and are equally likely to be present in a cervical smear in which they appear better preserved. Exfoliation of tumour cells may not occur, or it may be sparse. The cells may undergo necrotic change *in vivo* or after they have been shed and may not be easily identifiable. The sensitivity of diagnosis of endometrial carcinoma is consequently considerably lower than of cervical tumours which are generally scraped under vision. Direct sampling of the endometrial cavity by jet wash or aspiration has been advocated for cases of postmenopausal bleeding and for screening women receiving hormone replacement therapy. The techniques are not always acceptable to a woman with an atrophic genital tract and this has limited their application.

Adenocarcinoma of the fallopian tube is extremely rare. Tumour cells may find their way into the vagina or cervical canal; whilst their malignant character is usually obvious, the site of origin cannot be determined from the cellular appearance.

Malignant cells from an ovarian carcinoma are occasionally seen in a vaginal or cervical smear. These are generally from a disseminated cancer, but on rare occasions, cells from a carcinoma limited to the ovary may pass down the oviducts and uterus and appear in an otherwise normal smear.

Except in the case of the fallopian tube, it is often possible to suggest the likely source of the adenocarcinoma cells from the smear pattern and so direct attention to the site requiring further investigation. There is, however, a considerable overlap of histological variants seen in the different parts of the genital tract. Endometrioid-type cells are characteristic of a corpus carcinoma, but may form tumours in the endocervix and ovary. Mucous tumours, common in the endocervix and ovary, may develop in the endometrium. For this reason, clinical considerations are of particular importance in the diagnosis and localization of a genital tract adenocarcinoma.

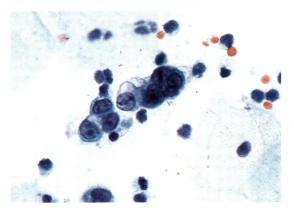

Fig. 1.38 Endometrial adenocarcinoma

Papanicolaou ×525

Compare the size of the tumour cells from this case of a
well-differentiated endometrial carcinoma with neutrophils
and with the malignant endocervical cells in the preceding
micrograph, and note their smaller size. The arrangement is
essentially similar to that in Figure 1.35. There are,
however, many more cells in the endometrial cluster and the
drawing-in of the outer border at the several points of cell
junction has produced a scalloped outline, often seen in a
typical group of adenocarcinoma cells. The degree of
cytoplasmic distension is variable and is reflected in the
variation in the nuclear-cytoplasmic ratio. Small but distinct
nucleoli are present.

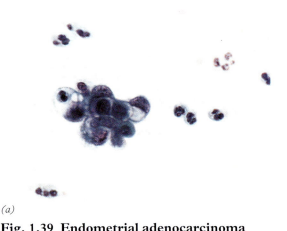

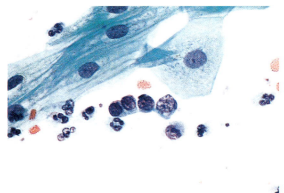

(a)

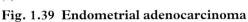

(b)

Fig. 1.39 Endometrial adenocarcinoma

Papanicolaou ×525: (a) secretory cells (b) same smear; another field

A closely similar malignant cluster with a scalloped border is
seen in (a). Note again that several nuclei are displaced by
secretory vacuoles to the edge of the cluster. Nucleoli are
absent or insignificant. A neutrophil is seen within one cell.
Foci of leukocytic infiltration are common in endometrial
carcinomas. A tumour cell packed with and obscured by
numerous neutrophils should not be included in a
diagnostic assessment as benign inflammatory disease may
show a similar appearance.

A different pattern of exfoliation is seen in (b). Five

tumour cells with a high nuclear-cytoplasmic ratio and
granular chromatin are streaked across the centre. In size,
they appear slightly larger than neutrophils. The partially
detached cell at lower right has an eccentric kidney-shaped
nucleus and resembles a small histiocyte. Cells from a
benign endometrial hyperplasia with cellular atypia have a
similar appearance and pattern of exfoliation and in the
absence of a typical adenocarcinoma cluster, distinction
between malignancy and benign hyperplasia is often
difficult.

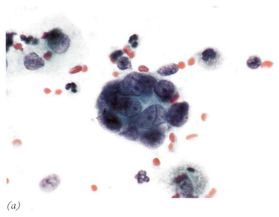

(a)

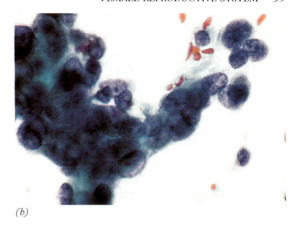

(b)

Fig. 1.40 Endometrial adenocarcinoma

Papanicolaou ×525 (a) secretory cells (b) same smear; another field

A less well-differentiated endometrial carcinoma is illustrated in these micrographs. The rosette-shaped arrangement of the cells in (a) is indicative of a glandular tumour. The individual cells are larger than in the two preceding examples of endometrial carcinoma; the nuclei are more variable in size and display a moderate degree of polychromasia. The nuclear-cytoplasmic ratio is very high and nucleoli, although not as large as in a non-keratinized invasive squamous cell carcinoma, are prominent.

In the other group (b), the cells are arranged in a sheet and the three-dimensional appearance of a round cluster is absent. Cytoplasmic vacuolization is not evident. The smooth outlines of several nuclei and their eccentric location on the edge of the sheet are suggestive of an adenocarcinoma.

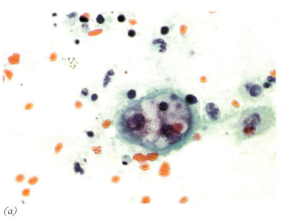

(a)

(b)

Fig. 1.41 Endometrial adenocarcinoma

Papanicolaou ×525 (a) large secretory cells (b) small cells: same smear; another field

The cells in (a) are typical of an adenocarcinoma. In size and in the abundance of mucous vacuoles, they resemble the malignant endocervical cells shown in Figure 1.35.

The clump of tightly packed, degenerate endometrial cells with hyperchromatic granular nuclei seen against a background of neutrophils, erythrocytes and breakdown products of blood (b) is not dissimilar to cells seen in a menstrual smear. Exfoliation of identifiable endometrial cells in association with adenocarcinoma cells is suggestive of involvement of the endometrium in the disease process. Assumption of a primary endometrial carcinoma would be reasonable, although secondary deposits which have destabilized the endometrium cannot be ruled out.

In the absence of typical tumour cells (a), a diagnosis of malignancy, based on the cells in (b) is less certain, even in a case of postmenopausal bleeding. In a case of dysfunctional bleeding, it would be hazardous.

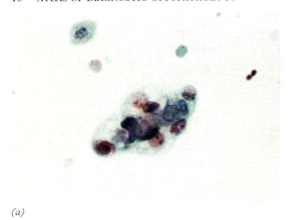

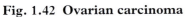

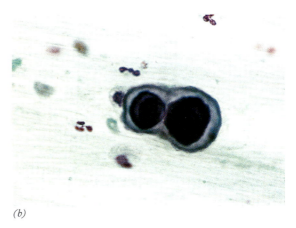

(a)   *(b)*

Fig. 1.42 Ovarian carcinoma

Papanicolaou ×525 (a) adenocarcinoma cells (b) psammoma bodies

A cluster of adenocarcinoma cells is seen in (a) and psammoma bodies in (b). A psammoma body or a calcospherite is an organized structure, somewhat variable in appearance, but usually consisting of a central area of density surrounded by dark, often wavy, concentric rings separated by pale zones. It is formed when minerals, chiefly calcium, are deposited in a focus of necrotic cells, and occurs commonly in papillary tumours. In the genital tract, they may occur in a papillary endometrial carcinoma; this type of tumour is, however, relatively uncommon. The ovary, on the other hand, is the most frequent site of a papillary carcinoma and the commonest source of psammoma bodies. A cytological diagnosis of a probable primary ovarian carcinoma was proved correct in this case.

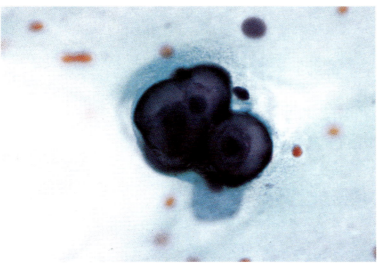

(a)

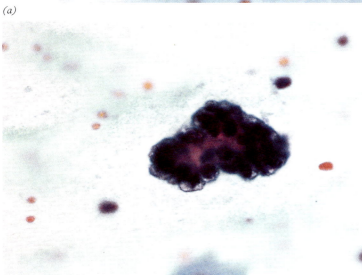

(b)

Fig. 1.43 Ovarian carcinoma

Papanicolaou (a) ×720: vaginal smear; psammoma bodies (b) ×720: vaginal smear; papillary tumour cells

A vaginal vault smear, shown in these micrographs, carries evidence of a recurrence of a serous cystadenocarcinoma of the ovary, treated 10 years earlier. Psammoma bodies are seen in (a). The tumour cells in (b) are ringed round pale fibrous tissue. A papillary tumour forms fronds which consist of a central fibrovascular core with an external lining of neoplastic cells. In a smear, the tips of the fronds may be seen and are identified by the presence of the fibrous core. Psammoma bodies are often abundant in serous papillary tumours of the ovary; these may be benign or malignant.

OVARY: FINE-NEEDLE ASPIRATION

Functional cysts

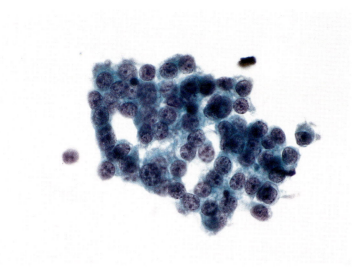

Fig. 1.44 Follicular cyst

Papanicolaou ×1810

A follicular cyst occurs in the premenopausal years. It may be single or multiple and varies in size from the microscopic to 10 cm or so in diameter; the average is 2–3 cm, and its size may be assessed in the laboratory by the volume of fluid aspirated. It develops in a follicle which, having reached a partial stage of maturation, undergoes regression and atresia. The cyst fluid is generally clear and colourless and contains a small number of follicle or granulosa cells from the lining. The cells are small with scanty cytoplasm and a high nuclear-cytoplasmic ratio. The nuclei, which appear hyperchromatic in sections, may be somewhat depleted of chromatin and hypochromatic in free-floating cells obtained from the cyst fluid.

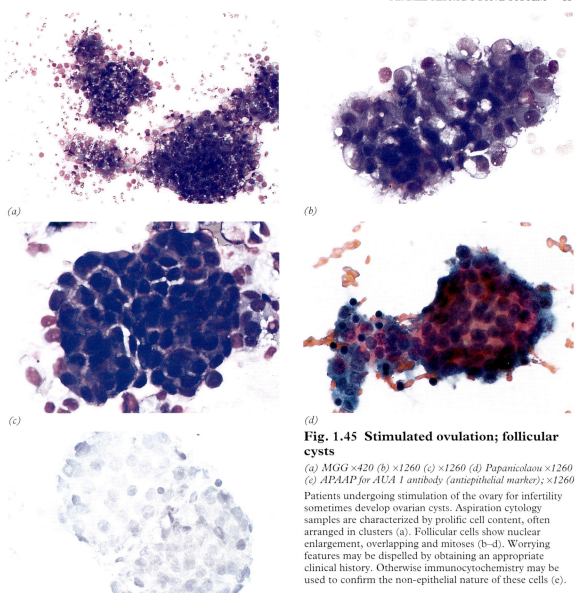

(a)

(b)

(c)

(d)

(e)

Fig. 1.45 Stimulated ovulation; follicular cysts

(a) MGG ×420 (b) ×1260 (c) ×1260 (d) Papanicolaou ×1260 (e) APAAP for AUA 1 antibody (antiepithelial marker); ×1260

Patients undergoing stimulation of the ovary for infertility sometimes develop ovarian cysts. Aspiration cytology samples are characterized by prolific cell content, often arranged in clusters (a). Follicular cells show nuclear enlargement, overlapping and mitoses (b–d). Worrying features may be dispelled by obtaining an appropriate clinical history. Otherwise immunocytochemistry may be used to confirm the non-epithelial nature of these cells (e).

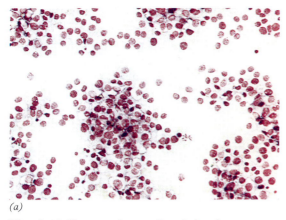

(a)

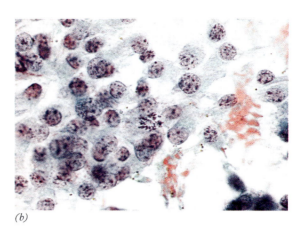

(b)

Fig. 1.46 Postovulatory luteinized cyst

(a) MGG ×133 (b) Papanicolaou ×525: another case

The cells surrounding an ovum in a maturing follicle multiply and become multilayered; mitoses are frequently seen at this stage. After discharge of the ovum, they enlarge under the influence of LH and their cytoplasm is filled with a yellow pigment; hence they are referred to as granulosa lutein cells. Fluid from a cyst which develops at this stage is yellow in colour, occasionally blood-stained and contains numerous cells (a). Morphological detail of granulosa lutein cells is seen in (b). The cytoplasm is moderately abundant, the nuclei are monomorphic and the nuclear chromatin is granular and regularly distributed. A mitotic figure is seen in the centre of the field. On occasion, several mitotic figures are seen and this, coupled with high cellular content, may create a false impression of a benign neoplasm.

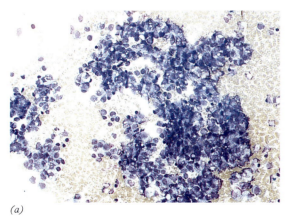

(a)

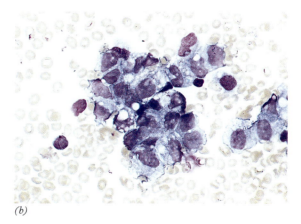

(b)

Fig. 1.47 Corpus luteum cyst

(a) MGG ×420 (b) ×1260: ovarian cyst aspirate

As luteinization progresses, the granulosa lutein cells acquire more cytoplasm and the nuclear-cytoplasmic ratio is reduced. Cytoplasm appears thin and vacuolated. The nuclei are homogeneous and hypochromatic. The cyst fluid is yellow and the cell content moderate or low.

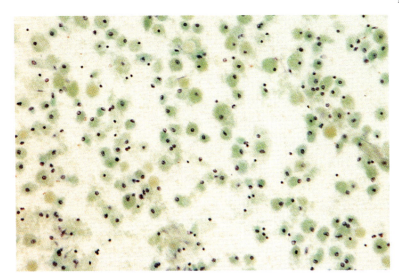

Fig. 1.48 Germinal inclusion cyst

Papanicolaou ×183

The external covering of the ovary is of mesothelial origin. It is referred to as germinal epithelium and consists of a single layer of cuboidal cells. These cells may invaginate the ovarian cortex, become separated from the external germinal layer, and form the lining of an inclusion cyst. The condition occurs most commonly in the perimenopausal years. The fluid is usually clear and colourless or straw-coloured. The mesothelial cells are degenerate and appear as large foamy histiocytic cells. The appearance is similar to that of long-standing cysts in other organs such as the breast or the kidney (see Figs 2.7 and 8.17).

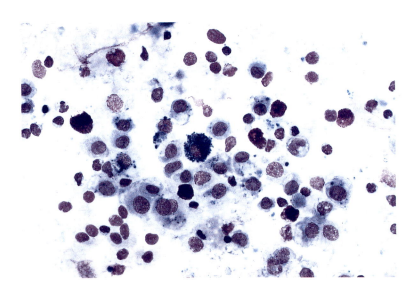

Fig. 1.49 Endometriotic cyst

(a) MGG ×1740

This term is applied to cystic degeneration in an area of endometriosis in the ovary. The fluid is chocolate-coloured, and contains altered blood, a few leukocytes and many iron-laden macrophages. A few cuboidal epithelial cells may persist. The appearance of the cells is compatible with that of endometrial cells, but cannot be distinguished from endometrioid cells that occur in the ovary and from which tumours may develop. Degenerate follicle cells may be similar in size and a diagnosis of a chocolate cyst is essentially a clinical or/and a histological one.

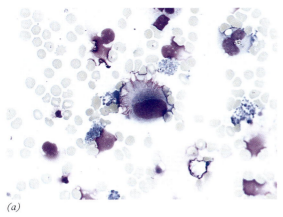

(a)

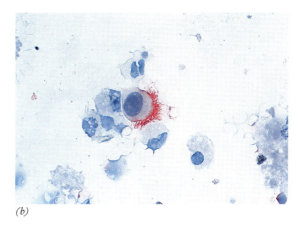

(b)

Fig. 1.50 Fimbrial cyst

(a) MGG ×1260 (b) APAAP for AUA 1 ×1260

Fimbrial cysts contain fallopian tube epithelium which is ciliated (a). The epithelial nature of the cells can be confirmed with immunocytochemical staining for epithelial antigens.

Neoplastic cysts

Epithelial tumours of the ovary, both benign and malignant, are derived from cells of the germinal epithelium, either on the surface or in sequestrated foci included within the stroma. The epithelium, which is of Müllerian origin, retains the capacity for differentiation along the various pathways taken by the glandular mucous linings of the genital tract. Differentiation to tubal-type epithelium is the most common and is seen in the serous group of tumours; endocervical-type or occasionally intestinal-type epithelium is found in the mucinous tumours; endometrioid cell tumours are relatively rare.

Fine-needle aspiration of a suspected ovarian carcinoma needs to be undertaken with care, and spillage avoided as these tumours are believed quickly to form peritoneal seedlings. The aspiration is carried out under direct vision, usually during a laparotomy, but may be repeated through a laparoscope as part of an assessment procedure. Collection of peritoneal washings for cytological examination has been recommended as an essential part of the staging of ovarian carcinoma and to provide a basis for therapy and future management. The washings first performed during open operation may also be repeated at subsequent laparoscopy. The cyst fluid and peritoneal washings are processed for cytological examination in the same manner as a serous effusion (see Chapter 4).

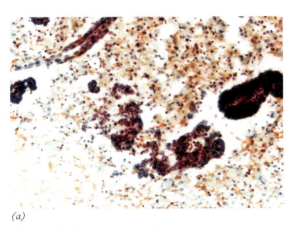

(a)   *(b)*

Fig. 1.51 Serous cystadenoma

(a) Papanicolaou ×133 (b) MGG ×420

The cytological presentation of a benign serous tumour of the ovary is extremely variable. A papillary tumour may be immediately recognizable in some cases (a), the only problem remaining being to determine whether it is benign or malignant.

The volume, colour and consistency of the fluid may contribute to the diagnosis and should be noted. Whereas colour and consistency of the fluid from a serous tumour may be no different from that of a corpus luteum or a germinal inclusion cyst, the volume may be significant. An inclusion cyst is arbitrarily divided into non-neoplastic if 3 cm or less in diameter and neoplastic if it exceeds this size.

The numerous fronds of tissue in (a) are immediately diagnostic of a papillary tumour. At high magnification (b) the cells that line the fronds are seen to be regular and small. The nuclei resemble each other and contain the odd clump of chromatin.

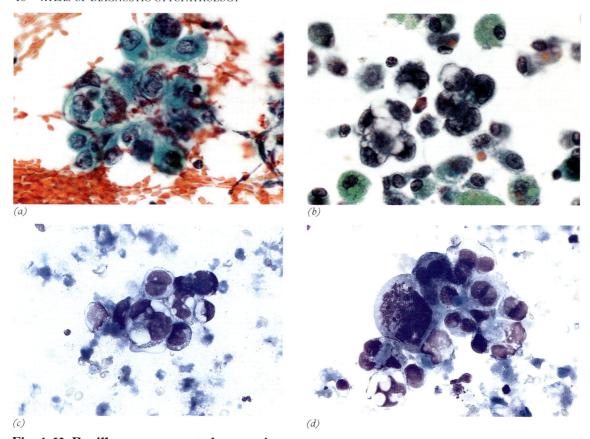

(a)   *(b)*

(c)   *(d)*

Fig. 1.52 Papillary serous cystadenocarcinoma

Papanicolaou (a) ×525 (b) ×525 MGG (c) ×840 (d) ×1260

Compare the cells from the two malignant serous tumours illustrated in these micrographs with the cells of benign serous tumours (Fig. 1.50) and note that the carcinoma cells are larger and display variations in cell size, nuclear size and nuclear-cytoplasmic ratios. The arrangement of cells in cluster is typical of an adenocarcinoma (a–d). The nuclei are distorted in shape, the cytoplasm is vacuolated and uniformly stained. Intracytoplasmic vacuoles with hard edges are seen (b, c).

The appearance is suggestive of mucous vacuoles and this was confirmed with Alcian blue. A serous cystadenocarcinoma may be heterogeneous and contain foci of mucous metaplasia. Unlike true mucinous tumours which secrete large amounts of extracellular mucin, secretion in serous tumours is usually sparse and evidence of scattered intracellular mucin does not alter the classification of the tumour.

Fig. 1.53 Mucinous cystadenoma

(a) Papanicolaou ×1260 (b) MGG ×840 (c) PAS-diastase ×840

The consistency of the fluid aspirated from a mucinous tumour often provides a clue, whereas colour is non-contributory. The extracellular mucin responsible for the viscosity of the fluid may be seen in the stained smear as a homogeneous translucent deposit which forms streaks or swathes in the background. The intracellular mucin, which is also present, may push the nucleus to one pole of the cell, which acquires a signet-ring appearance. The nuclei of the tumour cells are small, but the nuclear-cytoplasmic ratio varies with the degree of cytoplasmic vacuolization.

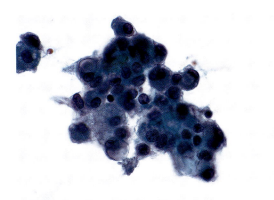

(a)

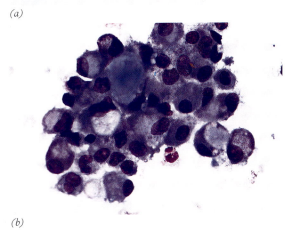

(b)

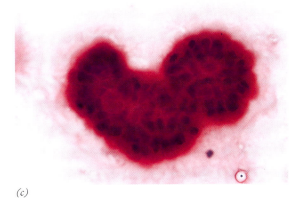

(c)

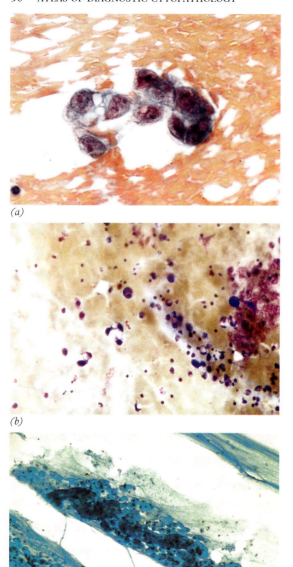

(a)

(b)

(c)

Fig. 1.54 Mucinous cystadenocarcinoma

(a) Papanicolaou ×525 (b) MGG ×133: same case; another smear (c) Alcian blue ×133: same case; another smear

Intracellular mucin vacuoles are evident in the cells in (a) which show stigmata of malignancy such as a variable chromatin pattern, anisonucleosis and disproportionately large nuclei. Note the hypochromasia of the nuclei, the prominent eosinophilic nucleoli and the smooth contours characteristic of a clump of exfoliated glandular cells. In the low-power view of another smear from the same specimen, stained with May–Grünwald–Giemsa, a streak of cells is seen embedded in an amorphous violet-stained deposit (b). This is free mucin and abundant intra- and extracellular mucin is confirmed in the Alcian blue-stained smear (c).

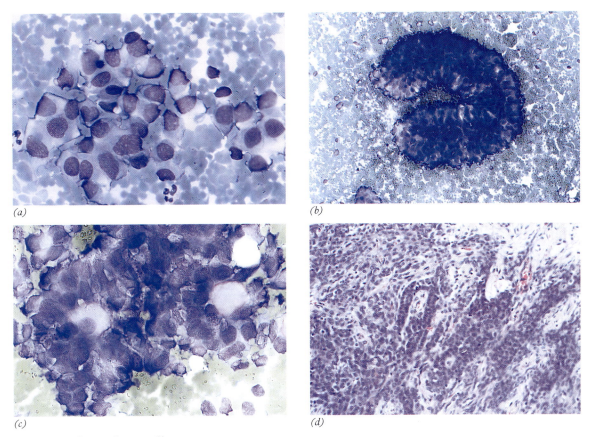

(a)   *(b)*

(c)   *(d)*

Fig. 1.55 Granulosa cell tumour

(a) MGG ×1260 (b) ×420 (c) ×1260 (d) H&E ×420

Ovarian sex cord stromal tumours are only rarely seen in fine-needle aspirates. This is an example of an infiltrating tumour which has extended beyond the ovary into the anterior abdominal wall. Aspirates show medium-size cells with no definite grooves (seen on histology) with a moderate amount of cytoplasm and no visible nucleoli (a). These are arranged in papillary clusters around capillaries (b) or can be seen to form acinar structures resembling Call–Exner bodies (c). Histological section of the tumour reveals solid cords of granulosa cell tumour, adult-type (d).

2. Breast

FINE-NEEDLE ASPIRATION OF THE BREAST

Four types of specimen may be obtained from the breast: nipple discharge, fine-needle aspiration (FNA) of cyst fluid or of a solid lesion and imprint smears of the nipple or the cut surface of a resected mass.

FNA of the breast is increasingly used as a rapid, reliable and inexpensive method for accurate diagnosis of malignancy. FNA will be successful if the following requirements are met:

   1 Aspiration technique.
   2 Optimal smear preparation and staining.
   3 Clinical history.
   4 Cytology report/diagnosis.

Aspiration technique

The aim of the FNA is to obtain maximum material from the representative site with minimum trauma to the patient. It is performed by a dedicated aspirator, either cytopathologist or clinician. Palpable lumps are immobilized between the two fingers, usually index and third finger, depth of the needle pass is assessed by the maximum diameter of the lesion as judged by the two fingers. This stereotactic skill of localizing the depth of the lesion improves with experience. Local anaesthetic (2% lignocaine) may be applied subcutaneously. FNA is performed by passing a fine needle (27, 25, 23, 22 or 21-G) either alone without suction or more commonly, attached to a syringe and syringe holder, into the lesion. The needle is moved within the lesion in a fan-shaped fashion, at the same time applying negative pressure either continuously or by repeated suction. Before exiting the lesion negative pressure is released. Blood in the syringe is undesirable and suction should stop at the appearance of blood in the hub of the needle. After exiting the lesion, the needle is detached from the syringe, air is taken and the contents of the needle expelled onto glass slides.

In cases of sclerotic or necrotic lesions where cell yield is poor, aspiration is repeated, aiming at the margins of the lesion which are usually representative of the sample.

Preparation and staining

Material obtained from the FNA needle on the glass slide is spread by using another glass slide. Spreading should be even and gentle, not using the ridge of the glass. FNA smears should be thin, contain no blood clots and no smearing (mechanical) artefacts. For special smearing techniques please refer to a cytopathology methods textbook. Smears are then fixed in 95% ethanol (immersed or sprayed) or air-dried. Stains used routinely are May–Grünwald–Giemsa (MGG) and Papanicolaou.

Clinical history

This should include the patient's age, sex, localization, clinical findings, previous therapy, pregnancy and lactation. The ultimate diagnosis should fit the clinical context even if the smears are examined blindly. Mammographic findings (e.g. ductal carcinoma-*in-situ*) may influence the cytodiagnosis.

Reporting

Providing that the above components are met as regards the technical quality and clinical history, the cytopathologist is expected to provide a diagnosis on the FNA smears. This can be expressed in five main categories, as recommended by the NHS Breast Screening Programme:

C 1 No diagnosis (too few cells, inadequate material).
C 2 No evidence of malignancy (cytologically benign cells, adequate material).
C 3 Atypia, probably benign (cytological features of both benign and atypical cells). Biopsy is advised.
C 4 Suspicious of malignancy (cells almost certainly malignant but due to the small number and/or suboptimally preserved cell detail caution is indicated). Biopsy is advised.
C 5 Malignant cells. Definite cytological evidence of malignancy on a representative cell sample.

If the cytological diagnosis confirms the mammographic and clinical findings (triple approach), definitive treatment can proceed on the basis of cytology. *Under no circumstances should a definitive treatment proceed without the agreement of all three modalities.* The diagnostic accuracy of combined clinical assessment, mammography and FNA cytology in diagnosing breast carcinoma is 98.8%.

BENIGN CONDITIONS

General cytological criteria for benign breast lesions are:
1 Monomorphic nuclei with smooth membranes.
2 Aggregates (monolayers) of epithelium with evenly distributed nuclei and myoepithelial cells.
3 Many naked bipolar nuclei.
4 Apocrine metaplasia, macrophages, leukocytes and clean background.

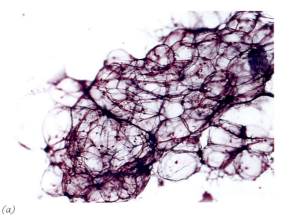

(a)   *(b)*

Fig. 2.1 Fibrofatty tissue

(a) MGG ×420 (b) Papanicolaou ×1260

Needle aspiration of a normal area of breast yields loose fibrofatty tissue and it is unusual to recover cells from a normal duct system. The breast has a rich blood supply and capillaries may occasionally be seen as ramifying channels in the fibrous tissue; red blood cells may be present in the channels.

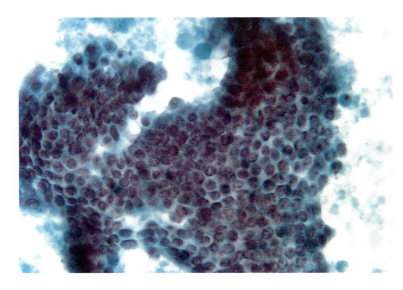

Fig. 2.2 Benign duct epithelium

Papanicolaou ×580

Aspirate of the breast usually yields a few clusters of benign duct epithelium. The presence of epithelium is considered to be one of the main criteria of smear adequacy in breast FNA. Breast epithelium has small oval nuclei with a regular chromatin pattern and nuclear outline, inconspicuous cytoplasm and nucleoli. It usually presents in tightly cohesive sheets and may have myoepithelial cells amongst it. These are small darker cells with no cytoplasm which appear to be on a slightly different plane from the epithelium (see Fig. 2.14d, e).

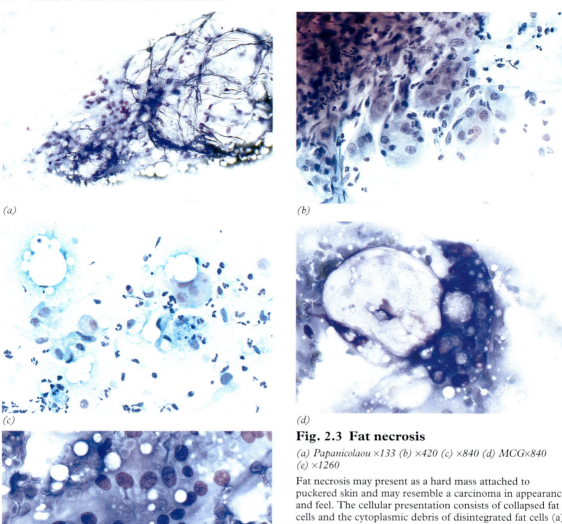

(a)

(b)

(c)

(d)

(e)

Fig. 2.3 Fat necrosis

(a) Papanicolaou ×133 (b) ×420 (c) ×840 (d) MCG×840 (e) ×1260

Fat necrosis may present as a hard mass attached to puckered skin and may resemble a carcinoma in appearance and feel. The cellular presentation consists of collapsed fat cells and the cytoplasmic debris of disintegrated fat cells (a). Polymorphs, lymphocytes, plasma cells and macrophages, including the multinucleate giant cells, follow soon (b, c).

Other causes of granulomatous response of breast tissue include foreign body granulomas (as a reaction to talc, suture, silicone implant, d, e), although tuberculosis and fungal infections are possible.

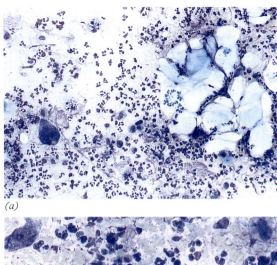

(a)

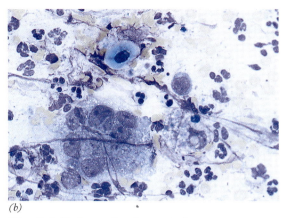

(b)

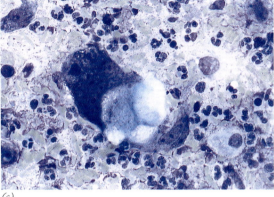

(c)

Fig. 2.4 Subareolar breast abscess

(a) MGG ×420 (b) ×1260 (c) ×1260

Fine-needle aspirate yields purulent material in which a mixture of numerous polymorphs, anucleate squames and multinucleate giant cells of foreign body type are seen (a–c). The lesion arises as a result of blockage of the main ducts with keratin; subsequent inflammatory reaction provoked by the blockage and keratin attempts to clear it (c). The lesion is benign and is usually excised surgically.

Benign breast lesions

The normal female breast is dependent on a variety of hormones which affect its structure and function. While the most dramatic changes are seen at puberty, pregnancy, lactation and menopause, the breast also undergoes subtle alterations during each menstrual cycle.

Disturbances or imbalance of the hormones or an altered or uneven response of the different elements in breast tissue results in the condition known as benign breast lesions. The disorder is also variously referred to as cystic mammary dysplasia, benign mammary dysplasia, fibrocystic disease and benign cystic mastopathy.

Fibroadenosis is the commonest disorder of the female breast. It simultaneously involves the ductal, lobular and stromal elements of the breast. The affected ducts show areas of dilatation (duct ectasia), which may appear as cysts containing fluid (cyst formation). The lobular ductules undergo hyperplastic proliferation (adenosis) and are surrounded by proliferating stroma (fibrosis). In one variant of fibroadenosis, the hyperplastic ductules are separated and compressed into tubular shapes by bands of dense fibrous tissue (sclerosing adenosis). Hypertrophy and multiplication of the lining epithelium may occur (epitheliosis).

A single component of fibroadenosis never occurs in isolation, but the term applied to the condition may be determined by the histological preponderance or the clinical presentation of one component. The disorder may produce a vaguely lumpy breast or present as a solitary mass. It occurs in the mature woman, particularly in the premenopausal years.

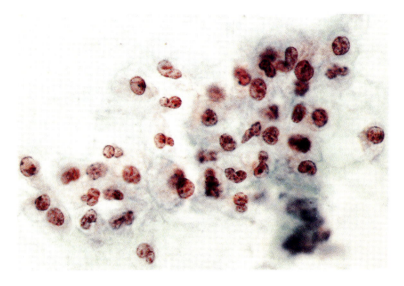

Fig. 2.5 Duct ectasia

Papanicolaou ×720: nipple discharge

Duct ectasia consists of dilatation of the mammary duct system and may be associated with a nipple discharge. This is usually clear, or may be slightly turbid. Duct epithelial cells are often seen, although some secretions are acellular and consist only of amorphous debris and a few leukocytes. The epithelial cells are usually swollen and foamy, and may occur as small aggregates or single forms. The nuclei are degenerative and may be round or indented. The foamy cells with reniform nuclei closely resemble large histiocytes.

A nipple discharge may also be associated with galactorrhoea, papillary hyperplasia of ductal epithelium, benign papilloma, intraduct or invasive carcinoma with an intraduct component. The nipple discharge associated with benign or malignant tumours generally contains a fair number of red blood cells or fibrin. These therefore serve as useful signals and merit full investigation as to the cause and source of the blood.

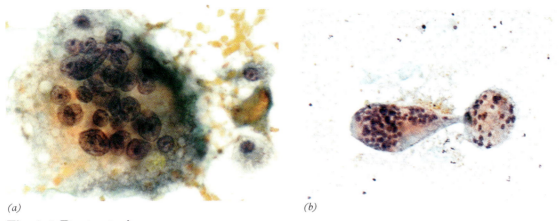

(a)   *(b)*

Fig. 2.6 Duct ectasia

Papanicolaou (a) ×525: nipple discharge; foreign body giant cell (b) ×133: same smear as (a). Fibrous tissue: foamy epithelial cells

Duct ectasia may present as a subareolar mass. The duct lumen is filled with detritus and lipid; chronic inflammatory cells infiltrate the periductal tissue. The duct-lining epithelium may become eroded and lipid enter the stroma and initiate a foreign-body giant-cell reaction (a). The illustration also shows small mononuclear macrophages and amorphous debris. Fragments of fibrous tissue and foamy epithelial cells may appear in the discharge (b).

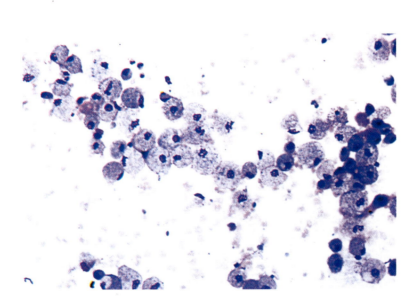

Fig. 2.7 Breast cyst

MGG ×183

A breast cyst may be small and microscopic or it may form a palpable tensile mass. A woman may present with one or more cysts in one or both breasts. The cyst collapses on aspiration of its contents and disappears altogether or recurs, or new cysts may appear. A solid lump overshadowed by the cyst may become apparent and it is customary to palpate the breast after the cyst has been aspirated and separately needle any residual lump.

In one type of cyst formation due to duct ectasia, the aspirated fluid contains mainly large foam cells, either single or cohesive. The foam cells are considered to have several different origins. Some are histiocytic, others are degenerate duct epithelial cells (compare with Fig. 2.5), yet others have residual morphological characteristics which suggest degenerative forms of apocrine metaplasia cells.

Neutrophils enter the cyst fluid and may be so numerous as to create an impression of pus.

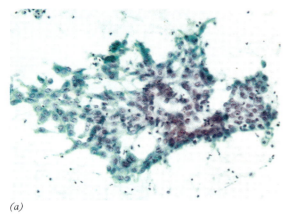

(a)

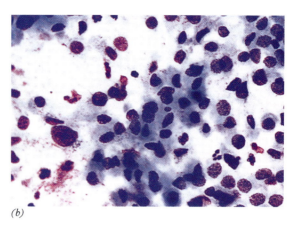

(b)

Fig. 2.8 Simple breast cyst

(a) Papanicolaou ×133 (b) MGG ×333

The lining of a breast cyst may consist of normal ductal epithelium which is shed into the fluid in loose aggregates; single forms are also seen. The cells are cuboidal or low columnar. If well-preserved, they have cyanophilic cytoplasm with the Papanicolaou stain and vesicular nuclei with pinpoint nucleoli (a). Degenerative changes in exfoliated cells include shrinkage of nuclei, irregularity of nuclear shapes and an impression of anisonucleosis (b). A few neutrophils are usually present.

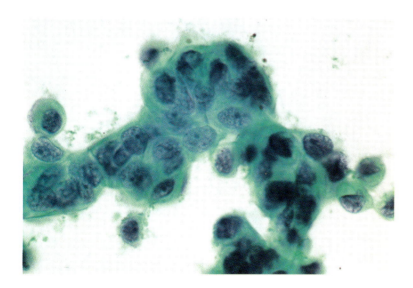

Fig. 2.9 Papillary cyst

Papanicolaou ×720

Occasionally, the epithelium lining a cystically dilated duct hypertrophies and forms papillary ingrowths into the cyst cavity. Branching fronds of epithelial tissue are seen in the cyst fluid. The cells show morphological features of proliferative activity. They are larger than their normal counterparts, basophilic and optically dense. The nuclei show some enlargement, but the nuclear:cytoplasmic ratio remains within the limits of benign cells. Slight enlargement of the nucleolus is usually apparent. Hyperplastic epithelial cells in cysts may occasionally contain mucous vacuoles.

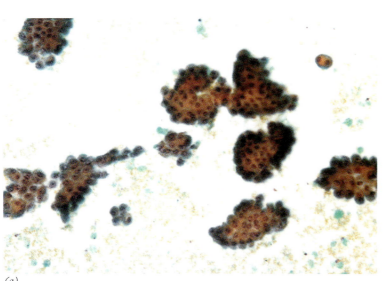

(a)

Fig. 2.10 Breast cyst: apocrine metaplasia

Papanicolaou (a) ×183 (b) MGG ×580 (c) MGG ×1740

Approximately one-third of breast cysts are lined by large cells, referred to as apocrine metaplasia cells because of their resemblance to cells of apocrine sweat glands. Fully formed apocrine metaplasia cells have a distinctive and striking appearance. They are amongst the largest epithelial cells seen in breast specimens and appear in smears in aggregates; a few single cells are also usually present (a). Apocrine metaplasia cells contain numerous coarse granules which impart an eosinophilia to the cytoplasm (b). In a Papanicolaou-stained smear, the cell may be uniformly pink or a variable amount of green or blue cytoplasm may be seen between the granules (b, c). The distal edge of the cell has a luminal fringe traversed by fine vertical lines (c). The fringe represents well-developed microvilli seen by electron microscopy. The round vesicular nucleus occupies a small part of the cell and the nuclear:cytoplasmic ratio is low; binucleation is not uncommon (a, b). Each nucleus has a prominent nucleolus.

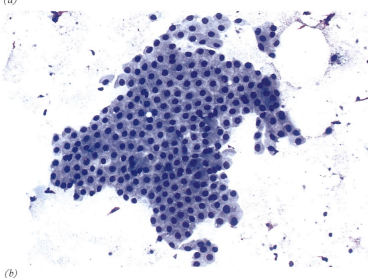

(b)

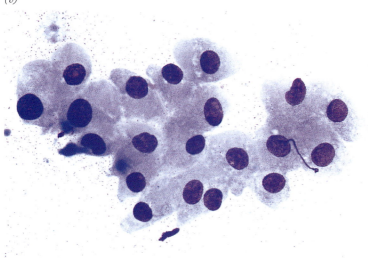

(c)

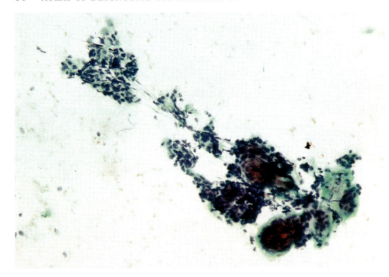

Fig. 2.11 Benign breast lesions

Papanicolaou ×183

The cellular presentation of fibroadenosis is variable. Dense fibrous tissue is resistant to aspiration and when fibrosis is the predominant component, the sample may be virtually acellular. In cases of marked adenosis, the smear may show only epithelial cells. The cytological diagnosis is therefore necessarily incomplete. In a few cases, fragments of hyperchromatic epithelial cells and cyanophilic connective tissue with few nuclei (lower right) may be recovered. The appearance is indistinguishable from that seen in fibroadenoma. However, samples from fibroadenosis may contain evidence of other components of the pathological complex, such as foam cells, apocrine metaplasia cells and neutrophils.

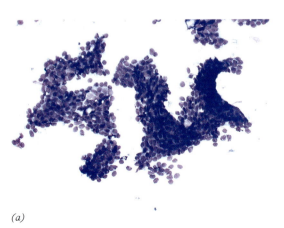

(a)

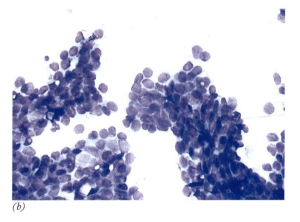

(b)

Fig. 2.12 Gynaecomastia

(a) MGG ×420 (b) MGG ×840

The normally rudimentary breast of the male may, under the effect of endogenous or exogenous hormones, undergo proliferative hyperplasia of ductal epithelium with a concomitant increase in periductal stroma. The condition is known as gynaecomastia. Certain therapeutic agents, notably cimetidine and spironolactone, oestrogens administered for carcinoma of the prostate, and ectopic hormone production by some neoplasms may induce hypertrophy of the male breast.

A case of gynaecomastia is illustrated from a man with small cell anaplastic carcinoma of the lung and a breast lump. Aspiration of this is invariably painful and the mass is often very rubbery, yielding scanty cellular material despite optimal aspiration technique. Smears show tightly cohesive branching fragments of epithelium (a) which is composed of small uniform oval cells with bland nuclear chromatin (b). Myoepithelial cells may be seen; stromal cells and amorphous background material are often present. Features are reminiscent of fibroadenoma in females.

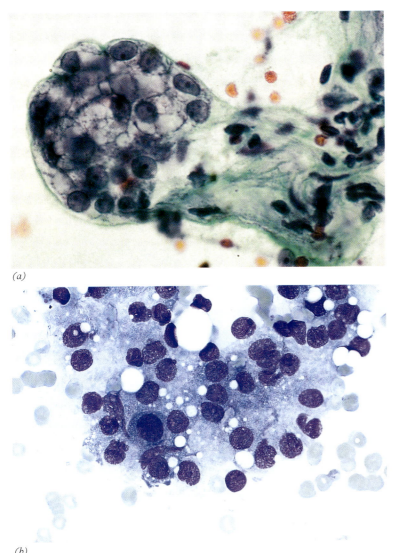

(a)

(b)

Fig. 2.13 Lactating breast

(a) Papanicolaou ×720 (b) MGG ×1740

Breast lumps during pregnancy or lactation are difficult to evaluate clinically or mammographically. FNA may be helpful if lactation changes are recognized. These are: moderate cellularity, small monolayers or clusters, hyperchromatic nuclei, nucleoli, no anisonucleosis, cytoplasmic vacuolation, macrophages and smearing artefact in the background.

Fig. 2.14 Fibroadenoma

*(a) MGG ×210 (b) ×580 (c) ×183
(d) ×1160 (e) Papanicolaou ×720
(f) ×840 (g) ×1260*

Fibroadenoma is composed of branching monolayers of epithelium (a) with well-defined outlines and stromal elements represented by amorphous background material which stains fuschia red in MGG stain (c) and also by numerous naked oval nuclei of stromal cells in the background (b). Bipolar (twin) nuclei are particularly characteristic of fibroadenoma. Epithelium is bland and regular. Within it, there are myoepithelial cells. These are small darker cells well visible on Papanicolaou-stained preparations (e) but can also be seen in the MGG stain (d, arrow). They appear on a different plane of focus to the epithelium (e). Aspirates from fibroadenoma are amongst the commonest causes of false positive breast cytology. This is almost invariably due to poor smear preparation including fixation and air drying as well as smearing artefacts. We show an example of a cellular fibroadenoma where the distinction between epithelium and stroma is imperceptible (f), particularly when the cells are mixed with fat vacuoles (g). Immunocytochemistry may be necessary to make the distinction.

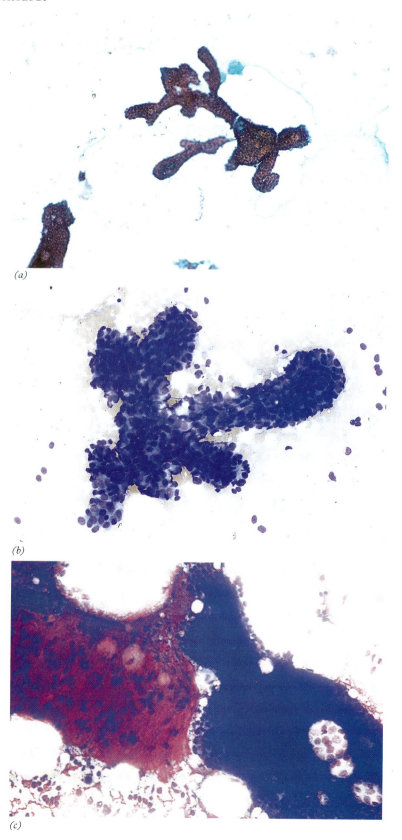

(a)

(b)

(c)

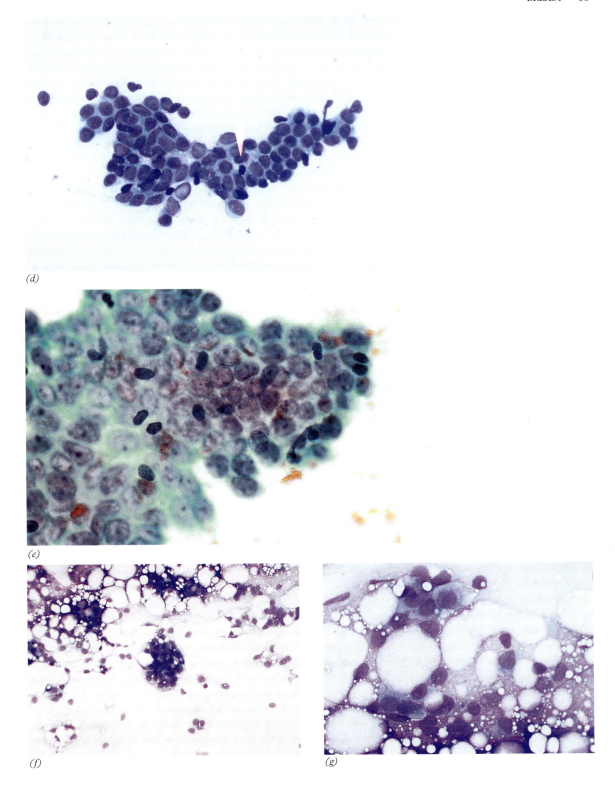

(d)

(e)

(f)

(g)

Variants of fibroadenoma

Fig. 2.15.1 Juvenile fibroadenoma

(a) MGG ×420 (b) ×1260 (c) ×1260

Relatively large well-defined mobile lumps in the breast of young women often prove very cellular on FNA smears. The general pattern is that of a fibroadenoma with a prominent stromal cell component (a). Macrophages and apocrine metaplasia may also be present (b). Epithelium is usually more crowded and less regular, its outlines being more ragged than in usual fibroadenoma. The general pattern and the patient's age as well as the clinical presentation must be considered when analysing the cytological details.

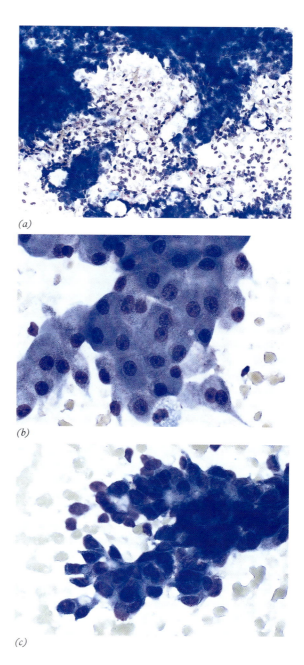

(a)

(b)

(c)

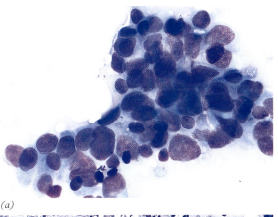

(a)

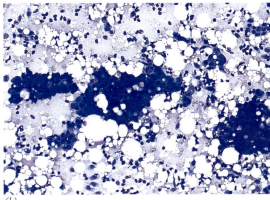

(b)

Fig. 2.15.2 Fibroadenoma in pregnancy and lactation

(a) MGG ×1260: 8 weeks' pregnancy (b) ×420: lactating breast

Aspirates of fibroadenoma in pregnancy and lactation can often show worrying features if a clinical history is not given. The epithelium shows a marked anisonucleosis and lactation changes similar to that described in Figure 2.13. The background contains fatty milk vacuoles, giving the stromal cells a disturbed appearance.

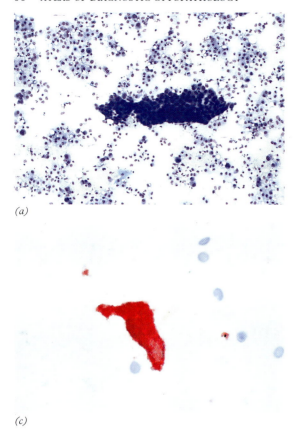

(a)

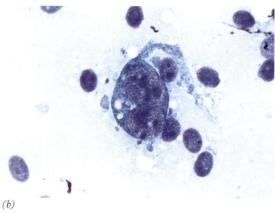

(b)

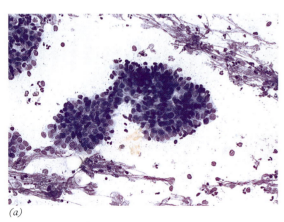

(c)

Fig. 2.16 Phyllodes tumour

(a) MGG ×420 (b) ×1260 (c) APAAP MIB I ×1260

Fibroadenomas occasionally have a very prominent stromal cell component, in which case, particularly in women over 35 years, a suspicion of phyllodes tumour may be raised. Epithelium is usually unremarkable (a). Stromal cells may contain occasional bizarre forms, raising suspicion of malignancy (b). Adequate assessment of stroma is usually not possible on FNA smears, although attempts are made to identify proliferating stromal cells with immunocytochemistry (c). The definitive diagnosis of phyllodes tumour and prediction of its biological behaviour remain the domain of histology.

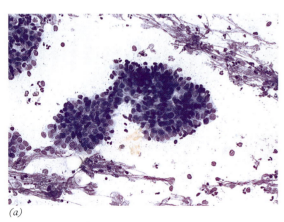

(a)

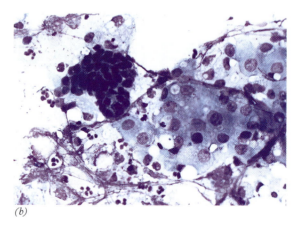

(b)

Fig. 2.17 Breast papilloma

(a) MGG ×420 (b) ×840

Breast aspirate contains papillary three-dimensional cell clusters composed of small duct-type cells. These are usually crowded and can vary in shape and size. They are surrounded by the content of a dilated duct: macrophages, debris, inflammatory cells (a). Differentiation from papillary carcinoma may be difficult. Areas of apocrine metaplasia (b) may be helpful in suggesting the benign nature of the lesion.

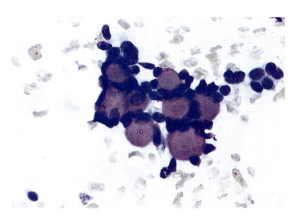

Fig. 2.18 Collagenous spherulosis

FNA breast; MGG ×1260

This rare, benign and incidental finding in the breast tissue of women between the age of 25 and 50 is usually found adjacent to foci of benign breast disease: sclerosing adenosis, radial scar and intraduct papilloma. Aspirates contain small hyaline globules within lobular acini which may show simple epithelial hyperplasia but generally appear bland. There are myoepithelial cells in the background. Globules (spherules) are composed of type I collagen and laminin: cells surrounding them show myoepithelial differentiation. Similar change may be seen in pleomorphic adenoma and low grade adenoid cystic carcinoma of the salivary glands. Adenoid cystic carcinoma usually has hyperchromatic nuclei with coarse granular chromatin and sometimes prominent nucleoli. Finger-like projections of hyaline material may be seen in adenoid cystic carcinoma. Both conditions may have dispersed single cells in the background with ill-defined cytoplasm. In cases of doubt, excision may be advised to exclude the possibility of adenoid cystic carcinoma.

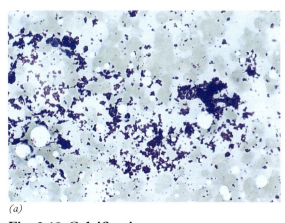

(a)

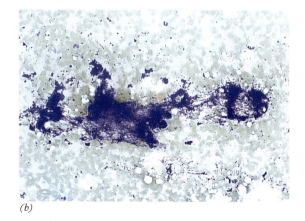

(b)

Fig. 2.19 Calcification

(a) MGG ×420 (b) ×840

Calcium deposits can be seen in benign and malignant breast lesions. Their finding on cytological material is significant in that it confirms to the aspirator that the sample is from the area corresponding to the imaging abnormality. Morphologically, on MGG-stained slides, it appears as tiny blue granules, either scattered (a) or clustered (b) in one area of the slide. They can be overlooked or mistaken for stain deposit from a poorly filtered Giemsa stain.

PRIMARY CARCINOMA

Cytology has an important role to play in the primary diagnosis of breast carcinoma. Together with imaging and clinical diagnosis, it forms part of a 'triple approach' in the diagnosis of carcinoma whereupon no definitive treatment should be done on the cytology report alone, i.e. without consideration for imaging and clinical diagnosis.

The histological classification of breast carcinoma into ductal, lobular and special types is only partially reflected in cytological preparations. Similarly, the concept of *in situ* and invasive carcinoma can only rarely be claimed on cytological preparations. Histological grading of tumours (Bloom and Richardson) is not applicable in its full form (i.e. mitoses and tubule formation) to cytology.

The cytological grading of tumours is based on nuclear grading. This may be performed by using criteria embodied in Fisher's modification of Black's system and the Scarff–Bloom–Richardson scheme (see descriptions given with Fig. 2.20).

The diagnostic accuracy of FNA cytology in diagnosis of breast carcinoma is 95% as compared with clinical examination (86%), mammography (86%), and ultrasonography (82%). Triple assessment is the combination of clinical examination, imaging and FNA cytology. By combining the three methods, only 0.2% of carcinomas are considered benign.

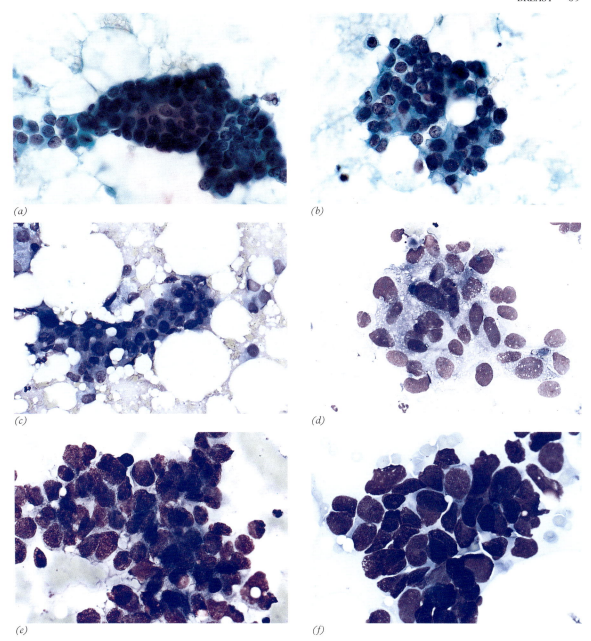

Fig. 2.20 Ductal carcinoma

(a) Papanicolaou ×1260 (b) ×1260 (c) MGG ×1260 (d) ×1260 (e) ×1260 (f) ×1260

The appearances of ductal carcinoma cells vary from very monotonous (low nuclear grade) to moderately and severely pleomorphic (high grade). Some centres apply nuclear grading to the diagnosis. Nuclear grade 1 (NG 1) has a nucleus similar to that in normal duct epithelium with minimal enlargement, round smooth nuclear membranes, uniform fine chromatin, and no nucleoli (a, b). NG 2 indicates a nucleus that may be up to twice the size of that of NG 1 (overall moderate anisonucleosis), with smooth nuclear membranes and uniform chromatin. Uniformity in size is the rule, even though nuclei are enlarged. Small nucleoli may be present (c, d). NG 3 is readily distinguishable by virtue of marked anisonucleosis in which the nuclei invariably show at least a threefold variation in diameter (e, f). They show marked hyperchromatism, irregular nuclear contours and macronucleoli may be present. They are arranged in clusters and dispersed singly in the background.

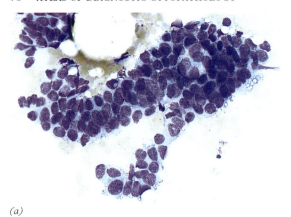

(a)

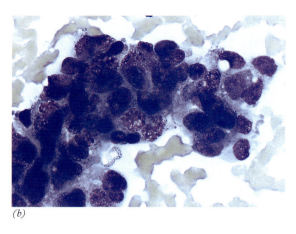

(b)

Fig. 2.21 Ductal carcinoma-*in-situ*

(a) MGG ×420 (b) MGG ×1260

Occasionally ductal carcinoma cells appear in cohesive clusters of small cells showing variable pleomorphism, some loss of polarity and prominent nucleoli. These features may be the indication of ductal carcinoma-*in-situ*. In view of the morphological similarity to benign breast disease such lesions are best biopsied.

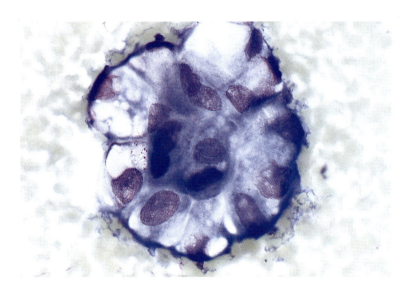

Fig. 2.22 Intracystic carcinoma

MGG ×1740

Less than 3% of breast cysts are malignant; the fluid from these is generally tinged or heavily stained with blood. The cells in this micrograph, seen against a background of fibrin, are variable in size. Much of the intense hyperchromasia is due to nuclear pyknosis, but in the cells in the centre of the field, it is due to condensed coarsely granular chromatin. Palpation of the breast after aspiration of the fluid did not disclose a solid lump, and the carcinoma was found to be limited to the cyst-lining epithelium. This type of tumour is classified as non-invasive intracystic carcinoma.

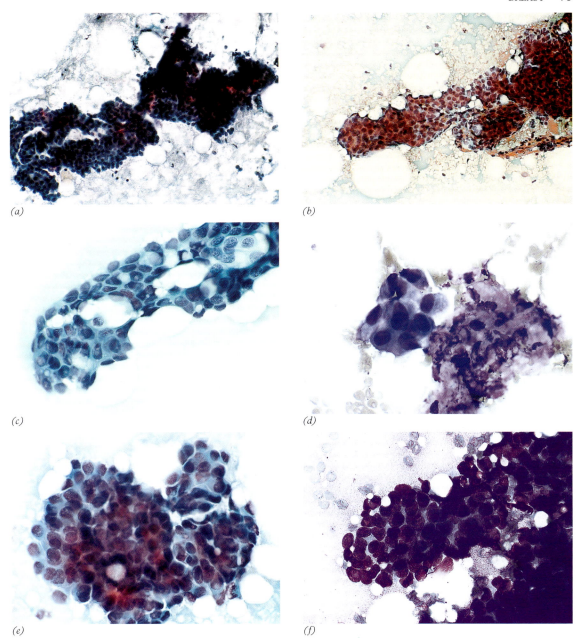

Fig. 2.23 Lobular carcinoma

(a) Papanicolaou ×420 (b) ×420 (c) ×1260 (d) MGG ×1260 (e) Papanicolaou ×1260: lobular carcinoma-in-situ (f) MGG ×1260: same case

Lobular carcinoma can be difficult to diagnose cytologically, both as a tumour type but also sometimes as malignancy. Classical cytological features of lobular carcinoma are: sparse cellularity, small atypical cells lying singly, in files or in small groups, the nuclei may be regular in size but irregular in shape (lack of uniformity). The cytoplasm may be absent, scanty or may show the presence of intracytoplasmic lumina. Diagnosis may be missed because the small cell size may mimic inflammatory process. Sometimes, most of the tumour cells present in tightly cohesive aggregates of uniform cells resembling fibroadenoma (a). These often represent either lobular carcinoma in situ or pagetoid tumour spread along the ducts (b, c). In these cases myoepithelial cells may be seen outlining the aggregates. Great care must be given to the background where single epithelial cells must be distinguished from stromal cells. Not infrequently, the background in lobular carcinoma aspirates may contain fragments of amorphous stromal material (d) and fat, sometimes infiltrated by tumour cells. This feature does not predict invasive nature of the tumour. Cell morphology (anisonucleosis, pleomorphism, nucleoli) and nuclear crowding are often the only indication of malignancy (e, f), particularly in the pleomorphic lobular carcinoma.

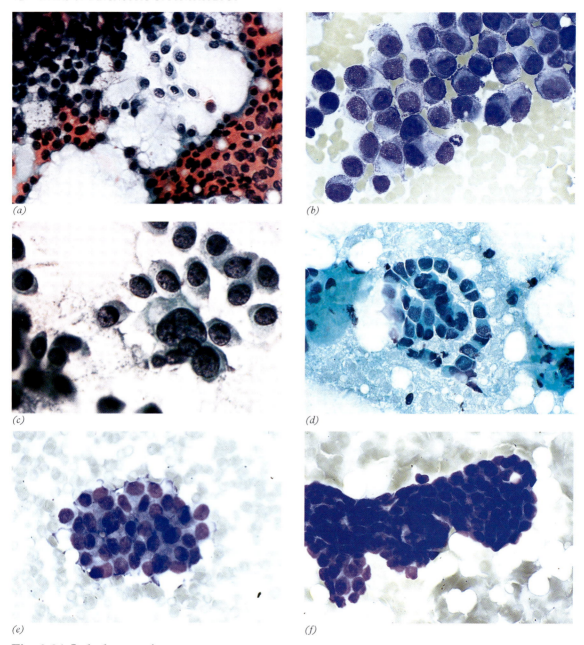

Fig. 2.24 Lobular carcinoma

(a) Papanicolaou ×333 (b) MGG ×1260 (c) Papanicolaou ×832 (d) Papanicolaou ×1260 (e) MCG ×1260 (f) ×1260

A case of infiltrating lobular carcinoma with a focus of carcinoma-*in-situ* is illustrated. The cells of a lobular carcinoma are generally small and monomorphic (a). The dispersed pattern of monomorphic epithelial cells with eccentric nuclei and relatively abundant cytoplasm suggests lobular carcinoma (b–d). Indian file arrangement, which is helpful in histology, is only rarely seen (d).

Lobular carcinoma may cause diagnostic difficulties due to the lack of cell pleomorphism, particularly when the cells are in tightly cohesive clusters as in this example of lobular carcinoma in situ (e) with pagetoid spread along the ducts (f).

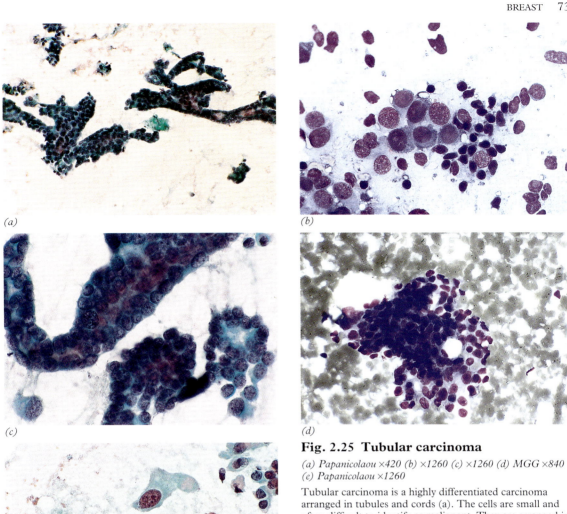

(a)

(b)

(c)

(d)

(e)

Fig. 2.25 Tubular carcinoma

*(a) Papanicolaou ×420 (b) ×1260 (c) ×1260 (d) MGG ×840
(e) Papanicolaou ×1260*

Tubular carcinoma is a highly differentiated carcinoma arranged in tubules and cords (a). The cells are small and often difficult to identify as malignant. They are arranged in tightly cohesive clusters and single cells. Cells in clusters may have a beaded appearance with well-defined outer margins and occasional lumina (b–d). They have disproportionately large nuclei and mostly little cytoplasm. Apical snouts seen on histology are only rarely present (e). Nuclear chromatin is finely stippled. Mitoses can be seen.

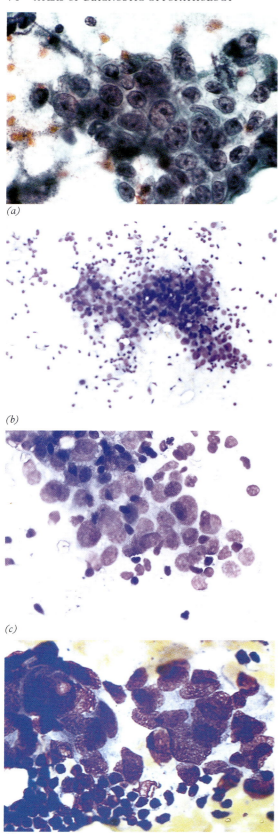

(a)

(b)

(c)

(d)

Fig. 2.26 Medullary carcinoma

(a) Papanicolaou ×525 (b) MGG ×1260 (c) ×1260 (d) ×525

A medullary carcinoma has distinctive clinical, cytological and histological features. The tumour is soft to palpation and lacks the serpiginous hard edges of the usual infiltrating duct carcinoma. Macroscopically, it appears circumscribed; the cut surface tends to bulge outwards and the tumour is referred to by surgeons as encephaloid carcinoma. The histological pattern is of sheets and broad anastomosing cords of tumour cells without a discernible glandular structure or desmoplastic reaction. Aspirates contain clusters and single, large cells with mainly round, smooth-bordered, vesicular nuclei and with prominent nucleoli and resemble the cells of a seminoma (a). Infiltration by lymphoid cells is a feature of medullary carcinoma (b, c) and may be mistaken for dual cell population of benign conditions, e.g. fibroadenoma.

Prominent lymphoid infiltration may occur in invasive ductal carcinoma, not of medullary type. The nuclei are angular and nucleoli are inconspicuous. Cell morphology is not that of medullary carcinoma (d).

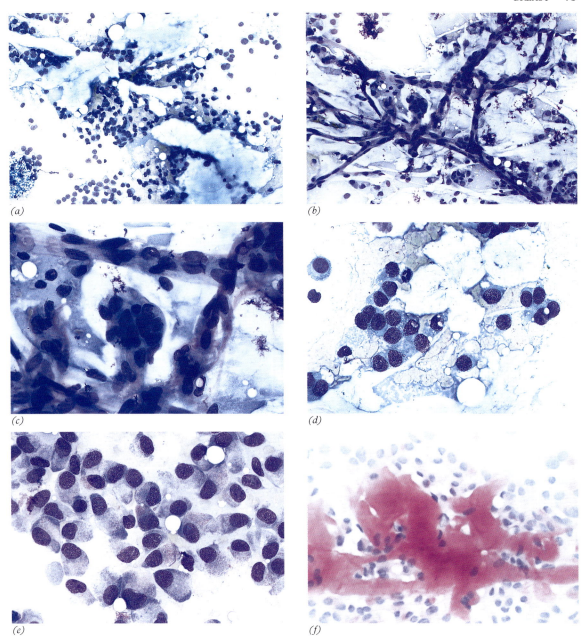

(a) *(b)* *(c)* *(d)* *(e)* *(f)*

Fig. 2.27 Mucinous carcinoma

(a) MGG ×420 (b) ×420 (c) ×1260 (d) ×1260 (e) ×1260 (f) PAS diastase ×840

The term mucinous carcinoma is applied to breast tumours which have a large amount of extracellular mucin. Tumours are associated with a better prognosis (10% mortality over 20 years) compared to other tumour types. They are often admixed with ductal carcinomas and the proportion of ductal element can only be assessed on excision of a specimen of the tumour. This can, according to various authors, be up to 25%. Cytology therefore, whilst able to give a diagnosis, is not a definitive method of diagnosing mucinous tumours.

Morphology of mucinous carcinoma is striking in that even on low power there are cells immersed in the background material (a) traversed by cords and nests (b, c). Islands of well-differentiated carcinoma are seen near the lakes of extracellular mucin (d). Cells are usually very bland and uniform with eccentric nuclei (e). Staining for mucin is only rarely necessary to prove the nature of background material (f).

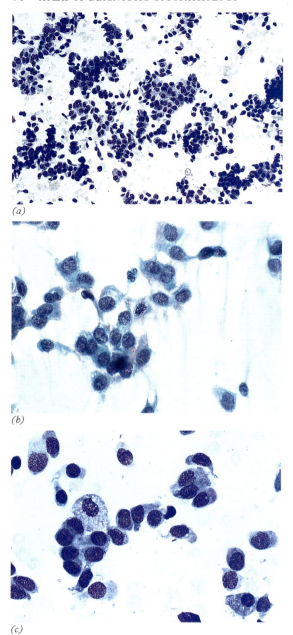

(a)

(b)

(c)

Fig. 2.28 Papillary carcinoma

(a) MGG ×420 (b) Papanicolaou ×1260(c) MGG ×1260

This rare tumour presents in FNA smears as a monotonous cell population of single and aggregated cells (a) which on higher power have a columnar appearance with a suggestion of apical 'snouting' seen on histological sections (b, c). Anisonucleosis is minimal and, although the chromatin is granular, the monotony of the cell population as well as the presence of macrophages (c) in the aspirates may mislead one into making a diagnosis of benign disease.

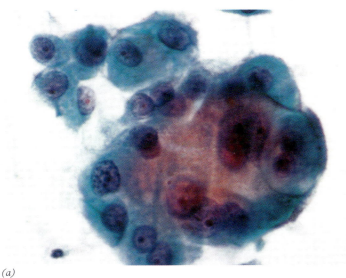

(a)

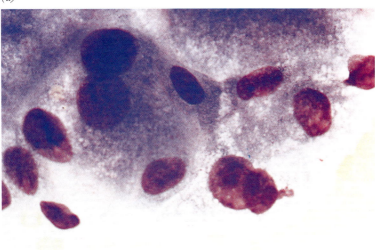

(b)

Fig. 2.29 Apocrine carcinoma

(a) Papanicolaou ×720 (b) MGG ×720: another case

An apocrine carcinoma is composed of large cells, eosinophilic with haematoxylin and eosin, reminiscent of apocrine metaplasia cells. The variable-sized malignant cells in (a) are mainly large, the nuclear-cytoplasmic ratio is low and nucleoli are prominent. The cytoplasm is amphophilic. Intracytoplasmic granules are not seen. The overall morphology is suggestive of apocrine carcinoma and was reflected exactly in sections of the mastectomy specimen. The cells in (b) are also devoid of granules but show all the other features of apocrine metaplasia cells. The histological diagnosis was apocrine carcinoma.

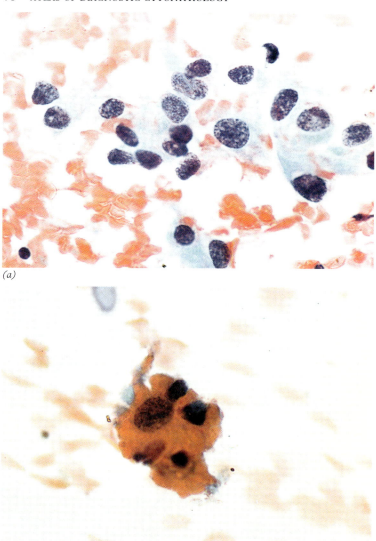

(a)

(b)

Fig. 2.30 Paget's disease of the nipple

Papanicolaou (a) ×720 (b) ×183: nipple scrape

In Paget's disease of the nipple, an underlying ductal carcinoma which may be invasive (but is more often intraepithelial) spreads through the mammary ducts and infiltrates the squamous epithelium of the nipple. The areola is reddened and thickened, develops fissures and later usually ulcerates; it may appear eczematous. The carcinoma cells (a) are large and pleomorphic with abundant cytoplasm and granular nuclei. The squamous cells from the affected nipple and areola generally appear dyskaryotic and dyskeratotic in smears (b).

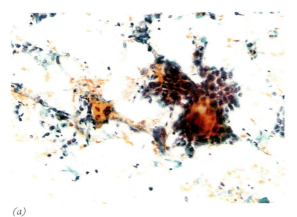

(a)

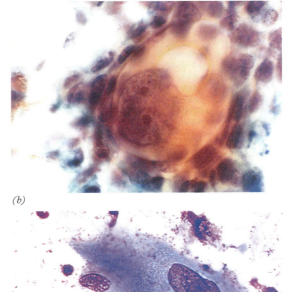

(b)

Fig. 2.31 Ductal carcinoma with squamous metaplasia

Papanicolaou (a) ×133 (b) ×525: same field (c) MGG ×525: same specimen; another smear

The World Health Organization classification of breast carcinoma includes the category 'carcinoma with metaplasia'. Foci of squamous cells, spindle cells, cartilage and osseous tissue may be seen in a recognizable ductal carcinoma. Small cyanophilic malignant ductal cells and a few large opaque orangeophilic cells are seen attached to each other in (a). At a higher magnification (b), the large cell with two giant nuclei and macronucleoli is seen to be of a different type from the surrounding ductal carcinoma cells. The squamous character of the cell is indicated by the size, texture and pale cytoplasm in the MGG smear (c).

(c)

Fig. 2.32 Carcinoma of the male breast

Papanicolaou ×720

Carcinoma of the male breast is extremely uncommon. The malignant cells are of ductal origin, moderately large and moderately pleomorphic with hyperchromic granular nuclei and an occasional nucleolus.

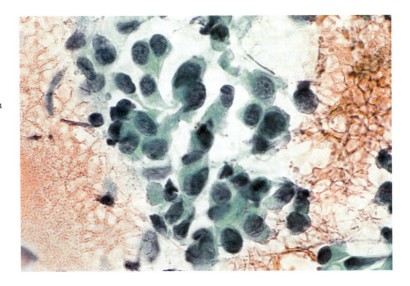

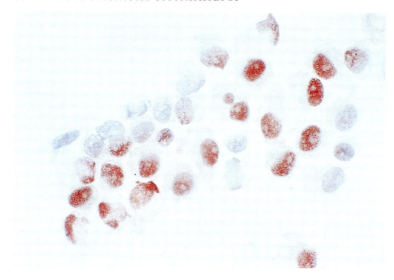

Fig. 2.33 Oestrogen receptor status

APAAP staining for oestrogen receptors ×1740

This can be determined on cytological preparations provided there is a good nuclear staining. Technique is particularly useful in cases where surgery is not contemplated or where it is to be preceded by another treatment (laser, chemotherapy).

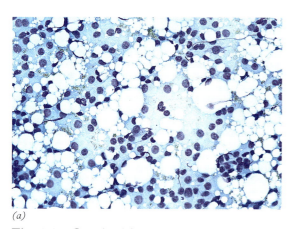

(a)

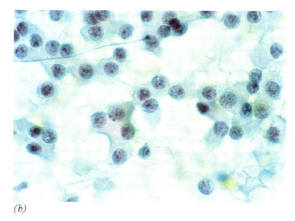

(b)

Fig. 2.34 Carcinoid tumour

FNA breast: (a) MGG ×840 (b) Papanicoloau ×1260 (courtesy of Dr P. Wilson)

Mammary carcinoid is an uncommon tumour with characteristic histological, ultrastructural and immunocytochemical features. Fine needle aspirate yields a cellular sample with cells mostly dispersed singly with very few clusters and acinus-like structures or sheets (a). The cells are small, regular and have uniform round or oval, often eccentric nuclei, stippled chromatin and abundant cytoplasm which may contain granules (b). The cells may give a 'plasmacytoid appearance'. No necrosis is seen in the background. Immunocytochemistry shows positive staining for neuroendocrine markers. Ultrastructural features include membrane-bound dense core particles in the cytoplasm consistent with neuroendocrine secretory granules.

Cytologically, differential diagnosis in the breast includes lobular carcinoma, non-Hodgkin's lymphoma and metastatic carcinoid tumour. The features of the latter are the same as primary breast carcinoid and distinction has to be made on clinical grounds. Primary breast carcinoid is usually argyrophil positive so that whenever an argentaffin tumour is seen, diagnosis of carcinoid metastatic to the breast has to be considered. Lobular carcinoma usually has lesser cell yield, 'Indian file' arrangement, some cell pleomorphism, intracytoplasmic vacuole and does not show stippled chromatin typical of carcinoid tumours. Non-Hodgkin's lymphoma has dispersed population of monotonous cells. However, careful scrutiny of cell detail reveals characteristics of lymphoid cells: clumped chromatin and a variable amount of cytoplasm depending on the cell type and maturity.

Prognosis of mammary carcinoma with carcinoid features is comparable to that of conventional carcinoma. There are no reliable morphological features that could predict the biological behaviour of this tumour.

MESENCHYMAL LESIONS

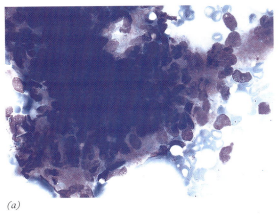

(a)

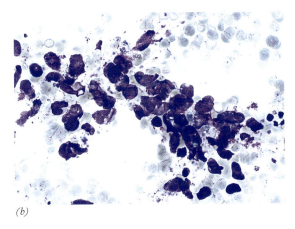

(b)

Fig. 2.35 Dermatofibrosarcoma protuberans

(a) MGG ×1260 (b) MGG ×1260

This is a cutaneous lesion of borderline malignancy. It tends to recur if incompletely excised. Unlike its benign or malignant counterparts (benign and malignant fibrous histiocytoma), it does not show a mixture of histiocytes, inflammatory cells and pigment, although occasional Tauton giant cells may be seen. Instead, it is composed of irregularly shaped spindle cells which mainly appear as bare nuclei immersed in dense background stromal material (a, b). This material is at the same time the clue to the lesion's mesenchymal origin. Staining for endothelial markers (CD 34) is weakly positive, making distinction from angiosarcoma difficult.

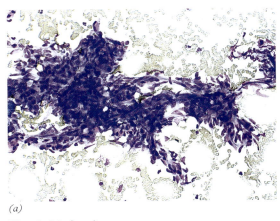

(a)

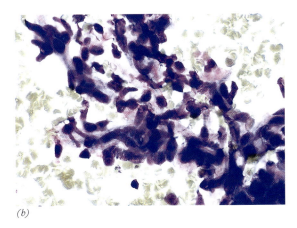

(b)

Fig. 2.36 Angiosarcoma

(a) MGG ×420 (b) ×1260 (courtesy of Dr A. Rubin)

This highly malignant tumour often presents in young women as a large mass clinically mimicking carcinoma. FNA of the high-grade angiosarcoma illustrated in our case shows cellular smears composed of interweaving spindle cells immersed in background material (a). They show anisonucleosis and cell pleomorphism. Occasionally tramtrack cellular fragments mimicking capillaries are seen connecting the fragments (b). Cytological features as well as negative epithelial markers should alert the observer to angiosarcoma.

METASTATIC TUMOURS

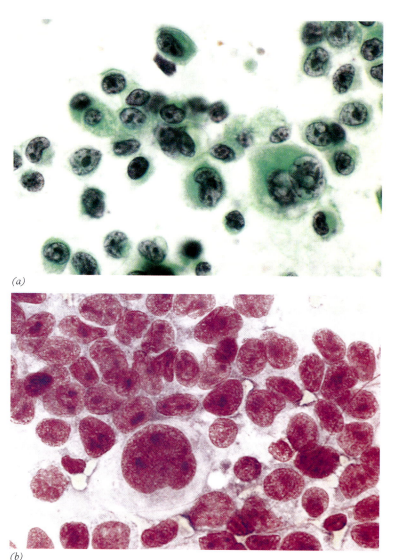

(a)

(b)

Fig. 2.37 Metastatic amelanotic melanoma

(a) Papanicolaou ×720 (b) MGG ×720 same specimen; another smear

Metastatic spread of extramammary cancer to the breast is exceedingly rare. The commonest source of metastatic deposits is primary carcinoma of the contralateral breast. Next most frequently seen is metastatic, non-Hodgkin's lymphoma, followed by oat-cell carcinoma of the lung. A case of metastatic amelanotic melanoma is illustrated. Fluid aspirated from a fluctuant cystic mass in the breast of a young woman in the 28th week of pregnancy was found to contain pleomorphic malignant cells with prominent nucleoli and several mononuclear and binucleate large forms. The cells were unlike any of the usual variants of breast carcinoma generally seen. A history of an amelanotic melanoma on the back excised a year earlier was obtained. The solitary mass was resected and found to be a metastasis from the melanoma.

3. Respiratory tract

Exfoliative cytology of sputum and bronchial secretions for the diagnosis of bronchogenic carcinoma has a time-honoured history. The wider use of sophisticated interventional radiology and of the flexible fibreoptic bronchoscope which allows examination of the bronchial tree as far as the pulmonary parenchyma has increased the variety of diagnostic specimens obtainable and extended the scope of cytopathology.

The specimens selected and the sequence in which they are examined are determined by the presumptive pathology under investigation.

SAMPLING TECHNIQUES

Sputum

This must be an early-morning 'deep cough' specimen from the lower respiratory tract, collected before food and drink, other than water, are taken and before the teeth are cleaned. As not every specimen is informative, it is common practice to examine three specimens, obtained on consecutive days; a persistent search may be indicated in cases in which invasive methods are contraindicated. Sputum expectorated in the few days following bronchoscopy may contain diagnostic material, not previously identified.

The specimen is poured into a Petri dish and examined for suggestive fragments such as opaque grey threads or blood-streaked strands. These are transferred to a glass slide, smeared and fixed.

Fibreoptic bronchoscopy specimens

Trap

Bronchopulmonary secretions are trapped in a tube interposed between the bronchoscope and a suction pump. The specimen is processed in the same manner as sputum.

Bronchial washings

Warm sterile buffered saline (10 ml) is introduced in small aliquots into the bronchi and reaspirated. Washings may be obtained from different bronchopulmonary segments. Smears are made from centrifuged deposit.

Bronchoalveolar lavage

The tip of the bronchoscope is impacted in a peripheral bronchus. Two to three aliquots of 50–60 ml buffered saline are injected and reaspirated. Smears are made as from bronchial washings.

Bronchial brushings

These are collected following washings and biopsies. The brush can be extended beyond the tip of the scope and material obtained from a lesion not easily visualized or biopsied. Rapid fixation is essential to avoid dehydration and the smears are spread and fixed one at a time in the operating theatre.

Transbronchial biopsy

This is obtained at bronchoscopy with a fine needle introduced through the bronchial wall into adjacent lung tissue. The material obtained is usually sufficient for one or two smears.

Percutaneous fine-needle aspiration (FNA)

The needle is introduced through locally anaesthetized skin and subcutaneous tissue into the lesion under imaging control. A syringe is attached to the needle which is moved in different directions whilst steady suction is applied. Resistance is met when tissue enters the needle lumen. At this point, the piston must be released to equalize pressure before the withdrawal of the needle. Smears are made immediately and may number up to 10 or more. The syringe and needle are rinsed out in saline, or alcohol or a cell culture medium; this is held in reserve for analysis.

The recommendations laid down for the handling of class B pathogens should be observed in the processing of respiratory tract specimens.

Romanowsky stains are not satisfactory for sputum, trap and bronchial washings on account of their mucus content, and the Papanicolaou method is preferred by most cytopathologists. Both techniques are applicable to bronchoalveolar lavage and aspiration smears. In the author's laboratory, both methods are routinely employed and are found to be complementary.

Nasal secretions may be examined for eosinophils in allergic rhinitis and a maxillary sinus carcinoma may be identified in washings. Pharyngeal carcinoma may be scraped or brushed. Pathological lesions of the nasopharynx however are not commonly met with in routine diagnostic cytology and emphasis in this section has been laid on disorders of the lower respiratory tract.

BENIGN CONDITIONS

Oral mucosa

Squamous cells from the upper respiratory tract are present in all respiratory tract specimens except transbronchial or percutancous FNAs. In specimens from the lower respiratory tract, they are accompanied by macrophages and bronchoalveolar epithelial cells.

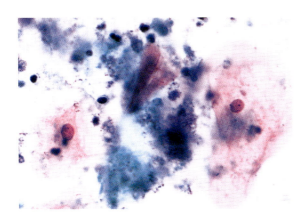

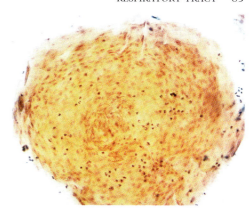

Fig. 3.1 Squamous cells

Papanicolaou ×525: saliva

A salivary specimen consists mainly of large polyhedral superficial squamous cells. Bacteria from the mouth and a few neutrophils are generally present; alveolar macrophages are conspicuous by their absence. Saliva is unsuitable for cytopathological assessment of diseases of the respiratory tract.

Fig. 3.2 Squamous cells

Papanicolaoux ×133: bronchial washings

Instrumentation of the respiratory tract may dislodge a fragment of stratified squamous epithelium from the upper part of the tract. The tightly packed, normal squamous cells are identified by their large size, delicate translucent cytoplasm and the small regular nuclei.

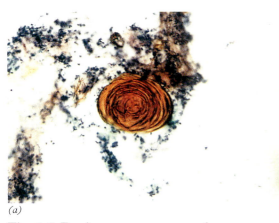

(a)

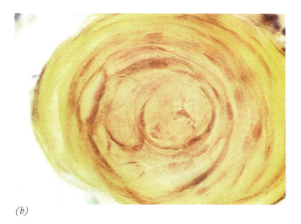

(b)

Fig. 3.3 Benign squamous pearl

Papanicolaou (a) ×133: bronchial washings (b) ×525: same field

Similarly dislodged hyperkeratotic epithelium may be arranged in a concentric manner and simulate a malignant epithelial pearl (a). At a higher magnification, the pearl is seen to consist of layers of anucleate keratinized cells rolled round intermediate squamous cells with bland nuclei and keratohyaline granules in the cytoplasm (b).

Respiratory epithelium

The respiratory epithelium lining the trachea and the major bronchi consists of ciliated columnar cells and mucus-secreting goblet cells. As the bronchi divide into smaller branches, the lining cells undergo a gradual transition into non-ciliated cuboidal cells; the goblet cells which are abundant in the trachea gradually diminish in number and are absent from the terminal bronchioles. A fourth type of cell which is non-ciliated and non-mucus-secreting, the Clara cell, makes its appearance in the terminal bronchioles. It can be identified by its distinctive ultrastructure and is probably involved in the synthesis of surfactant. The alveolar epithelial lining has been shown by electron microscopy to consist of the type 1 pneumocyte which has an attenuated cytoplasm and which cannot be seen by light microscopy, and the type 2 pneumocyte, which is a rounded cell, the nucleus of which is visible by light microscopy. The type 2 pneumocyte may acquire phagocytic properties. Scattered through the bronchial mucosa is the endocrine Kulchitsky or Feyrter cell, characterized by neurosecretory dense core granules, derived from the APUD system.

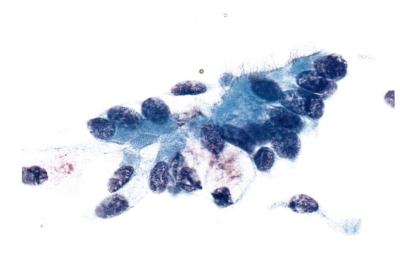

Fig. 3.4 Bronchial epithelial cells

Papanicolaou ×720: bronchial brush

This micrograph shows a sheet of normal bronchial mucosa. The ciliated bronchoepithelial cell is tall and slender. Its free luminal end has a clearly defined terminal bar or end-plate to which the cilia are attached. The end anchored to the basement membrane tapers to a fine point or tail and gives the cell a pyramidal or triangular shape. The oval nucleus, nearer the apical end, is the same width as the cell and the lateral cell borders coincide with the lateral nuclear borders. The goblet cell is larger. Its cytoplasm is distended with secretory vacuoles and the nucleus lies at the base of the cell.

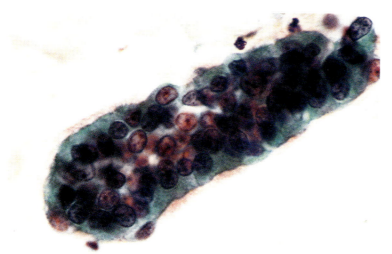

Fig. 3.5 Ciliated columnar cells

Papanicolaou ×720: sputum

Ciliated columnar cells may be shed in clusters, generally following mechanical or chemical irritation. The pseudopapillary arrangement seen here is due to a strip of bronchial epithelium being folded back on itself. Neither the arrangement nor the physiological variation in nuclear size is of significance.

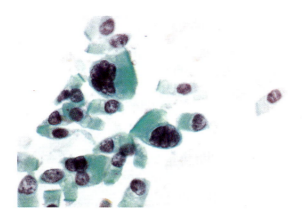

Fig. 3.6 Ciliated columnar cells

Papanicolaou ×525: bronchial brush

Multinucleated forms of ciliated bronchial cells are uncommon but normal. The cilia, being fragile, are easily lost; the cell type is nevertheless easily identified by the persistence of the end-plate. Recognition of the end-plate in a hypertrophic or otherwise morphologically abnormal cell can be of paramount diagnostic importance, as it is not elaborated by a malignant cell.

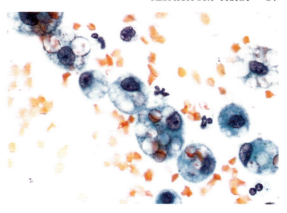

Fig. 3.7 Mucus-secreting goblet cells

Papanicolaou ×525: sputum

Goblet cells tend to become spheroidal when exfoliated into a fluid or semifluid secretion such as mucus. The cytoplasm is distended with single or multiple secretory mucous vacuoles. These are clearly outlined, often with a dark rim, have some depth of focus and, not infrequently, indent the nucleus. Condensed mucus appears as an eosinophilic inclusion within the vacuole.

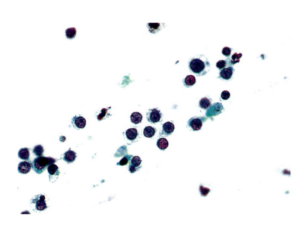

Fig. 3.8 Cuboidal bronchiolar cells

Papanicolaou ×525: sputum

The non-ciliated, non-mucus-secreting cuboidal cells that line the smaller bronchi and bronchioles are not often exfoliated in sputum. They are a little larger than lymphocytes and have round nuclei surrounded by a narrow zone of transparent or translucent cytoplasm.

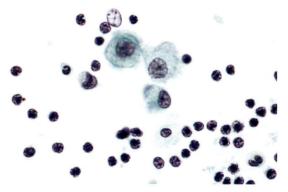

Fig. 3.9 Bronchoalveolar cells: lymphocytes

Papanicolaou ×525: bronchoalveolar lavage

Moderately large cells with hypochromic nuclei and a fair amount of translucent cytoplasm are a feature of bronchoalveolar lavage specimens. The cells may be discrete or they may be attached to each other in the manner of epithelial lining cells. They also frequently contain phagocytosed inclusions and are probably the source of alveolar macrophages. The small cells are mature lymphocytes. The lavage specimen was from a patient with pulmonary sarcoidosis, a disease in which lymphocytes constitute a high proportion of cells in the alveoli.

Macrophages

The presence of alveolar macrophages is mandatory for the identification of a deep cough sputum suitable for cytology. Microscopic examination is necessary to establish this fact as not every mucoid specimen is derived from the lower respiratory tract, nor every thin watery specimen merely saliva. Indeed, small-cell carcinoma of the lung is occasionally associated with thin, clear secretions. Alveolar macrophages are frequently present in bronchial brush and FNA smears, but their presence in these specimens is not essential.

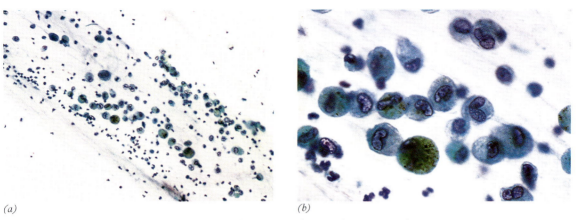

(a)   *(b)*

Fig. 3.10 Pulmonary alveolar macrophages: anthracotic macrophages

Papanicolaou (a) ×133: sputum (b) ×525: same field

Macrophages are usually seen in streaks against a background of mucus, accompanied by neutrophils. As a rule, they are round and the average size approximates to that of a rounded goblet cell. The nuclei, usually eccentric, are remarkable for wide variations in shape and size; they may be round, oval, indented or lobulated. Each nucleus

has one or more small nucleoli. The cytoplasm is finely vacuolated and foamy. Phagocytosed material, most notably black carbon, is a common feature (anthracotic macrophage). However, not all macrophages contain inclusions.

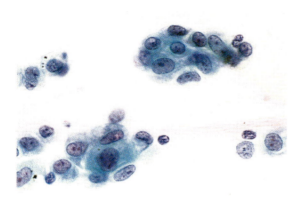

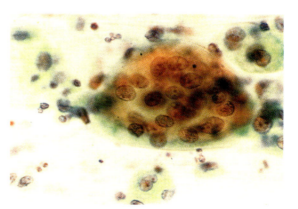

Fig. 3.11 Cohesive alveolar macrophages

Papanicolaou ×525: sputum

Whereas macrophages derived from blood monocytes are always discrete and generally smaller, pulmonary macrophages often appear in cohesive sheets and resemble epithelial cells. The presence of phagocytosed particles identifies the histiocytic nature of the cells illustrated. Compare these with the bronchoalveolar cells shown in Figure 3.9. The similarities in cytoplasmic texture and nuclear characteristics support the hypothesis that some of the pulmonary macrophages are derived from the type 2 alveolar cell.

Fig. 3.12 Multinucleated macrophages

Papanicolaou ×525: sputum

Giant multinucleated epithelioid macrophages are present in a wide variety of benign pulmonary disorders, particularly granulomatous lesions. Since they also occur in the absence of such diseases, their presence in a respiratory tract cytology specimen is non-contributory to any consistently reliable diagnosis.

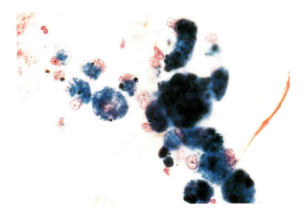

Fig. 3.13 Iron-laden macrophages: siderophages

Perl's Prussian blue ×525: sputum

Macrophages which have ingested haemosiderin released by the lysis of erythrocytes (siderophages) contain iron pigment which can be correctly identified with an appropriate stain, such as Prussian blue. Their presence in a respiratory tract specimen is indicative of either past intrathoracic bleeding or extravasation of red blood cells into the alveoli due to a sluggish blood flow, as in congestive cardiac failure; hence they are referred to as heart failure cells. Large numbers of siderophages are seen in Goodpasture's syndrome, a condition in which antiglomerular membrane nephritis is associated with pulmonary haemorrhage. The presence of siderophages together with considerable extracellular haemosiderin is of considerable value in establishing a diagnosis of the rare disorder, idiopathic pulmonary haemosiderosis.

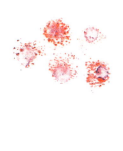

Fig. 3.14 Fat-laden macrophages: lipophages

Sudan II (oil scarlet) ×525: tracheal suckings

Macrophages containing many fat globules have been reported in lipoid pneumonia. Their presence in carefully collected bronchial suckings from neonates suspected to have aspiration pneumonia has proved useful in the author's laboratory. Once again, in order to establish the true nature of the diagnostic inclusions, the use of specific stains such as oil scarlet or Sudan black is mandatory. A duplicate smear from which the fat has been extracted by exposure to a lipid solvent such as chloroform acts as a control.

Obstructive airway disease

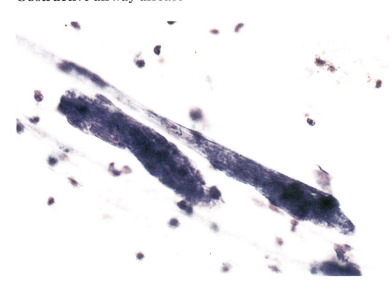

Fig. 3.15 Mucus

Papanicolaou ×720: sputum

Mucus derived from goblet cells is present in every respiratory tract specimen, as a thin film or in small streaks. Mucosal oedema in acute asthma and marked mucous gland hyperplasia in chronic bronchitis and asthma result in excess mucus production; the problem is compounded by loss of ciliary activity. The sputum of such subjects generally has few cells and consists mainly of thick irregular masses of viscid mucus showing varying degrees of inspissation.

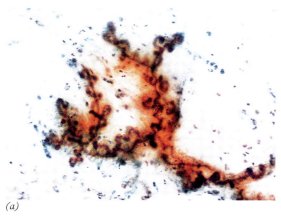

(a)

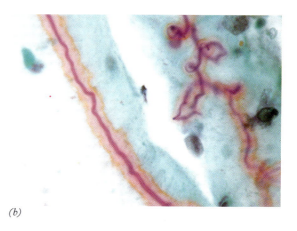

(b)

Fig. 3.16 Curschmann spiral

Papanicolaou (a) ×133: sputum (b) ×1260

Inspissated mucus plugging the smaller bronchi forms a complex branching spiral or corkscrew-shaped cast known as the Curschmann spiral; such a structure is diagnostic of bronchial obstruction and is very common in sputum from cases of obstructive airway disease. Malignant cells should be looked for in the more feathery part of the mucus that fans out from the dense central axis of a Curshmann spiral when a neoplasm is the suspected cause of bronchial occlusion.

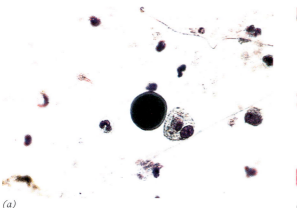

(a)

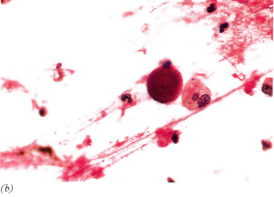

(b)

Fig. 3.17 Corpora amylacea

(a) Papanicolaou ×525: bronchial washing (b) PAS ×525: same field

Small structures composed of concentric rings of varying density may be formed in the bronchopulmonary passages (a). One of these, the corpora amylacea, is composed mainly of glycoproteins which give a positive reaction with periodic acid-Schiff (PAS; b). There is some uncertainty about the origin of this structure. In view of its positive reaction with PAS, it seems likely that it is an organized form of inspissated mucus.

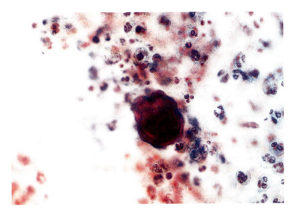

Fig. 3.18 Calcospherite (psammoma body)

Papanicolaou ×525: sputum

The terms calcospherite and psammoma body are considered to be synonymous. Somewhat similar in structure to the corpora amylacea but dissimilar in its chemical composition, the calcospherite consists of various minerals. These bodies are commonly formed when the minerals, mainly calcium, are deposited in degenerating tips of tumour tissue. They are also seen in large numbers in the extremely rare condition, pulmonary alveolar microlithiasis. The structure illustrated was non-reactive with PAS.

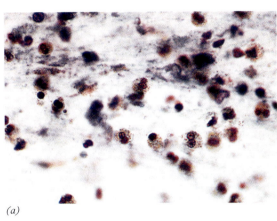

(a)

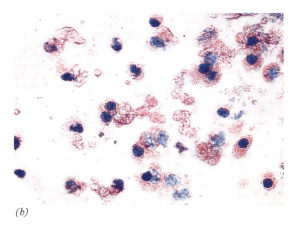

(b)

Fig. 3.19 Eosinophils

(a) Papanicolaou ×525: sputum (b) Hansel's stain ×525: sputum; another specimen

Eosinophils in respiratory tract specimens are usually associated with a component of hypersensitivity. These include chronic bronchitis with or without wheezing, Wegener's granuloma, primary pulmonary eosinophilia, helminthic infections, some types of interstitial airway disease and, occasionally, malignant tumours. However, by far the commonest cause of pulmonary eosinophilia is bronchial asthma. A high percentage of eosinophils in sputum is of considerable value in discriminating bronchial asthma which causes reversible airway disease from the irreversible type caused by chronic bronchitis.

The characteristic bi-lobed 'pair of spectacles' nucleus of the eosinophil is easily recognized, but the less mature mononuclear eosinophil, often seen in sputum in asthma, is difficult to identify in a smear stained by the Papanicolaou method (a). Correct identification is facilitated by the use of special stains such as a Romanowsky stain, carbol chromatrobe and Hansel's stain (composed of methylene blue and eosin) which highlight the specific granules of this polymorphonuclear leukocyte (b).

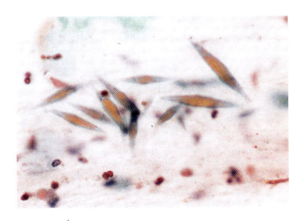

Fig. 3.20 Charcot–Leyden crystals

Papanicolaou ×525: sputum

The cell membrane of the eosinophil contains several enzymes. One of these, lysolecithinase (together with phospholipase A and D) spontaneously forms rhomboid-shaped structures termed Charcot–Leyden crystals. Often associated with intact eosinophils, the crystals may persist when the eosinophils have disintegrated, and remain the only clear indication of an allergic condition. With the Papanicolaou stain, they are bright orange and sometimes have green borders and apices.

Pneumoconioses

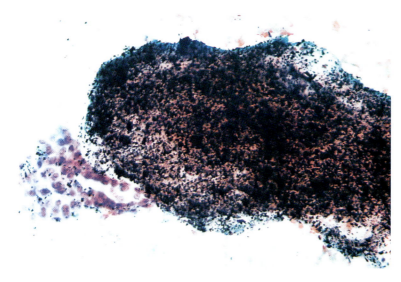

Fig. 3.21 Coal miner's lung

Papanicolaou ×183: FNA; lung

Exposure to silica dust which cannot be seen in routine cytological and histological preparations is an occupational hazard of miners. Chronic irritation by the inhalant provokes a multifocal fibrotic reaction; the alveoli and the alveolar macrophages are filled with black-staining carbon.

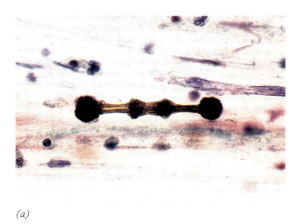

(a)

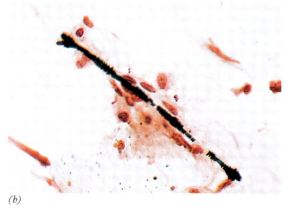

(b)

Fig. 3.22 Ferruginous body: asbestos body

(a) Papanicolaou ×525: sputum (b) Perl's Prussian blue ×525: same specimen; another smear

A variety of long, needle-like mineral fibres inhaled into the lung become coated with proteinaceous material derived from bronchial secretions. Contraction of the bronchial muscles as the coated fibre is propelled forward is believed to produce the curious coiled structure with transverse corrugations and club-shaped ends. Haemosiderin is gradually incorporated into the coat and gives the ferruginous body a typical golden-brown colour (a). The iron in the haemosiderin is specifically stained by Perl's method (b). Note that the fibre is clearly visible where it has not yet acquired the proteinaceous coat (b). Ferruginous bodies were formerly known as asbestos bodies in the belief that the reaction was specific to asbestos, a complex silicate. While this is now known not to be the case, asbestos remains the most significant source of the fibres to result in the formation of these structures. Exposure to the uncommon blue asbestos is the main aetiological factor in the causation of mesothelioma, and exposure to the common white asbestos when coupled with cigarette smoking plays a major role in the development of bronchogenic carcinoma.

Flora and fauna

Investigation and confirmation of the common bacterial and viral infections of the respiratory tract generally lie within the province of a microbiologist. Some parasitic infestations and primary mycoses of the lung have, however, been successfully diagnosed by sputum, bronchoscopic and aspiration cytology.

The immunosuppressed host is particularly prone to pulmonary complications with high morbidity and mortality rates. Accurate diagnosis and prompt treatment are essential in such a life-threatening situation, and in recent years, identification of several of the opportunistic infective agents has been added to the cytopathologist's more traditional role of diagnosing malignant disease. Some of the pathogenic fungi, such as *Histoplasma*, *Coccidioides*, and *Blastomyces* are common in the Americas, but virtually unknown in Europe. The reader is referred to specialist literature on these. The pathogenic and opportunist infective agents met with in the author's laboratory are illustrated below.

Fig. 3.23 *Mycobacterium tuberculosis*

Zieh–Neelsen ×1144: FNA; lung

The acid-fast bacilli shown in this micrograph were recovered from a patient with a lung mass; the differential diagnosis included pulmonary tuberculosis and primary carcinoma. The organism was subsequently identified as *M. tuberculosis* by culture studies. Since saprophytic varieties of mycobacterium found in water and soil and the avian type may act as opportunists in humans, laboratory investigation of pulmonary complications in an immunodeficient subject should include a search for acid-fast bacilli. The tubercle bacillus may appear as a slender rod or it may be finely beaded.

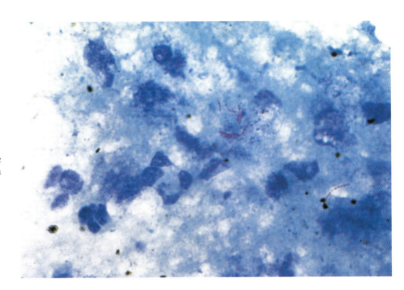

Fig. 3.24 *Nocardia*

Papanicolaou ×720: FNA; lung

Nocardia is an aerobic member of the Actinomyces family which has a filamentous appearance, but is, in fact, a bacterium. The two strains responsible for human nocardiosis are *N. asteroides* and *N. brasiliensis*. The disease may, rarely, be primary, but is more frequently an opportunistic infection. Actinomycetes-like organisms may colonize the mouth and their presence in a sputum or bronchoscopic specimen is of no significance. The lung aspirate illustrated was obtained from a middle-aged man with an immunodeficiency state consequent on alcohol abuse.

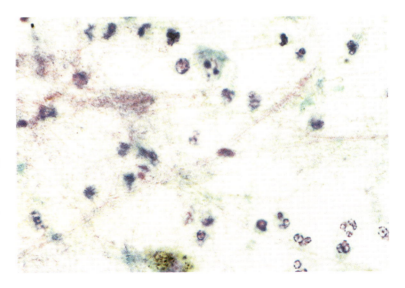

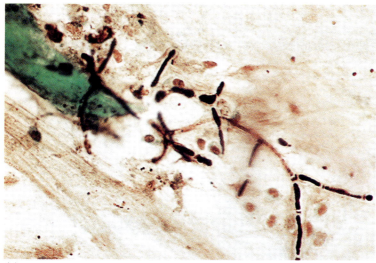

(a)

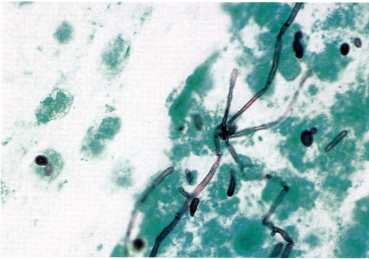

(b)

Fig. 3.25 *Candida* spp.

Grocott's silver methanamine (a) ×720: sputum; C. albicans (b) ×720: bronchoalveolar lavage; C. parapsilosis

Candidiasis is the most widespread of mycotic diseases. Mucocutaneous and cutaneous infections are common, systemic infections less so. Primary pulmonary candidiasis is rare, but secondary infections of the lower respiratory tract are frequent in immunocompromised subjects and in patients with some other primary lung disease such as neoplasm, tuberculosis, bacterial or viral pneumonia.

The most common pathogenic species is *Candida albicans*, one of the natural flora of the body. The other species are essentially saprophytes, but opportunistic infections are caused by *C. glabrata, C. guilliermondi, C. krusei, C. parapsilosis* and *C. tropicalis*.

C. glabrata consists only of yeast forms. All the other species form astrospores, pseudohyphae and true hyphae. A blastospore is a round or oval asexual spore, 3–5 mm in diameter, produced by budding of the yeast cell or along a hypha. A psuedohypha is a filament-like chain of successive blastospores that elongate, but do not separate. The hypha is the vegetative filament that makes up the body of the fungus. The hyphae of the *Candida* species are septate and branch freely in various directions.

The clinical significance of *Candida* in a respiratory tract specimen requires fine judgement. *Candida* seen in sputum frequently comes from the mouth and must on no account be taken to indicate bronchopulmonary infection. The sputum sample shown in (a) came from a young woman with legionnaire's disease and oral and vulvovaginal candidiasis acquired prior to the respiratory tract infection.

In the case illustrated in (b), the *Candida* sp. present in the bronchoalveolar lavage of an immunodeficient patient treated for leukaemia with a bone marrow transplant indicates opportunistic candidiasis. Culture of the lavage specimen yielded a growth of *C. parapsilosis*.

Fig. 3.26 *Aspergillus fumigatus*

(a) Papanicolaou ×1160, bronchoalveolar lavage; (b) ×183, sputum (c) ×720 same field

Four types of pulmonary infections are caused by the *Aspergillus* species: three are invasive, one is non-invasive. Primary invasive infection is rare, but may occur in a normal individual subjected to a massive exposure of the fungus. A sensitized individual may develop primary allergic bronchopulmonary aspergillosis. Secondary invasive infection is common in an immunodeficient or debilitated host. Non-invasive colonization of a pre-existing cavity results in an aspergilloma or fungus-bronchoalveolar lavage. Most cases of aspergillosis are caused by *A. fumigatus*; some are due to *A. flavus*, *A. niger* and *A. terreus*.

Colonization of the upper respiratory tract by this fungus can occur but is extremely rare. The presence of *Aspergillus* in a sample of sputum is consequently of clinical significance.

The fungus is seen as a tangled mycelium formed by hyphae which show characteristic dichotomous branching at about 45°. Secondary and tertiary branches radiating in one direction create the typical sunburst pattern or the actinomycetoid form. The hyphae are septate, fairly uniform and between 4 and 6 µm wide. Variable staining of the hyphae is due to alterations of rapid and slow growth phases.

The diagnostic feature that absolutely identifies *Aspergillus* is the fruiting head from which the fungus derives its name (*Aspergillus*: a kind of brush used to sprinkle holy water). A stalk arises from a specialized cell, the foot cell, of the mycelium; the stalk expands at its upper end to form a club-shaped vesicle; peglike structures develop from fertile areas of the vesicle to give rise to unbranched chains of conidia. The vesicle and the conidia constitute the fruiting head or conidiophore, which requires air for its development. It may be seen in an aspergilloma in an aerated cavity, but does not develop in invasive aspergillosis. Calcium oxalate crystals, which are birefringent by polarized light, may be formed from oxalic acid produced by the fungus.

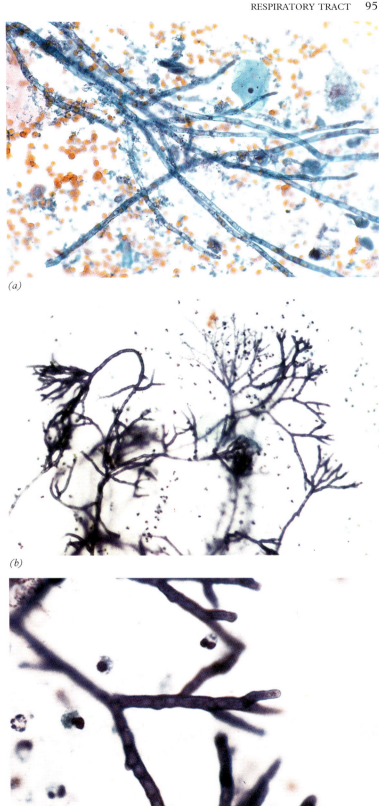

(a)

(b)

(c)

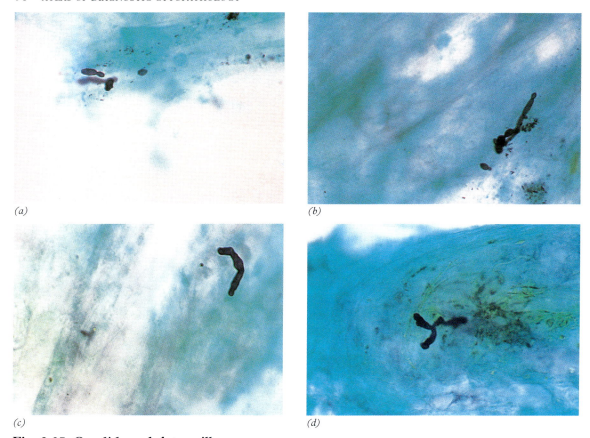

(a)

(b)

(c)

(d)

Fig. 3.27 *Candida* and *Aspergillus*

Grocott's silver methanamine (a) ×525: sputum; Candida albicans (b) same smear as (a) (c) ×525: sputum; Aspergillus (d) same smear as (c)

Aspergillus is, as a rule, easily recognized by its dichotomous branching, but may, on occasion, be confused with other fungi that form hyphae, one of which is *Candida*. Both fungi were present in the sputum of a patient who developed an allergic bronchopulmonary condition of sudden and rapid onset.

C. albicans was isolated from the sputum and, although there was no clinical evidence of oral candidiasis, its pathogenicity could not be assumed. The serum immunoglobulin E was markedly elevated and precipitins to *Aspergillus* were present.

Compare the *Candida* in (a) and (b) with the *Aspergillus* in (c) and (d). The *Candida* is seen in the form of blastospores (a) and (b) and pseudohyphae (b), neither of which is formed by the *Aspergillus* spp. Note also the budding blastospore at the segmental line of the hypha (b); this is another characteristic of *Candida* and is never seen in *Aspergillus*. The latter consists of a thicker septate hypha (c) and shows dichotomous branching (d).

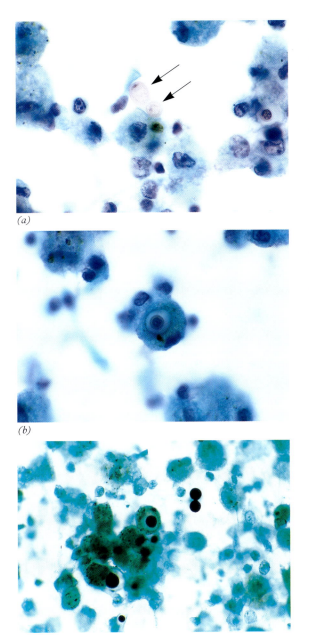

(a)

(b)

(c)

Fig. 3.28 *Cryptococcus neoformans*

Papanicolaou ×1100 (a) FNA: lung; capsulated budding yeasts (b) same smear; another field; pseudohypha

The lung is the principal portal of entry for the yeast *C. neoformans* found in the excreta of birds, particularly the pigeon. The primary lesion may consist of subpleural fibrotic nodules, a single large solid granulomatous lesion known as cryptococcoma, or a cavitating lesion. Occasionally, the yeast causes miliary disease with blood-borne dissemination. Cryptococcal meningitis is frequently the first manifestation of infection.

In the case of a cryptococcoma such as the one shown, large numbers of the yeasts are seen in extracellular collections (a) or within giant cells. The individual yeast is round or has a single bud and is surrounded by a capsule which does not stain with the Papanicolaou stain or haematoxylin and eosin (H&E; a). The outline of its refractile capsule can be seen in the extracellular or intracytoplasmic position (a, b). Capsule stains with mucopolysaccharide stains (PAS) or methenamine silver (Grocott stain; c). Short chains of two or typically three budding yeasts may be seen.

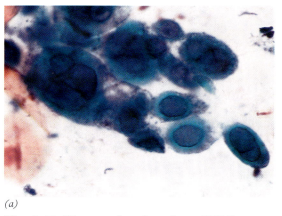

(a)   *(b)*

Fig. 3.29 Herpes simplex virus (HSV)

Papanicolaou ×525 (a) sputum (b) bronchial washings; another case

The cytopathic effects of HSV, a DNA virus, are seen characteristically in the nucleus; the cytoplasm shows non-specific degenerative changes. The nucleus is filled with homogeneous inclusions and acquires a ground-glass appearance; a heavy deposit of chromatin on the margin sharply defines its outline. A dense intranuclear inclusion, seen in the occasional cell (a) or not at all (b) in the early stages of infection, is usually present in the majority of cells in later stages or in recurrent infections. The number of nuclei varies from one to several; in the multinucleated cells, the nuclei adjoin and typically mould one another (a).

The diagnostic relevance of herpesvirus cytopathia has to be assessed with reference to the clinical status of the patient and the type of specimen. Superficial mucocutaneous lesions are not uncommon in susceptible subjects and are of little clinical significance. The sputum specimen illustrated in (a) came from a man with bronchopneumonia and herpetic vesicles round the lip margin. There was no evidence of viral involvement of the lower respiratory tract.

Immunocompromised and debilitated individuals, on the other hand, are more susceptible to tracheobronchial and pulmonary infections. A bronchial wash specimen from an elderly woman with bilateral pneumonia and respiratory failure which required intensive therapy is shown in (b). There were no vesicles on the lips or the oropharyngeal mucosa; herpetic infection of the tracheobronchial mucosa was suggested by the cytopathic effects seen in sheets of bronchial mucosal cells.

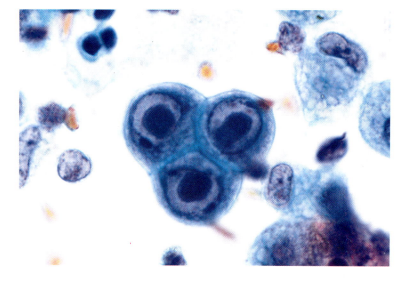

Fig. 3.30 Cytomegalovirus (CMV)

Papanicolaou ×2900 (oil): bronchoalveolar lavage

The diagnostic feature of infection with CMV, a member of the Herpes family of viruses, is the presence of a large intranuclear inclusion surrounded by a clear halo. A punctate deposit of chromatin marks the outline of the ghost nucleus. The intranuclear inclusion is basophilic with the Papanicolaou stain, green or black with silver methanamine. It is neither necessary nor customary to use a silver stain to demonstrate CMV. However, familiarity with this appearance is useful, as CMV is often associated with *Pneumocystis carinii*, which is best demonstrated by the Grocott method.

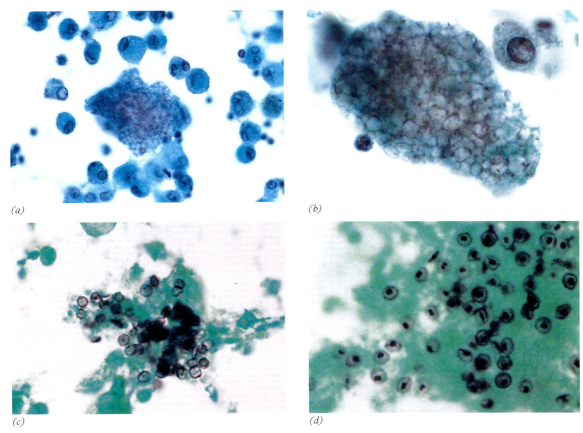

(a)

(b)

(c)

(d)

Fig. 3.31 *Pneumocystis carinii*

(a) Papanicolaou ×1260 (oil) bronchoalveolar lavage (b) ×2100 (oil) (c) Grocott ×525: bronchoalveolar lavage; same case as in Fig. 3.30 (d) ×832: bronchoalveolar lavage: another case

The parasite, *Pneumocystis carinii*, has long been known to cause chronic interstitial pneumonia in premature and malnourished infants. It has become increasingly important in recent years, as a common opportunistic pathogen in subjects of all ages whose immune mechanism is deficient. The deficiency may be due to congenital causes, acquired immune deficiency syndrome (AIDS), malignant disease, particularly that of lymphoid cells, or it may be iatrogenic for purposes of organ transplant or cytotoxic therapy.

The organisms can be detected by routine staining in the induced sputum, bronchoalveolar lavage fluid (a, b) or percutaneous needle biopsy (in the cases of limited, granulomatous presentation, pneumocystoma, where bronchoalveolar lavage may be negative). More recently, organisms have been described in the pleural effusion and head and neck lymph nodes. They present as three-dimensional clusters of extracellular foamy, well-outlined material, resembling alveolar casts (a, b) Grocott's silver stain stains the wall of thin-walled round or crescentic cysts and trophozoites (c, d).

Pneumocystis has not been completely classified but it is considered to be a protozoon, class Sporozoa. By the Grocott method, it is seen as a thin-walled black cyst, round or crescentic. Within the cyst are the trophozoites, 1–6 in number; these may be close to or applied to the cyst wall, when they resemble Barr bodies (a). In some preparations, the trophozoites are close together in the centre of the cyst and resemble a very small safety pin (b). The cyst wall collapses when the trophozoites are extruded (a).

The parasites illustrated in (a) are from the same case with CMV shown in Figure 3.30. The lavage specimen show in (b) came from a male who presented with atypical pneumonia and was found to have serum antibodies to human T-lymphotrophic virus III (HTLV III).

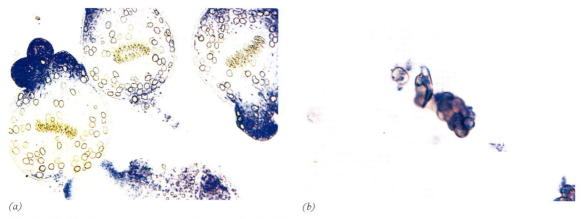

(a)   *(b)*

Fig. 3.32 Echinococcus granulosus (Hydatid)

Methylene blue (a) ×133: hydatid cyst fluid; scolices (b) ×525: same specimen: another preparation; hooklets

The causative agent of hydatid disease is Echinococcus granulosus, a 5-mm-long tapeworm which has a head, a neck and three proglottides. The dog and other canines act as definitive hosts, harbour the adult worm in the jejunum and excrete numerous eggs. The usual intermediate hosts are sheep, cattle and camels. Man becomes an intermediate host, usually in childhood, by ingesting eggs present in contaminated food and water, or in faecal dust on the coats of dogs. The embryo (oncosphere) is liberated in the stomach and upper small intestine, penetrates the bowel mucosa and enters the portal circulation. From here it is carried to the liver (50%), lung (25%) and bone, brain, kidney and other organs. The larva forms a typical cystic structure with an external laminated wall and an inner nucleated germinal layer. Brood capsules and second and third generation daughter cysts develop from the germinal layer and in turn give rise to the scolex or head. This has a distinctive structure with four sucking discs and a circlet of hooklets. Hydatid sand found in cyst fluid consists of scolices from ruptured brood capsules.

Leakage of hydatid cyst fluid into tissues and body cavities is likely to induce anaphylactic shock and aspiration of a suspected hydatid cyst is contra-indicated. The case illustrated was aspirated with care at thoracotomy.

Micrograph (a) shows typical scolices. In the absence of these, a firm diagnosis can be made by finding the flanged, sickle-shaped hooklet (b). The round or oval hyaline structures which stud the scolices in (a) and are seen in an aggregate next to the hooklet in (b) are known as calcareous corpuscles, and characterize cystircus larvae.

Squamous metaplasia and cell atypia

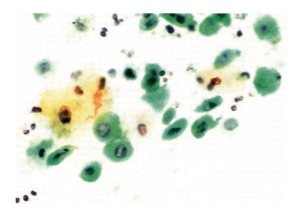

Fig. 3.33 Squamous metaplasia

Papanicolaou ×525: sputum

Metaplastic squamous cells tend to dissociate from each other and have the morphological features of the Malpighian-layer cells. They may be round or roughly ovoid; some retain the angular projections characteristic of prickle cells. The cytoplasm is generally cyanophilic and firm in texture.

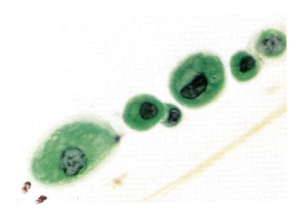

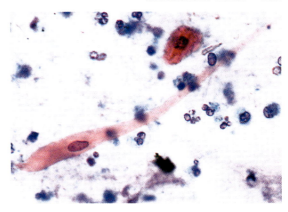

Fig. 3.34 Squamous metaplasia

Papanicolaou ×525: sputum

Degenerative changes are common in metaplastic cells and the cytoplasm frequently contains autolytic vacuoles which vary in number and size. The better preserved nucleus occupies a small part of the cell and is round and reticular. The degenerating nucleus may be hypochromic and blurred; more frequently it tends to pyknosis and intense hyperchromasia (Fig. 3.32). A heavy deposit of chromatin on the membrane which appears thick and crenation of the margin are two common and significant indications of early degenerative changes in the nucleus. Both characteristics are often seen in malignant cells which have a marked propensity to degeneration, but they are not criteria of malignancy *per se*.

Fig. 3.35 Atypical squamous metaplasia: caudate cell

Papanicolaou ×525: sputum

A disturbing aspect of an atypical metaplastic squamous cell is alteration of cell shape. Caudate forms with short or long tails (tadpole cell) occur. The nucleus of a benign caudate cell is very small relative to the cytoplasm and some of its structure is preserved. Compare the benign cell illustrated with the malignant caudate cells in Figure 3.47 (e, f).

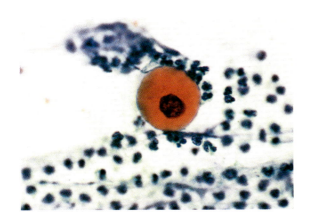

Fig. 3.36 Atypical squamous metaplasia: dyskeratotic cell

Papanicolaou ×525: sputum

Dyskeratosis is a common feature of the atypical metaplastic squamous cell. The cell which still retains its nucleus becomes partially or fully keratinized. Grossly atypical metaplastic squamous cells, suspicious of malignancy, may occur in the bronchial tree in the absence of squamous carcinoma or may coexist with bronchogenic carcinomas of all cell types. A diligent search for confirmatory evidence in further specimens is indicated, but a firm diagnosis of carcinoma should be made only when unequivocal malignant cells are identified.

Hyperplasia of bronchial mucosa

Reactive cells from hyperplastic bronchial mucosa are met with in a variety of pulmonary disorders, notably asthma, chronic bronchitis, slowly resolving pneumonia, bronchiectasis, and occasionally viral pneumonia.

Benign cells lining the bronchi are one layer deep or pseudostratified and may be expected to exfoliate in flat monolayers. While this is often the case, it is by no means universally true and this aspect of benign mucosal cells has been overstressed in some literature. The appearance seen is influenced to some extent by the nature of the specimen and the functional state of the cell. In sputum and bronchial secretions, hyperplastic mucosal cells (especially distended goblet cells) are not infrequently spheroidal and shed in clusters which have a considerable depth of focus. The overall appearance may resemble that seen in adenocarcinoma cells and pose a major diagnostic problem. In brush and aspiration smears, both types of cells tend to be flat. Unlike keratinized squamous carcinoma and small cell carcinoma (SCC), which are often recognizable at a glance, close attention to morphological detail is necessary to avoid a misdiagnosis of adenocarcinoma.

More often than not, benign clumps contain both goblet and ciliated cells. The most helpful feature in the identification of a group of hyperplastic cells is the presence of cilia, or, since these, being fragile, are easily lost, the persistence of the terminal bar.

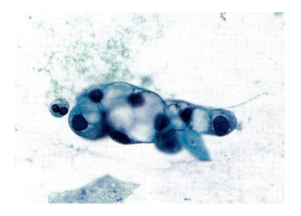

Fig. 3.37 Hyperplasia of bronchial mucosa

Papanicolaou ×525; sputum

Two features may be seen in both benign mucous hyperplasia and in adenocarcinoma. First, the nuclear-cytoplasmic ratio varies inversely with the degree of distension of the cytoplasm by the secretory product. Second, one of the nuclei is pushed to the periphery of the cell which has thereby acquired a signet-ring appearance.

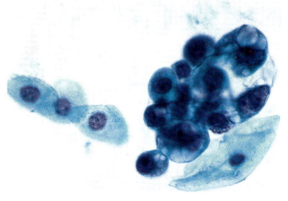

Fig. 3.38 Hyperplasia of bronchial mucosa

Papanicolaou ×525: sputum; same case as in Figure 3.37; another specimen

The prominent large nucleoli are indications of proliferative activity of these cells from hyperplastic bronchial epithelium. There is considerable variation in the size of the nuclei and in their relation to the periphery of the cluster. Several lie on the outer edge and there is loss of polarity and of an orderly surface configuration. The terminal plate on the one columnar cell within the group identifies the benign character of the entire group.

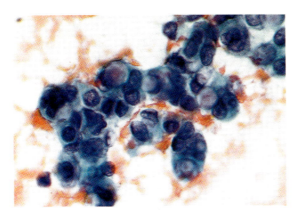

Fig. 3.39 Hyperplasia of bronchial mucosa

Papanicolaou ×525: bronchial brush; unresolved pneumonia

In brush smears, even large fragments of mucosa tend to spread flat. The sheet in this micrograph is composed of ciliated and goblet cells. Note the terminal plate at one edge and the scattered mucous globules. The variation in the shape and size of the cells and the nuclei is enhanced by intracytoplasmic vacuoles and compression of the cells. A suggestion of reticulation is evident in the chromatin.

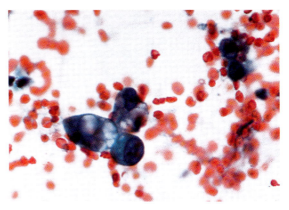

Fig. 3.40 Hyperplasia of bronchial mucosa

Papanicolaou ×525: bronchial washings; same case as in Figure 3.39

In bronchial washings, clumps of cells are likely to become rounded and three-dimensional. The nuclei are more liable to distortion and examination of the chromatin pattern may be unrewarding. A diagnosis of carcinoma should not be submitted unless single cells with unequivocal malignant features are identified.

An attempt should be made to visualize cilia which may only be visible under oil immersion. In the presence of cilia, a diagnosis of malignancy should not be made.

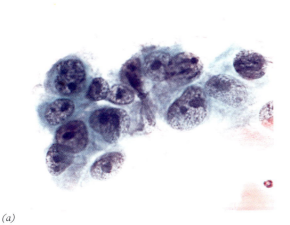

(a)

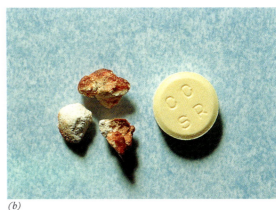

(b)

Fig. 3.41 Regenerative changes of the bronchial epithelium

(a) Papanicolaou ×1260 bronchial brushing (b) remnants of aspirated tablets; normal tablet on the left for comparison

Bronchial epithelium may undergo ulceration and show marked regenerative changes with prominent large nucleoli. These features should not be mistaken for malignancy. The clue to their nature is often a gradual transition between the worst-affected epithelium and adjacent 'normal' bronchial epithelium, often in the same sheet of cells. Despite the alarming size of the nuclei and nucleoli, the nuclear-cytoplasmic ratio remains relatively low compared to malignant cells.

The case illustrated was a bronchial brushing of a patient who has aspirated tablets.

Inflammatory and other benign conditions of the lung

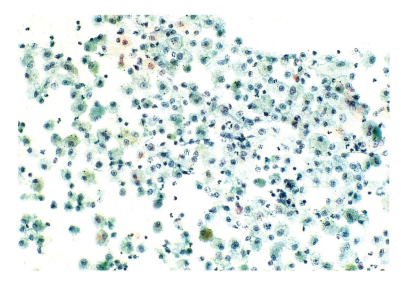

Fig. 3.42 Amiodorone-related changes

(a) Papanicolaou ×580 bronchoalveolar lavage fluid

Amiodorone may produce pulmonary toxicity in about 6% of patients taking the drug. Smears from bronchoalveolar lavage demonstrate a predominance of alveolar macrophages, most of them with carbon particles. Transbronchial biopsy reveals numerous large cells in adjacent bronchial epithelium. Some resemble alveolar macrophages and others are larger, pleomorphic with granular cytoplasm and one or more nuclei which may be large and have coarse chromatin pattern.

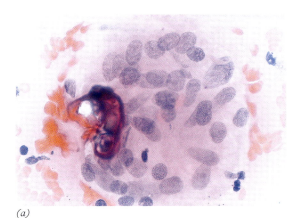

(a)

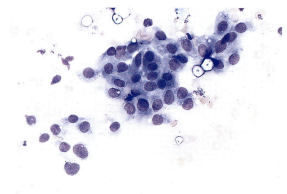

(b)

Fig. 3.43 Sarcoid: FNA of the lung

(a) Papanicolaou ×1260 (b) MGG ×840 (c) MGG ×1260

Granulomatous lesions of the lung include sarcoid. FNA material from these non-caseating granulomas contain clusters of epithelioid cells in the absence of necrosis. Inflammatory exudate may not be prominent. The main pitfall is mistaking the epithelioid cells for epithelium. They present in aggregates of randomly arranged nuclei and poorly outlined abundant cytoplasm (b). The nuclei show folds and grooves, fine chromatin pattern and inconspicuous nucleoli (c). Pleomorphism is absent. Immunocytochemistry and a clinical history may be important for confirming the diagnosis.

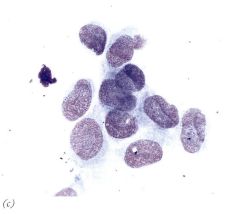

(c)

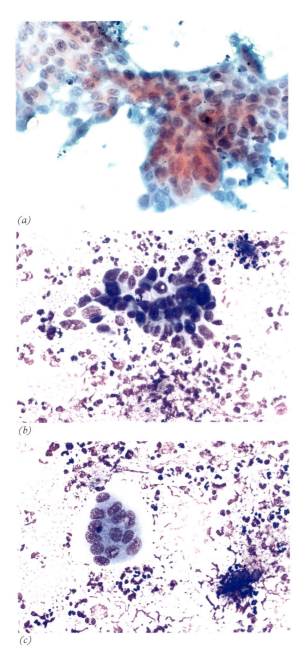

(a)

(b)

(c)

Fig. 3.44 Rheumatoid nodule: FNA of the lung

(a) Papanicolaou ×840 FNA lung (b) MGG ×840 FNA lung (c) MGG ×840

Aspirates from these lesions contain areas of acute and chronic inflammatory exudate, necrosis and multinucleate giant cells (c). The epithelium surrounding the nodule may show cuboidal metaplasia (a, b) and may mimic squamous cell carcinoma. A clinical history of rheumatoid should be sought in cases of doubt.

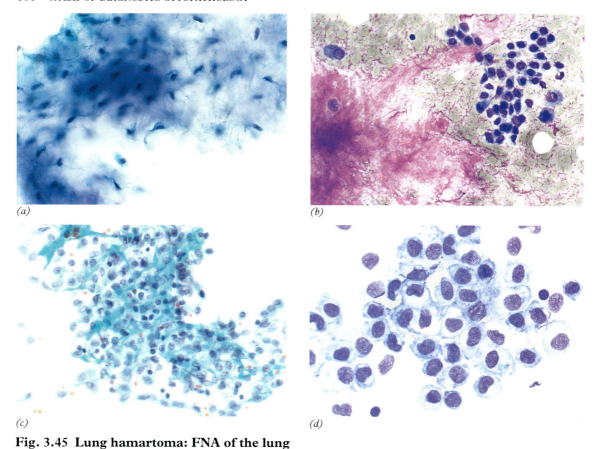

(a)   *(b)*

(c)   *(d)*

Fig. 3.45 Lung hamartoma: FNA of the lung

(a) Papanicolaou ×840 (b) MGG ×420 (c) ×840 (d) ×1260

Cytological diagnosis of hamartomas consists of a mixture of various mature mesenchymal components such as cartilage (a), fat, fibrous tissue, myxomatous tissue (b) and epithelial cells (b-d). Epithelial cells may have a 'histiocytic' inflammatory appearance (c) with plasmacytoid features and could be interpreted as inflammatory pseudotumour ('plasma cell granuloma'). The search for mesenchymal component is therefore important. Even the smallest amount of cartilage is significant since FNA of normal lung does not include cartilage.

Radiological appearances of hamartomas are characteristic with prominent central calcification.

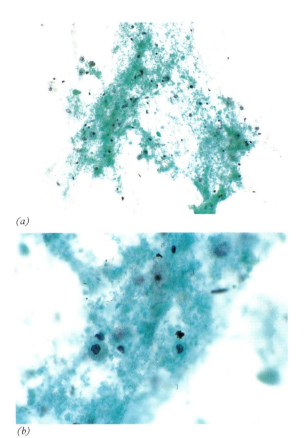

(a)

(b)

Fig. 3.46 Alveolar proteinosis

(a) Papanicolaou ×420 (b) ×1260

Bronchoalveolar lavage fluid in alveolar proteinosis contains dense fibrillary, background material trapping the cells and dominating the findings. Features are non-specific but can suggest the condition. Lung biopsy is mandatory for diagnosis.

PRIMARY BRONCHOGENIC CARCINOMA

Introduction

The three main types of primary bronchogenic carcinomas are squamous cell carcinoma, SCC and adenocarcinoma. A subtype of adenocarcinoma, which arises either from cells of the terminal bronchioles including the Clara cells, or less commonly from the type 2 pneumocyte, and forms either a localized mass or spreads laterally along the scaffolding provided by the alveolar walls, is designated by the World Health Organization as bronchoalveolar carcinoma. The very poorly differentiated adenocarcinoma or squamous cell carcinoma is sometimes difficult to classify by light microscopy; vestigial features which provide a clue to the cell type are identifiable only by electron microscopy. Such a tumour is classified as a large cell undifferentiated carcinoma. In a cytological specimen, the material available for analysis is relatively sparse and the pattern of cell arrangement less informative than in a histological specimen. The cytodiagnostic rate for large cell undifferentiated carcinoma tends to be higher than in histological series.

Squamous cell carcinoma

Squamous cell carcinoma is the commonest primary tumour of the lung. The majority develop in the main bronchi or their major divisions close to the hilum and most are visible through the bronchoscope. The small number of peripherally located squamous carcinomas not accessible to the biopsy forceps may, sometimes, be reached and sampled by the bronchial brush.

In histological preparations, the well-differentiated squamous cell carcinoma is characterized by a basic stratified pattern, distinct intercellular bridges and keratinization, progressing in several areas to epithelial pearl formation. The moderately differentiated tumour has features intermediate between the well-differentiated and the poorly differentiated squamous carcinoma, in which the intercellular bridges are barely discernible.

In cytological material, architectural structure is not evident. The diagnosis of malignancy is based on analysis of cell morphology.

Fig. 3.47 Well-differentiated squamous cell carcinoma

(a) Papanicolaou ×525: bronchial washings (b) MGG ×525: FNA; lung; another case (c) Papanicolaou ×525: same smear as (a) (d) Papanicolaou ×525: sputum; another case (e) Papanicolaou ×525: same specimen as (b); another smear (f) Papanicolaou ×525: sputum; another case (g) Papanicolaou ×525: sputum; another case (h) Papanicolaou ×133: FNA; lung; another case

A good proportion of the cells from a well-differentiated squamous cell carcinoma contain keratin, or, more often, prekeratin. This imparts a number of distinctive characteristics to the cell. In consequence, the cytoplasmic features are of particular importance in this type of carcinoma and contribute more to the correct diagnosis than does the nucleus.

Papanicolaou included the cytoplasmic counterstain Orange G to the compound stain he devised because of its affinity for keratin. The dyskeratotic cell, stained by his method, is strongly orangeophilic and conspicuous against the background of mucus, macrophages and bronchial mucosa (a, c–f). In a Romanowsky-stained smear, cytoplasm containing keratin is pale, has a bluish or violet tinge (b) or may be unstained and almost white.

The texture of the keratinized cell is sometimes hard, homogeneous and matt. This gives a sculptured look to the cell which will have a sharply defined outline (a, b). More often, the cytoplasm in a Papanicolaou-stained smear is bright and refractile; lowering the condenser enhances the refractility (c, d). Focal collections of smooth, glistening droplets are often present (c, d). Whether refractile or dull, the cell does not transmit light.

Variations of shape are another striking feature, and cells from a squamous carcinoma may have the most bizarre appearance (d). The cell often has cytoplasmic processes which may be short or long, single or multiple (c, f). The tail-like process may end sharply (c) or in a bulbous expansion (e, f). Forms with cytoplasmic tails are referred to as caudate or tadpole-shaped cells.

The number of nuclei and the nuclear-cytoplasmic ratio vary considerably in this type of tumour. The single nucleus or the total mass of the multiple nuclei is often disproportionately great, but small pyknotic nuclei may also be seen (d–f). Dyskeratosis of the cytoplasm is invariably associated with nuclear degeneration. The perinuclear membrane is crenated (a–c) and may be thick with a heavy deposit of chromatin. Progressive condensation of the chromatin results in marked hyperchromasia; eventually the nucleus shrinks into a small opaque smooth or jagged mass, with a black 'India-ink' staining reaction (e, f). Finally, the remains of the nucleus may be indicated only by a faint outline (d, g) or it may be altogether absent (d). Anucleate orange 'cell ghosts' are particularly abundant in cytological material from a squamous carcinoma which has undergone central necrosis (h). The high nuclear-cytoplasmic ratio characteristic of most malignant cells is irrelevant to the diagnosis of a keratinizing carcinoma cell.

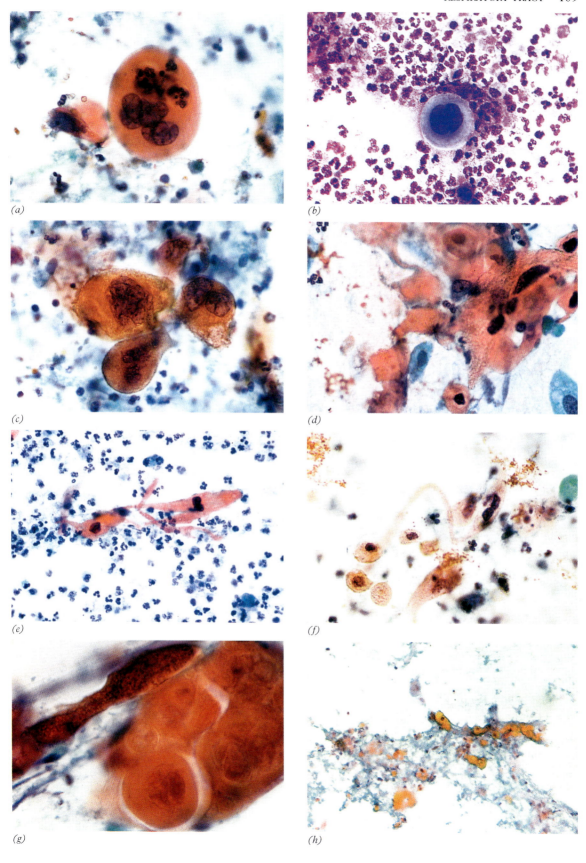

(a)

(b)

(c)

(d)

(e)

(f)

(g)

(h)

Fig. 3.48 Poorly differentiated squamous cell carcinoma

Papanicolaou ×720 (a) FNA; lung (b) same smear as (a) (c) sputum; another case (d) bronchial washings; another case (e) FNA; lung; another case (f) sputum; another case

Cells from the less differentiated squamous carcinomas cannot be graded or even typed with any consistency. Their cytoplasm is often delicate and translucent, and always cyanophilic. It may contain fine hydropic vacuoles.

The diagnosis of malignancy, based on nuclear abnormality, is seldom in doubt. The nuclei vary in size and staining intensity. A point to note is the relative hypochromasia of some of the aspirated nuclei (a, c). The nuclear-cytoplasmic ratio is high. Nucleoli, single or multiple, large and prominent (a, b) or small and inconspicuous (d), are generally present.

Two features, when present, aid in the recognition of a squamous origin. The more important is the arrangement and interrelationship of the cells. Unlike differentiated squamous cells, these remain cohesive and are recovered in small sheets which have ragged borders (a–e). Sharply angular projections of cytoplasm corresponding to intercellular bridges link the cells (a, b). Similar angular extensions may be seen at the free edge of a cell (a–c).

The other indication of probable squamous origin, although less reliable, is the relative firmness of cytoplasmic texture of some of the cells in a cluster.

In the absence of such fine points (c), discrimination between a poorly differentiated squamous carcinoma and a large cell carcinoma is not possible.

On occasion, poorly differentiated squamous cells may appear in clusters with smooth outlines; identification of the cell type is then even more difficult. The production of minute quantities of mucin does not, according to the World Health Organization, invalidate a diagnosis of squamous carcinoma. Degenerative cytoplasmic vacuoles coupled with smooth outlines (f) may result in an appearance rather more suggestive of adenocarcinoma.

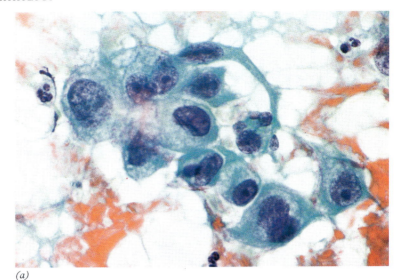

(a)

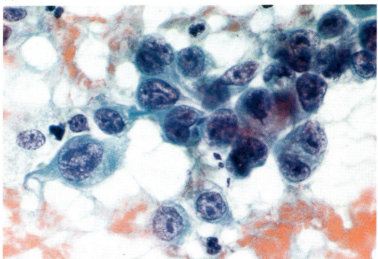

(b)

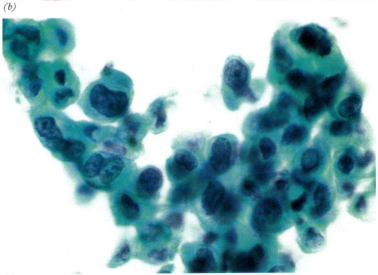

(c)

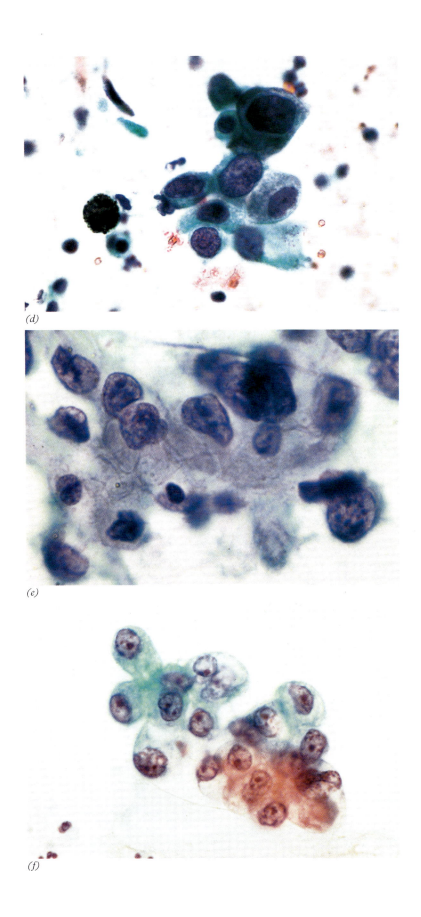

(d)

(e)

(f)

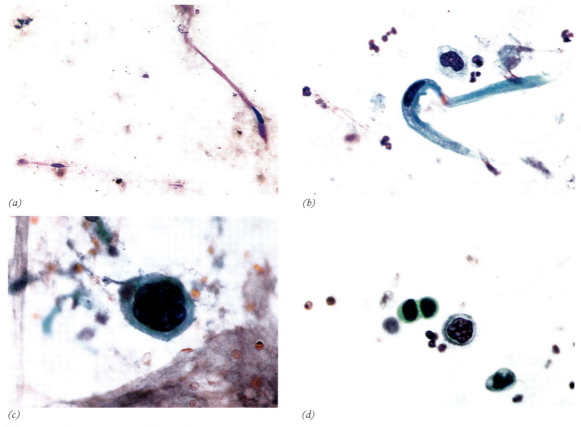

(a)

(b)

(c)

(d)

Fig. 3.49 Squamous cell carcinoma

(a) MGG ×525: FNA; lung (b) Papanicolaou ×525: sputum; another case (c) Papanicolaou ×525: bronchial washings; another case (d) Papanicolaou ×525: sputum; another case

Two morphological features indicative of squamous differentiation may be recognized in a cell that is not yet keratinized. One is a coiled fibrillary apparatus, seen in the tail of some caudate cells, and known as the Herxheimer spiral (a, b). The other is the presence, in a round cell, of one or more perinuclear lamellations (c, d) which resemble the rings in a cross-section of a tree trunk. Both probably represent closely packed thick tonofilaments.

Squamous cells as they begin to differentiate tend to dissociate from their neighbours, and appear as single forms.

Small cell carcinoma

SCC of the lung is a highly aggressive tumour which spreads rapidly, metastasizes early and most patients have disseminated disease when first seen. For this reason, surgical resection is contraindicated and combined chemotherapy with or without radiotherapy is the treatment of choice. For the same reason, identification of the cell type and discrimination from other small-celled tumours is of particular importance.

In light microscopic preparations, the cells of SCC are said to resemble oat grains. Its earlier name of oat cell carcinoma, based on this resemblance, is still in current usage in many centres as a generic term, but is used by the World Health Organization to denote one of three subtypes:

1. SCC, oat cell carcinoma: a malignant tumour composed of uniform small cells, generally larger than lymphocytes, having sparse cytoplasm, dense and inconspicuous nuclei.

2. SCC, intermediate cell type: a tumour of less regular appearance with fusiform, polygonal or round cells with more abundant cytoplasm. The nuclear characteristics are the same as in oat cell carcinoma. A large cell element may be present in some tumours.

3. Combined oat cell carcinoma: a tumour with a definite component of oat cell carcinoma with squamous cell and/or adenocarcinoma.

The origin of SCC is still a matter of debate. SCC and bronchial carcinoid were both considered to arise from the Feyrter or Kulchitsky (K) endocrine cell of the APUD (amine precursor uptake decarboxylation) system of cells which secrete peptide hormones. Ultrastructurally, APUD cells have membrane-bound dense core granules similar to granules present in some nerve endings, and they were considered to derive from the neural crest. More recently, it has been postulated that all benign and malignant bronchial mucosal cells have a common endodermal stem cell origin. The stem cell undergoes progressive differentiation along several different pathways, one of which is endocrine, and may switch from one pathway to another under different stimuli. This would explain the similarity and the difference between SCC and bronchial carcinoid, the presence within SCC of large cell elements, combined tumours and the not infrequent emergence of a different malignant cell type in patients treated with chemotherapy protocols appropriate to SCC. Tumour-related endocrinopathies are not uncommonly associated with SCC which may secrete a variety of ectopic hormones, notably adrenocorticotrophic hormone and antidiuretic hormone.

The cytoplasmic dense core granules of SCC are small in size, sparse in number or altogether absent. When seen, they are generally located near the cell membrane and are usually argentaffin with silver stains. In cytological materials, the size and shape of the SCC cell, the amount of cytoplasm and nuclear characteristic appear to be affected more by the nature and preparation of the specimen than by the histological subtype.

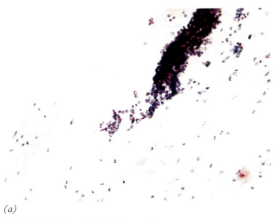
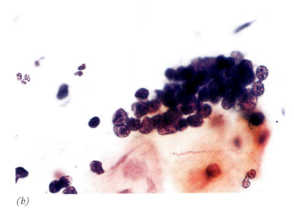

(a)   (b)

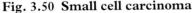

Fig. 3.50 Small cell carcinoma

Papanicolaou (a) ×133: sputum (b) ×525: sputum; another case

Sputum from a patient with SCC is often clear, or it may be flecked with blood. The tumour cells are seen aggregated in clumps or flat sheets, often against a clean background free of mucus and macrophages. The cluster often thins out at one or both ends, so that the cells appear in linear streaks (a). The individual cell appears to consist almost entirely of nucleus with virtually no cytoplasm (b).

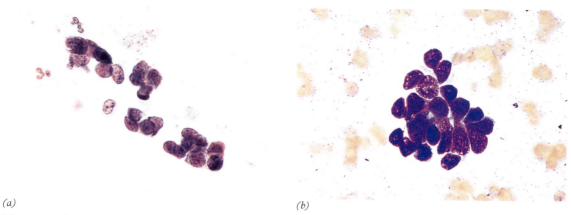

(a)   *(b)*

Fig. 3.51 Small cell carcinoma

(a) Papanicolaou ×525: sputum (b) MGG ×525: FNA; lung; another case

Compression of one or more sides of closely adjacent cells results in the characteristic moulding of oat cells. The space between two moulded nuclei is minimal, almost linear. However, it should be clearly seen—as overlapping nuclei or a wider space do not constitute the typical moulding of SCC. More often than not, one nucleus of a moulded pair is round while its neighbour has one semilunar margin (a). Nuclear moulding, considered to be virtually diagnostic of SCC, is almost always seen in bronchial secretions; it may be present in brush and aspiration smears (b), but is inconstant and often inconspicuous.

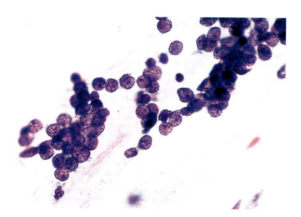

Fig. 3.52 Small cell carcinoma

Papanicolaou ×525 sputum

Nucleoli which are inconspicuous in sections may be seen in some of the better-preserved SCC cells in almost all types of cytological specimens. Generally, the nucleolus is basophilic, small and single (a). Occasionally, it is eosinophilic, large and prominent. As a rule, only one or two cells in an aggregate have large nucleoli. The presence of prominent red nucleoli in all the cells in one cluster in a specimen with classical oat cells is suggestive of an SCC with a large cell component.

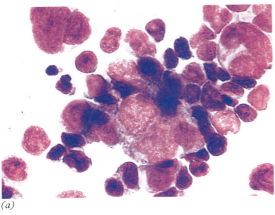

(a)   (b)

Fig. 3.53 Small cell carcinoma

(a) MGG ×525: FNA; lung (b) APAAP: UJ13A ×1260: same case

Some SCCs display considerable pleomorphism. A single tumour may be composed of small oat-like cells, spindle-shaped cells, small and large polygonal cells and a few multinucleated giant cells. The anisocytosis and anisonucleosis are enhanced by air-drying (a). These tumours may be examples of SCC with a large cell component. Note the cell within cell (b); this feature is frequently seen in all variants of SCC.

Immunocytochemistry for neuroendocrine cell markers (UJ13A) shows strong positivity, confirming the diagnosis (b).

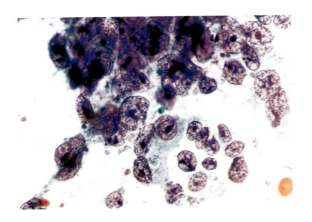

Fig. 3.54 Treated small cell carcinoma

Papanicolaou ×525: bronchial brush

Large undifferentiated malignant cells with prominent polymorphic nucleoli were recovered in a bronchial brush specimen from a patient who had shown a partial response to chemotherapy administered for a histologically confirmed SCC. Emergence of a refractory large cell element and even another malignant cell type after treatment for SCC has been well-documented.

Bronchial carcinoid

Bronchial carcinoids are neoplasms of low-grade malignancy. With few exceptions, they are centrally located and 90% are visible through a bronchoscope. They are generally circumscribed and present either as a fleshy endobronchial polyp or have a locally infiltrating 'iceberg' pattern of growth. Both types develop in the bronchial submucosa and are covered with epithelium which may be normal, but is more often metaplastic. The so-called atypical carcinoid is more anaplastic and may show a histological and clinical similarity to the highly malignant SCC.

Pulmonary carcinoids resemble intestinal carcinoids. Their most important secretory product is serotonin (5 hydroxytryptamine) and they may be associated with the carcinoid syndrome. Their relationship to SCC is not clear. Both tumours contain ultrastructural dense-core secretory granules with an endocrine function. The granules of a carcinoid are larger, variable in size and shape, abundant and are distributed through the cytoplasm. The majority are argyrophilic, i.e. they require an external reducing agent to convert a silver solution to metallic silver. They may also be demonstrated by the alkaline diazo method; a few are argentaffin. Immunocytochemistry shows cells to be positive for neuroendocrine markers (e.g. chromogranin).

Cells from a pulmonary carcinoid are not exfoliated in bronchial secretions unless the covering mucosa is ulcerated. Brush smears taken after a biopsy forceps has disrupted the epithelium and transbronchial and percutaneous needle aspirations are more likely to yield diagnostic material.

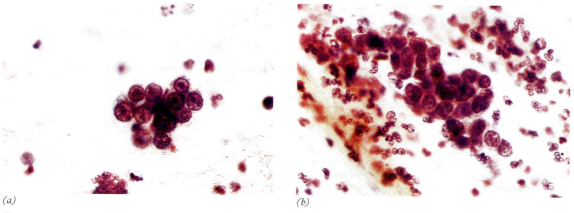

(a)   *(b)*

Fig. 3.55 Carcinoid tumour

Papanicolaou ×525 (a) sputum (b) sputum; another specimen from the same case

The cells illustrated were present in the sputum of a patient with local recurrence several months after resection of a circumscribed carcinoid tumour. They were abundant and formed clusters. The cells in (a) are typical of carcinoid tumours. They are small and uniform and have a narrow rim of cytoplasm. The round nuclei contain prominent nucleoli. The nuclear borders are thick and moulding is not seen. The cells in another sample of sputum from the same patient are less regular, the nuclei have a 'salt and pepper' chromatin, there is a suggestion of nuclear moulding and nucleoli are not seen. Further surgery was performed on the patient and the recurrent tumour was seen to be more anaplastic and had infiltrated the adjacent lung parenchyma.

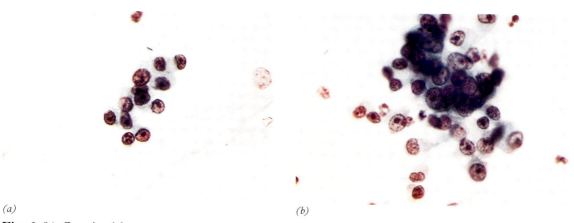

(a)   *(b)*

Fig. 3.56 Carcinoid tumour

Papanicolaou ×525 (a) bronchial brush (b) same smear; another field

These micrographs show a bronchial carcinoid with some atypia. The cells in (a) appear somewhat larger than in the preceding example, but are uniform. The eccentrically situated nuclei show minimal variation in shape and size and contain conspicuous nucleoli. Compare the normochromasia and the near absence of a chromatin deposit on the nuclear margin of these viable tumour cells with the hyperchromasia and thick nuclear membrane of the degenerating exfoliated cells shown in Figure 3.61 (a). Another field in the same smear is seen in (b). The variation in the size of the cells and nuclear pleomorphism is greater.

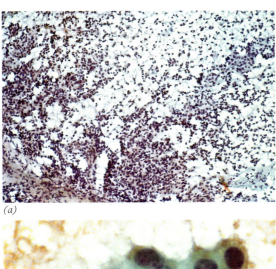

(a)

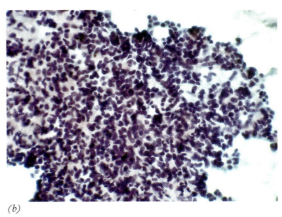

(b)

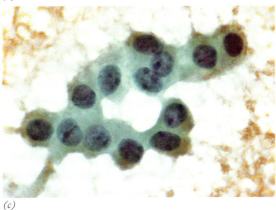

(c)

Fig. 3.57 Carcinoid tumour

(a) Papanicolaou ×210 FNA lung (b) ×420 (c) ×2100

Lung aspirates from carcinoid yield cellular material (a) giving an impression of an overall monotonous population composed of small uniform cells (b) in clusters but also dispersed (mimicking lymphoma). Material often includes large vessels. High power (c) reveals epithelial cells with relatively abundant cytoplasm in which granules may be seen. Nuclei are uniform, often eccentrically placed ('plasmacytoid') and have coarsely granular chromatin. Nucleoli are inconspicuous or may be visible.

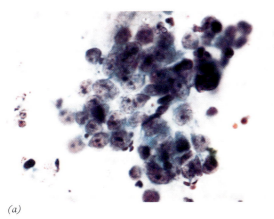

(a)

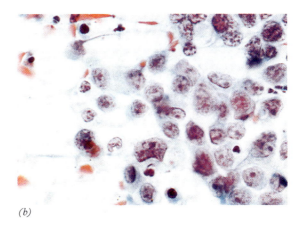

(b)

Fig. 3.58 Carcinoid tumour

Papanicolaou ×525 (a) sputum (b) FNA; lung; same case

This is an example of a pleomorphic, high malignant, atypical carcinoid which was diagnosed by aspiration and sputum cytology as a poorly differentiated adenocarcinoma. The correct diagnosis was established by histological and ultrastructural examination of the resected specimen. The patient developed widespread metastases and died of disseminated malignancy 14 months later.

Adenocarcinoma (including bronchoalveolar carcinoma)

Adenocarcinoma is the least common of the three major primary lung carcinomas and one that occurs in non-smokers. An increasing incidence has been reported in recent years, and it is now considered to be provoked to some extent by cigarette smoking.

Approximately three-quarters originate in the smaller bronchi at the periphery of the lung fields. They have a special propensity for scar tissue and most of the scar cancers that arise in chronic interstitial fibrosis (honeycomb lung) or in areas of focal fibrosis that result from pneumoconiosis or treated tuberculosis are adenocarcinomas.

Three basic histological patterns of growth are seen. The acinar type shows a predominance of glandular structures; the papillary type consists of fronds of tumour with cells covering a fibrovascular stalk; the solid carcinoma lacks a distinctive pattern but has many mucus-secreting cells. A tumour may exhibit mainly one pattern and may be typed accordingly, or it may have a mixed pattern.

Bronchoalveolar carcinoma is a rare subtype of adenocarcinoma and constitutes approximately 1% of all primary lung cancers. It may present as a single coin lesion or a mass in the vicinity of a pre-existing scar, as multicentric nodules or exhibit a diffuse extensive intrapulmonary spread and lobar consolidation. Bronchoalveolar carcinoma may have a papillary pattern, but typically uses the walls of the alveoli as a scaffolding along which it grows. Some arise in the mucus or the Clara cells of the terminal bronchioles, others in the type 2 pneumocyte.

Two histological and clinical patterns are observed. In one, thin alveolar septa are lined by tall mucus-secreting cells and bronchorrhoea of 1–4 litres of clear fluid may be a major and troublesome symptom. In the other, the cells are cuboidal and peg-like and contain little or no mucin.

It has been claimed that the acinar and papillary subtypes of adenocarcinoma can be identified by cytology. In the author's view, a papillary tumour, whether benign or malignant, can be diagnosed with certainty, only when a fibrovascular stalk covered with malignant cells is seen. Such an appearance is seen in FNA, but is exceedingly rare in other respiratory tract specimens. Similarly, cytological distinction between a localized bronchoalveolar carcinoma and the other adenocarcinomas is not consistent. The diffuse variety of bronchoalveolar carcinoma cannot be separated with certainty from primary large cell bronchogenic carcinoma or a metastatic gastrointestinal carcinoma that grows along the alveolar walls. In the absence of histological confirmation, a diagnosis of bronchoalveolar carcinoma can be suggested if cytological appearances are assessed in conjunction with radiological and clinical features.

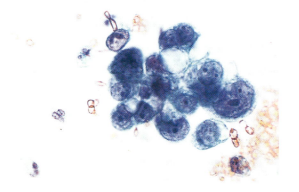

Fig. 3.59 Adenocarcinoma of the lung

Papanicolaou ×525: sputum

This micrograph shows several typical features of an exfoliated cluster of well-differentiated adenocarcinoma cells. An acinar space is seen in the right lower part. Several sharply circumscribed mucous vacuoles are present. There is a dipping down of the smooth outer margins to the points of junction between adjacent cells. This may be seen in cohesive benign glandular cells, but tends to be greatly enhanced in adenocarcinoma cells and gives a scalloped effect to the entire cluster (compare with Fig. 3.38). A wide variation is apparent in the size of the cells, the nuclei and the nucleoli and the nuclear-cytoplasmic ratio.

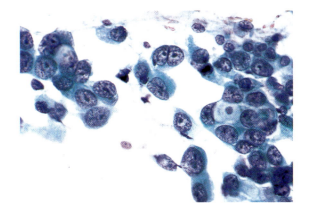

Fig. 3.60 Adenocarcinoma of the lung

Papanicolaou ×525: bronchial brush

A two-dimensional spread of adenocarcinoma cells is the rule rather than the exception in brush smears. Distinction from a large cell carcinoma can be difficult and the presence of intracytoplasmic mucin may be the only clue to cell type. Unlike a hydropic vacuole, a mucous vacuole often indents the nucleus and may consist of a sharply demarcated clear area with a central dense body.

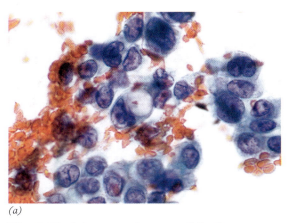

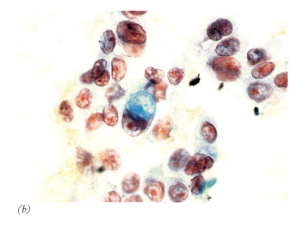

(a)　　　　　　　　　　　　　　　　　　　　*(b)*

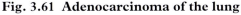

Fig. 3.61 Adenocarcinoma of the lung

(a) Papanicolaou ×525: FNA; lung (b) Alcian blue ×525: same field

A similar problem is encountered in aspiration smears. The cells shown formed flat sheets, several contained intracytoplasmic vacuoles, some with a central condensation (a). The smear was decolorized in 1% hydrochloric acid for 30 seconds, restained with 1.0% Alcian blue and the presence of mucin was confirmed (b). For a correct interpretation of this procedure, the cells examined should be clear of free background mucin which is often present in a respiratory tract specimen, and the Alcian blue-positive secretory product should be clearly delineated within the limits of the cytoplasm.

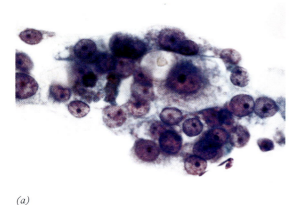

(a)

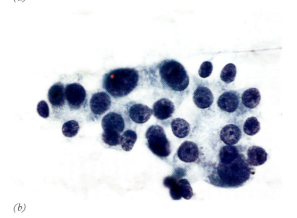

(b)

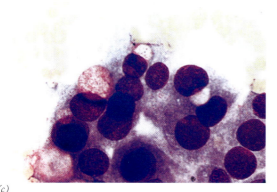

(c)

Fig. 3.62 Adenocarcinoma of lung

(a) Papanicolaou ×525: sputum (b) Papanicolaou ×525: FNA; lung; same case (c) MGG ×525: same specimen as (b) another smear

The large sheet of malignant epithelial cells with ill-defined intercellular borders and a haphazard distribution of nuclei shows an arrangement unusual in sputum (a). The thick nuclear membrane, the paucity of chromatin and the extreme hypochromasia of the main body of the nucleus are due to degenerative changes. Nucleoli are prominent against the pale nucleus. One mucous vacuole with a central condensation, resembling an erythrocyte, is seen. The same basic morphological features, namely a fragile cytoplasm which appears almost syncytial, the random distribution of variable-sized nuclei, differences in size and number of nucleoli, are seen in the lung aspirate (b). The chromatin pattern of the aspirated viable cells is significantly different. The chromatin is aggregated into granules, which vary in shape and size, some being exceedingly fine. Condensation of the chromatin on the nuclear membrane, an early indication of degeneration, is conspicuous by its absence. The relatively monomorphic malignant cells are identified as adenocarcinoma cells by the four finely stippled mucous vacuoles present in the Romanowsky-stained smear (c). The appearance seen in the sputum and the lung aspiration is suggestive of a poorly differentiated solid carcinoma with mucus secretion.

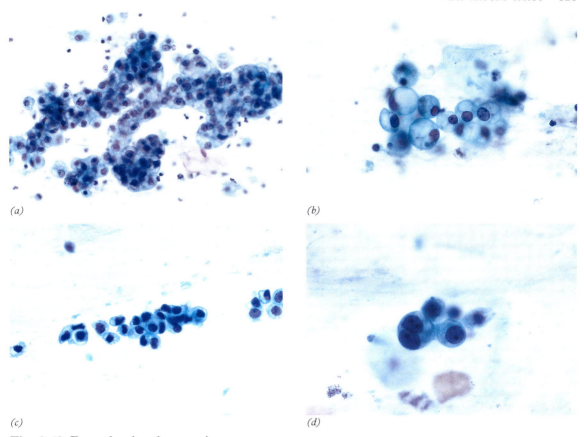

(a)

(b)

(c)

(d)

Fig. 3.63 Bronchoalveolar carcinoma

(a) Papanicolaou ×840: sputum (b) ×1260 same case (c) ×1260 bronchoalveolar lavage (d) ×1260 bronchoalveolar lavage

Because of the tendency of the cells from bronchoalveolar carcinoma to exfoliate freely, sputum is a very suitable medium for its diagnosis. As a rule, large numbers of cells are exfoliated, mostly in clusters (a), but single cells may be interspersed amongst macrophages. The cells are of similar size and appearance as alveolar macrophages and distinction may be difficult for the primary screener because tumour cells lack the established cytological criteria of malignancy. They have eccentric nuclei and relatively abundant, well-outlined, non-phagocytic cytoplasm. Nuclei are round and show minimal anisonucleosis and may have a prominent nucleolus. Distinction from macrophages is based mainly on the propensity of epithelium to form clusters, nuclear detail and cytoplasm without carbon particles.

Large cell anaplastic carcinoma

Electron microscopy studies of large cell carcinoma of the lung have shown that very few are completely undifferentiated and that the majority have poorly developed features of squamous or glandular cells. These are not appreciated at light microscopy level and large cell carcinoma is classified as a distinct entity. Two variants are recognized. The clear cell carcinoma is similar to renal cell carcinoma. The giant cell carcinoma has a looser pattern of growth and contains many pleomorphic giant cells.

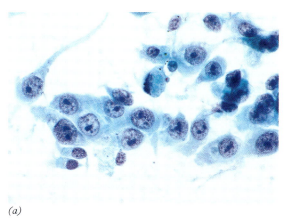

(a)

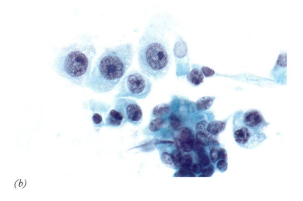

(b)

Fig. 3.64 Large cell anaplastic carcinoma

(a) Papanicolaou ×1260: bronchial brush (b) ×1260; same case

Cells from large cell anaplastic carcinoma, shown here in comparison with benign bronchial epithelium (a, b), are larger, have eccentric nuclei , abundant well-outlined cytoplasm and very prominent, often multiple nucleoli. They are reminiscent of malignant melanoma cells.

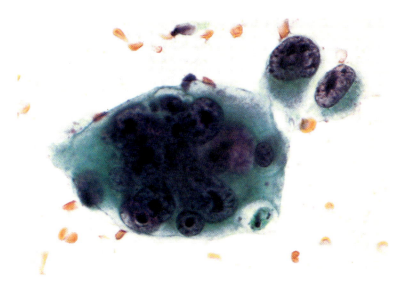

Fig. 3.65 Large cell anaplastic carcinoma: giant cell carcinoma

Papanicolaou ×720: bronchial brush

This micrograph shows another example of the giant cell variant. The specimen contained moderate-sized, mononuclear malignant cells which lacked definite cytological features of a squamous or glandular origin. Several giant cells with multiple large overlapping nuclei were present. Most of the nuclei contained prominent nucleoli which varied greatly in size and shape. Giant cells may be present in some poorly differentiated squamous cell carcinomas and adenocarcinomas, but do not usually have the appearance, as in this case, of giant sarcomatous cells.

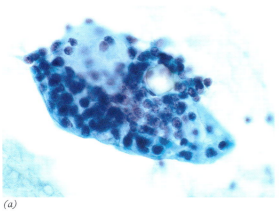

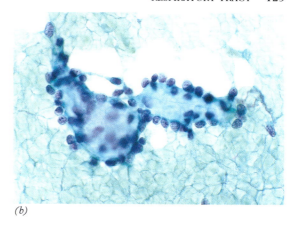

(a)   *(b)*

Fig. 3.66 Adenoid cystic carcinoma

(a) Papanicolaou ×1260: bronchial brush (b) ×1260 : same case (courtesy of Dr A Rubin)

The trachea and main bronchi may give rise to adenoid cystic carcinoma, identical to that found in the salivary glands. They may present as an endobronchial mass or circumferential tumours but are almost invariably in the submucosa and therefore unlikely to be detected by sputum examination.

In bronchial brushing and needle aspirates, tumour presents in three-dimensional clusters of small uniform cells which in 80% of cases characteristically surround spherical or cylindrical cores of homogeneous basement membrane material (a, b). Cells have oval nuclei, granular chromatin and moderately but definitely enlarged nucleoli.

METASTATIC CARCINOMA

The lungs have a vast capillary network through which the entire blood flow passes. They also possess an extensive network of lymphatics which have free anastomoses with the lymphatics of the upper abdomen. Cancer cells are easily carried to the lungs, which are common sites of metastatic tumours. It has to be remembered, however, that the lung is itself a frequent primary site of the commonest malignancies, namely adenocarcinoma, squamous cell and anaplastic carcinoma. In addition, many other tumours, including extragonadal germ cell tumours, a variety of sarcomas and assorted epithelial and mesenchymal neoplasms, benign or of borderline malignancy, develop in the lung. The cytopathologist required to give an opinion on a lung lesion needs to bear this in mind. Cytomorphological appearances seen in respiratory tract specimens may be diagnostic or suggestive of any of the lesions that occur in the lung, and may even direct attention to a silent extrapulmonary primary. In common practice, however, a cytopathological diagnosis of a metastatic pulmonary deposit is not made in isolation, but is correlated with clinical and radiological assessment.

A few examples of metastatic tumours and the associated diagnostic problems are illustrated and discussed below.

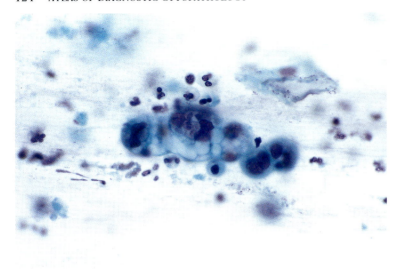

Fig. 3.67 Adenocarcinoma

Papanicolaou ×1160: bronchial brush

Adenocarcinoma diagnosed in the bronchial washings of a man with a history of colon carcinoma was confirmed by bronchial biopsy histology. Primary adenocarcinoma of the lung more usually arises in peripheral bronchi or scars. Secondary carcinoma occasionally presents as single or multiple endobronchial tumours. In this case, neither cytology nor histology was able to determine whether the tumour was bronchogenic or metastatic.

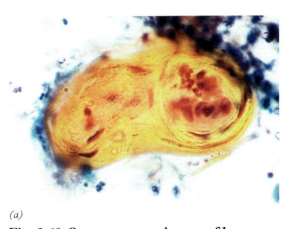

(a)

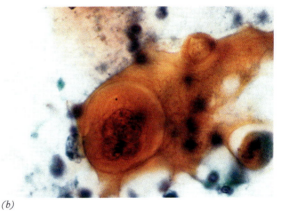

(b)

Fig. 3.68 Squamous carcinoma of larynx

Papanicolaou ×525 (a) sputum: secondary (b) sputum: primary; another case

Squamous carcinoma of the larynx is usually well-differentiated and epithelial pearl formation (a) is a notable feature. It may contain many refractile dyskeratotic cells, ghost nuclei and bizarre anucleate keratinized cells (b) indistinguishable from the cells of a keratinized bronchogenic carcinoma (see Fig. 3.47). The cells in (a) came from a patient who had multiple lung nodules, rheumatoid arthritis of long standing and a history of

carcinoma of the larynx treated by radiotherapy. The differential diagnosis, which lay between rheumatoid lung and metastatic disease, was resolved by the presence of numerous unequivocal squamous carcinoma cells in the sputum (a). The cells in (b) were found in the sputum of a patient with clear lung fields and a tumour seen through a laryngoscope to be confined to one vocal cord.

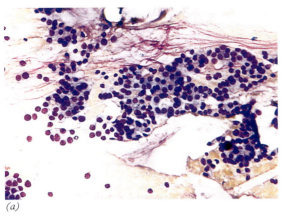

(a)

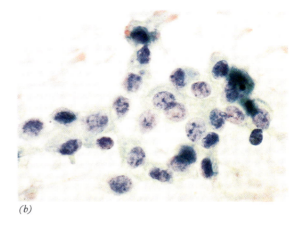

(b)

Fig. 3.69 Adenocarcinoma of breast

(a) MGG ×133: FNA; lung (b) Papanicolaou ×525: FNA; lung; another case

Carcinoma of the breast metastasizes readily to the pleural spaces. A deposit in the lung may develop from blood-borne tumour emboli direct from the primary site or via the pleural cavity. The tumour cells are often monomorphic, arranged in an acinar pattern and do not secrete much mucin but may contain an occasional intracellular mucin droplet. Both the patients whose cells are shown had undergone mastectomy for breast carcinoma; both had intrapulmonary masses with smooth contours. The chest X-ray appearances of these patients were highly suggestive of metastatic deposits and the cytological features were considered to be consistent.

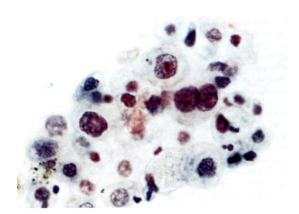

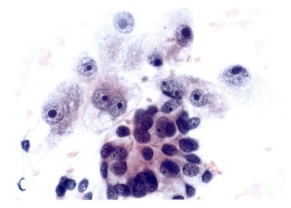

Fig. 3.70 Adenocarcinoma of pancreas

Papanicolaou ×525: sputum

The pancreas is probably the commonest source of a silent primary which spreads to the lung. An adenocarcinoma was diagnosed on sputum cytology, and bronchoalveolar carcinoma was suggested as the chest X-ray showed diffuse infiltration. Development of further symptoms in the patient led to the discovery of a pancreatic carcinoma.

Fig. 3.71 Renal cell carcinoma

(a) Papanicolaou ×1260: bronchial brushings (courtesy of Dr SS Kalra)

Large malignant cells, shown here in comparison with benign bronchial epithelium, have abundant clear cytoplasm, eccentric nuclei and prominent nucleoli. The radiological appearances of a 'cannon ball' mass on the chest X-ray and clinical history help to distinguish this tumour from the primary clear cell carcinoma of the lung.

LYMPHOPROLIFERATIVE DISORDERS

Fig. 3.72 Hodgkin's disease

(a) Papanicolaou ×720: FNA; lung (b) MGG ×720: same specimen; another smear (c) Papanicolaou ×720: same smear as (a)

The exact cell of origin of Hodgkin's disease, a lymphoproliferative disorder, is uncertain. The lymphocytes that accompany the neoplastic cells are benign and reactive. The diagnostic cell is the Reed–Sternberg (R-S) cell. In its classical form the R-S cell is binucleate (a, b) or appears multinucleated (c) in light microscopy preparations, although ultrastructural studies have shown a single polylobated nucleus in some instances. Each nucleus contains a prominent macronucleolus linked by fine strands of chromatin to the condensed chromatin on the nuclear margin. The cytoplasm is darkly staining and may be amphophilic. The mononuclear form, referred to as the Hodgkin's cell (a, b) is non-specific as it occurs in other lymphoproliferative malignancies. The treatment and prognosis of Hodgkin's disease are different from lymphocytic lymphomas and a diagnosis of Hodgkin's lymphoma should not be made in the absence of the R-S cell. Primary Hodgkin's lymphoma of the lung is rare, but secondary involvement of pulmonary tissue is common. The FNA illustrated was obtained from a new shadow which appeared in the lung of a patient with established extrapulmonary Hodgkin's disease.

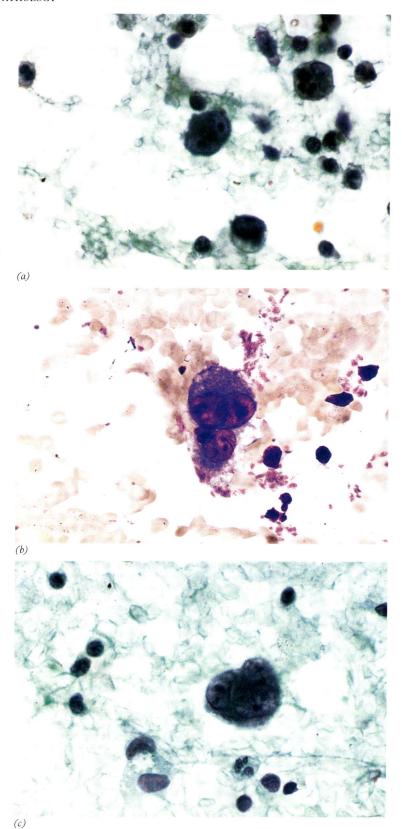

(a)

(b)

(c)

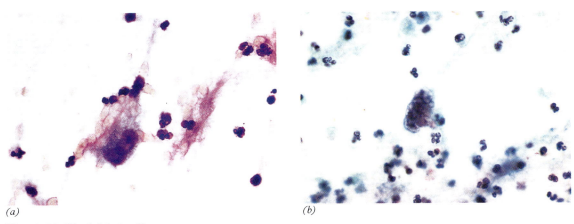

(a)   *(b)*

Fig. 3.73 Hodgkin's disease

(a) MGG ×525: FNA; lung (b) Papanicolaou ×525: same specimen; another smear

The binucleate (a) and polylobated (b) R-S cells illustrated are two of a dozen tumour cells identified in pus aspirated from a lung abscess in a 19-year-old male with a history of Hodgkin's lymphoma. Culture of the abscess fluid yielded a growth of *Streptococcus pneumoniae*, an infection to which patients with this disease are particularly prone. The

shadow diminished in size on antibiotic therapy but did not resolve completely and enlarged again shortly after. The flimsiness of the cytoplasm and the somewhat ragged appearance of the neoplastic cells are due to necrotic changes in a purulent specimen.

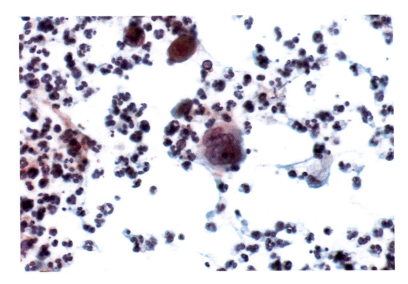

Fig. 3.74 Hodgkin's disease

Papanicolaou ×458: FNA; lung

The characteristic cell of nodular sclerosing Hodgkin's is a variant of the R-S cell, known as the lacunar cell. This type of cell has abundant pale cytoplasm, a polylobated nucleus and a smaller nucleolus than the classical R-S cell. The name derives from the tendency of the cell to shrink away from the surrounding structures in formalin-fixed tissues to lie within a clear lacuna. This appearance is not seen in alcohol-fixed cytological preparations and the cell is difficult to distinguish from other bizarre malignant cells of lymphoid origin. The diagnosis of primary nodular sclerosing Hodgkin's of the lung was established by open biopsy histology.

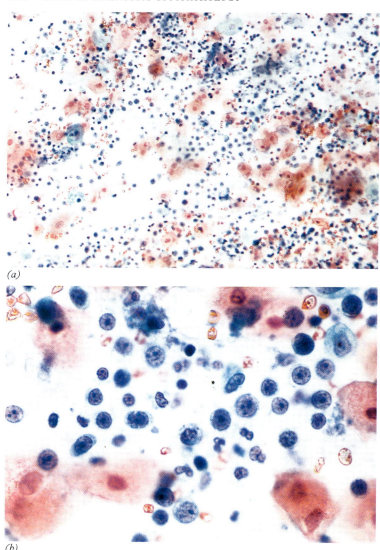

(a)

(b)

Fig. 3.75 Non-Hodgkin's lymphoma

Papanicolaou (a) ×183: sputum (b) ×720: same field

Precise classification of non-Hodgkin's lymphoma is established by combined immunocytochemical and morphological analyses of the malignant lymphoid cells. In the absence of the former, a reliable, if limited diagnosis is often possible in cytological material and an opinion may be given on the grade of the tumour. Small-celled lymphomas are generally of low-grade malignancy; larger neoplastic cells with nucleoli indicate a high-grade lymphoma. A shower of tumour cells (a) covered the smears made from the sputum of a woman with a bronchial biopsy diagnosis of SCC. High-power examination (b) shows discrete neoplastic cells with narrow rims of cytoplasm surrounding large nuclei. The majority of the nuclei are round; a few show the indentation or cleft seen in cells of lymph follicle centre origin. The nucleoli vary in size and number and are seen in all the cells in the field (b). A cytodiagnosis of a high-grade centroblastic lymphoma was confirmed by repeat biopsy histology.

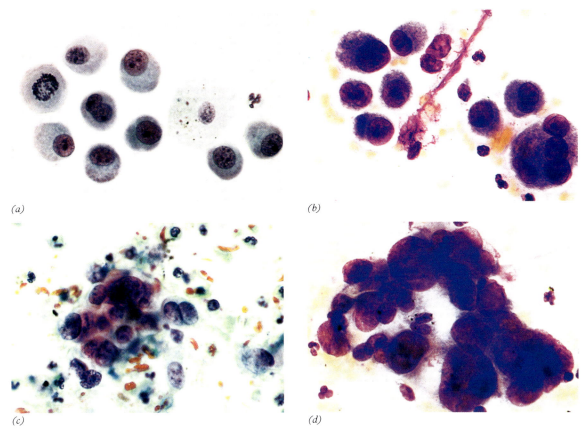

(a) *(b)* *(c)* *(d)*

Fig. 3.76 Multiple myeloma and primary bronchogenic carcinoma

(a) Papanicolaou ×525: FNA; lung; myeloma cells (b) MGG ×525: same specimen; another smear; myeloma cells (c) Papanicolaou ×525: same smear as (a); carcinoma cells (d) MGG ×525: same smear as (b); carcinoma cells

Two malignancies in the same organ are exceedingly rare, but not unknown. A diagnosis of double pathology should be based on clear-cut evidence, especially in cancers which can be extremely pleomorphic. The lung aspirate of an elderly patient contained two separate populations of malignant cells-myeloma and carcinoma cells.

Myeloma is a lymphoreticular neoplasm of plasma cells; it develops from a single clone and produces large quantities of a monoclonal antibody. It may form a solitary lesion (plasmacytoma) or present as multiple osteolytic foci or a diffuse infiltrate of marrow, lung and other organs. Light chains of the antibody may be excreted in the urine (Bence Jones protein). The tumour cells may be differentiated plasma cells or they may be immature and pleomorphic.

The cells in (a) and (b) are large and discrete, the cytoplasm is basophilic and the nuclei are eccentric in position. A cell in mitosis is seen in (a). Two binucleate forms and one large multinucleated cell are shown in (b). A kidney-shaped nucleus is seen in (a) and in (b). The prominent nucleoli indicate immaturity of the malignant plasma cells. The patient had dysproteinaemia and Bence Jones proteinuria.

Sheets of cohesive pleomorphic carcinoma cells with high nuclear-cytoplasmic ratios, granular chromatin and inconspicuous nucleoli were identified in the same smear (c, d).

In the terminal illness, the patient developed a pleural effusion which yielded mucin-positive adenocarcinoma cells, and heart failure induced by increasing viscosity of blood caused by a rapid rise in circulating myeloma proteins.

4. Serous effusions

The body cavities, the right and left pleural, the pericardial and the peritoneal have a common origin from the coelom. Each lies within a double-layered serous membrane derived from the embryonal mesenchyme. The inner layer of the membrane invests the organs within the cavity and is known as the visceral layer; reflected back over the internal wall of the body cavity, it becomes the outer parietal layer.

The three thoracic cavities containing the two lungs and the heart are self-contained. In the female the peritoneal cavity communicates with the genital tract through the fimbrial ends of the fallopian tubes; in the male, it consists of an additional small sac applied to the abdominal parietes. A potential space separates the closely apposed parietal and visceral layers of the pleura and pericardium; the distance between the outer layer of the peritoneum, which has a complex anatomical structure, and the serosal covering of the abdominal organs is greater.

The serous membrane is made up of loose connective tissue carrying capillaries, lymphatics and nerves, and is covered on its free surface by a simple pavement epithelium which is lubricated by a small quantity of serous fluid. The fluid between the two layers of the pleura is the result of the net hydrostatic oncotic pressure of the capillaries of the parietal pleura which favours flow of a relatively protein-free fluid from these capillaries into the pleural space and its reabsorption by the venous capillaries of the visceral pleura (80–90%) and the pleural lymphatics (10–20%). It is likely that a similar mechanism operates in the pericardium and peritoneum. Disturbances of the mechanism that normally maintains this dynamic flow may result in accumulation of excess fluid, i.e. a serous effusion. Free fluid in the peritoneal cavity is referred to as ascites (Greek *askos*, belly). Two types of effusions are recognized-transudates and exudates.

A transudate results when hydrostatic pressure is increased and oncotic pressure is reduced, as in congestive cardiac failure, cirrhosis, peritoneal dialysis, hypoproteinaemia of malnutrition or hypoalbuminaemia of the nephrotic syndrome. The fluid is generally straw-coloured and clear, occasionally opalescent, has a protein count of <3 g/dl, a specific gravity of 1015 or less and contains relatively few cells. Some long-standing transudates in heart failure and cirrhosis may be very cellular.

An exudate is formed when capillary permeability is increased, lymphatic flow is decreased, or both mechanisms operate. Malignant involvement of the serous membrane, which may, additionally, disrupt the capillary endothelium, is a common cause of an exudate. Other aetiologies include inflammatory disease due to infective agents, bacterial, viral, parasitic or fungal, connective tissue disease such as rheumatoid disease and lupus, pulmonary infarct, drug sensitivity and vasculitides such as Wegener's granulomatosis. The protein content of an exudate usually exceeds 3 g/dl, the specific gravity is greater than 1015 and the cell count is generally high.

Differences in the specific gravity and protein content are fairly useful in determining whether an effusion is a transudate or an exudate, but are unreliable in approximately 10% of cases.

METHODS OF PREPARATION

Most serous effusions will clot on standing, particularly exudates which have a high protein content and are rich in fibrin. The clot may be large and jelly-like in consistency or form one or more firm, thin strands. A considerable proportion of the cells are likely to become enmeshed in the clot. To prevent clot formation, an effusion should be placed immediately in a sterile container with an anticoagulant. Satisfactory anticoagulants for 20 ml of fluid are EDTA (ethylenediaminetetraacetic acid dipotassium salt) 20 mg; heparin, 2 mg or 200 units; 3.8% sodium citrate, 2 ml. Oxalate and liquoid are unsuitable as they distort cell morphology.

In the laboratory, the volume, colour and consistency should be noted. It is desirable but not essential to estimate the specific gravity and total protein content. A differential cell count is useful in a sterile, benign effusion. The usual methods of preparation are as follows:

1. The fluid is centrifuged in a conical tube at 600 **g** or approximately 1500 rpm for 5–10 min. The supernatant is discarded and smears made from the virtually fluid-free sediment, rapidly wet-fixed in 95% ethanol, for Papanicolaou and haematoxylin and eosin (H&E) staining, air-dried and fixed in methanol for a Romanowsky stain. Spare wet-fixed and air-dried smears are kept in reserve for any special staining procedures

that may be required. Some cytologists recommend resuspension of the cell button in normal saline, and a second spin to wash the cells free of protein before spreading the smear.

2. Cytocentrifugation.
3. Concentration of cells on membrane filters.
4. Preparation of cell blocks for histology.

A heavily blood-stained fluid can be treated with 1% acetic acid to lyse the cells. A preferable method is to make smears from the buffy coat of nucleated cells that separates out between the supernatant and the erythrocyte layer. If necessary, Wintrobe tubes may be used to obtain several buffy coats of reasonable depth. A clot in the fluid can be used to make a succession of dabs on one or more grease-free slides until all the fluid has been squeezed out. The last two or three imprint smears from the practically dry clot are usually satisfactory. Alternatively, it can be processed for histological sections.

BENIGN CONDITIONS

Mesothelial cells

The pavement lining of a serous membrane is formed by a single row of cuboidal mesothelial cells which are the only cells of epithelial origin native to a serous effusion. Other benign epithelial cells may, in rare instances, enter an effusion through a fistula or be accidentally introduced during a surgical procedure. A metastatic tumour is the most likely source of non-mesothelial epithelial cells. Almost all effusions, benign or malignant, also contain blood-derived cells.

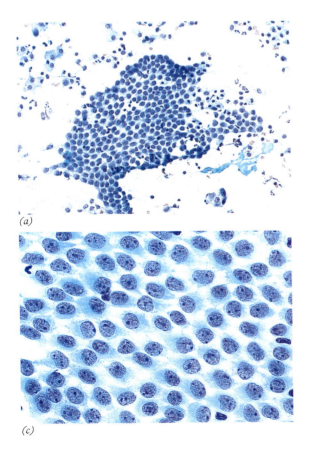

(a)

(c)

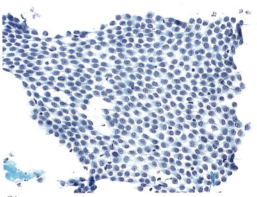

(b)

Fig 4.1 Mesothelial cells

(a) Papanicolaou ×420 (b) ×840 (c) ×1260: fluid from the pouch of Douglas

It is virtually impossible to obtain fluid from normal pleural or pericardial space. A small quantity of free peritoneal fluid is often present in the pouch of Douglas from which normal mesothelial cells may be recovered. These are often single or they may appear in a sheet of uniform cells with round or oval nuclei (a, b). Sheets of normal mesothelial cells may be dislodged by mechanical means which include washing the serous cavity with sterile normal saline. The cells are cuboidal in shape and have a translucent cytoplasm which sometimes contains small vacuoles. The nuclei are regular in size, finely reticulate and may have one to three small nucleoli (c).

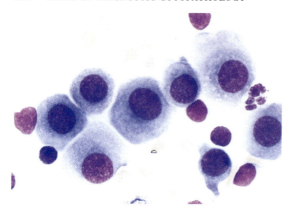

Fig 4.2. Mesothelial cells

MGG ×1740: pleural fluid

Mesothelial cells suspended in the fluid acquire a rounded shape with eccentrically placed round or oval nuclei and dense cytoplasm. Intercellular slit like spaces resemble those of squamous epithelium and reflect the presence of desmosomal junctions between the cells.

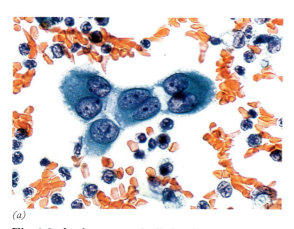

(a)

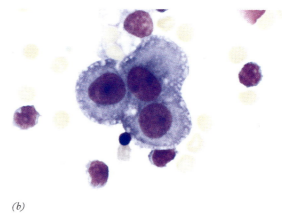

(b)

Fig 4.3 Active mesothelial cells

(a) Papanicolaou ×525 (b) MGG ×1260: pleural fluid; case of congestive cardiac failure

In a pathological collection of fluid, mesothelial cells display morphological changes which suggest that they have been shed from a hyperplastic mesothelium; these cells have many of the characteristics of proliferative cells and are referred to as active or reactive forms. The cells are larger than their normal counterparts. An increase in the amount of RNA is reflected in greater basophilia of the cytoplasm.

This may be uniform in colour or two-toned with a darker and a paler zone. In some cells, the zone of pallor is perinuclear while in others it is peripheral, often in blebs, representing glycogen deposits (b). Another indication of increased RNA is seen in the nucleoli. These are more prominent, may be increased in number and size and show variations of size and shape.

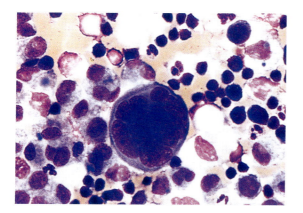

Fig. 4.4 Multinucleated mesothelial cells

MGG ×525: pleural fluid; case of left ventricular failure

The nucleus of the active mesothelial cell shows a proportionate increase in size and the nuclear-cytoplasmic ratio is relatively constant. The majority of cells have one nucleus but two or three nuclei are not uncommon (Figs 4.3, 4.5). Large multinucleated forms packed with 20 or more nuclei can occur; these show minor variations in size but have a comparable chromatin pattern.

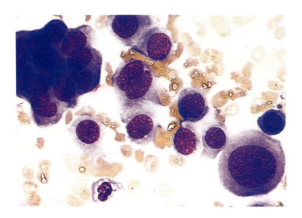

Fig. 4.5 Active mesothelial cells

MGG ×525: ascitic fluid; case of active chronic hepatitis

Variations in the size of the active forms within one specimen can be quite considerable. While a fair proportion of the cells are uniform, the odd cell may be disconcertingly large. A comparison of its nuclear and cytoplasmic characteristics with intermediate forms which progressively bridge the differences between it and a typical mesothelial cell is useful in identifying the cell.

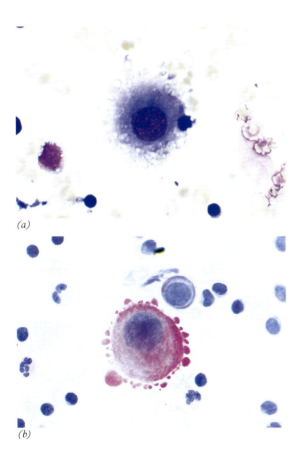

(a)

(b)

Fig 4.6 Active mesothelial cell

(a) MGG ×1260 (b) PAS ×1260: pleural fluid

Mesothelial cell surface carries small knobs or irregularly arranged microvilli, either all round or at one pole. They are better appreciated with periodic acid-Schiff (PAS) stain (b).

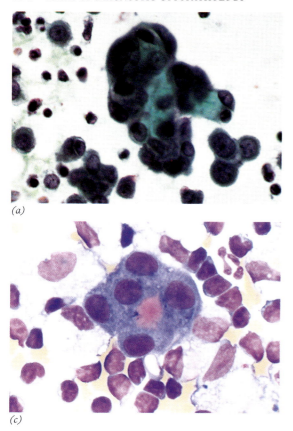

(a)

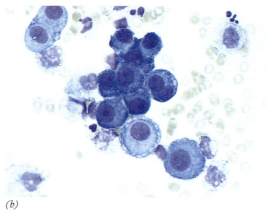

(b)

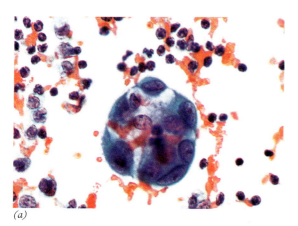

(c)

Fig 4.7 Active mesothelial cells

(a) Papanicolaou ×525 (b) MGG ×840 (c) ×1260

Mesothelial cells often adhere to each other in small collections. Larger clusters can occur and these are a source of diagnostic difficulty, even leading to a false-positive diagnosis of malignancy. Shed into a fluid, cells become rounded with some depth of focus. The fine vacuoles present in normal mesothelial cells may be enhanced in size and number. An overall impression of the glandular structure may be created. Occasionally, in May–Grünwald–Giemsa (MGG) preparations, mesothelial cells may surround pink eosinophilic material. This structure, mimicking glandular acinus, is yet another manifestation of reactive changes (c).

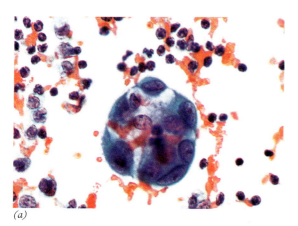

(a)

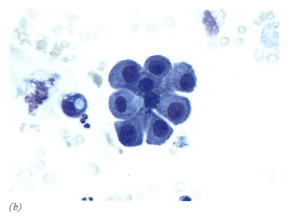

(b)

Fig 4.8 Active mesothelial cell

(a) Papanicolaou ×525 (b) MGG ×1260

The normal slit-like intercellular space may be widened between cells with well-developed microvilli into what is referred as a window. This is generally crossed by several hair-like bridges (presumably microvilli) connecting the neighbouring cells.

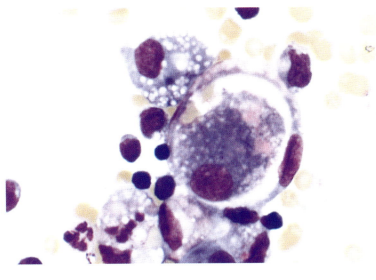

Fig 4.9 Active mesothelial cells

MGG ×1740: pleural fluid; pulmonary infarct

Fluids from patients with recent pulmonary infarcts are very cellular and include, amongst others, many reactive mesothelial cells and macrophages. These can engulf mesothelial cells.

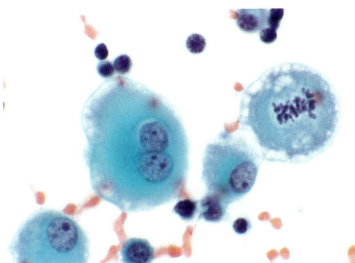

Fig 4.10 Mesothelial cells in mitosis

Papanicolaou ×1740

Mesothelial cells can be bi- and multinucleate; they can show mitotic figures since a sterile effusion can serve as a suitable culture medium and cells will continue to live and occasionally divide in it. Mitosis should not be taken as evidence of malignancy. Comparison with adherent typical benign mesothelial cells is helpful.

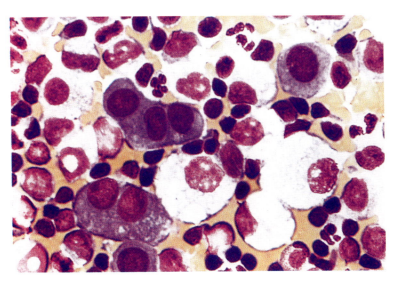

Fig. 4.11 Degenerate mesothelial cells

MGG ×720: same case as in Figures 4.3 and 4.10

While some mesothelial cells continue to proliferate in an effusion, others undergo degenerative changes. The degenerate forms are a shade larger than their viable fellows. Their foamy cytoplasm is distended with multiple hydropic and fatty vacuoles. The nucleus is usually eccentric, paler in colour and has a smudged chromatin. One or two nucleoli are generally visible. Foamy mesothelial cells may contain particulate matter and this has been attributed to phagocytic properties.

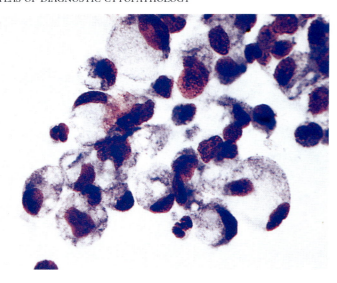

Fig. 4.12 Degenerate mesothelial cells: signet-ring forms

MGG: ×720: ascitic fluid; case of chronic hepatitis B and cirrhosis

In an extreme degree of degenerative vacuolization of the cytoplasm, the nucleus is compressed against the edge of the cell which acquires a signet-ring form. This type of cell occurs in any type of effusion, but is more plentiful and more often seen in ascites due to primary liver disease. A misdiagnosis of metastatic signet-ring carcinoma is avoided by careful assessment of the chromatin pattern.

INFLAMMATORY DISEASE

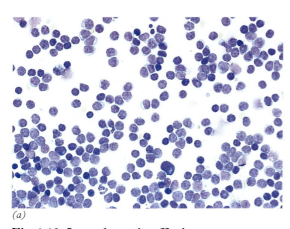

(a)

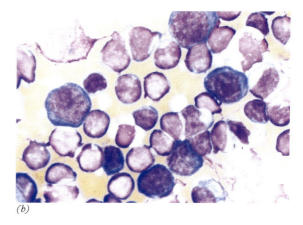

(b)

Fig 4.13 Lymphocytic effusion

(a) MGG ×420 (b) ×2100

Lymphocytes often constitute the largest single group of the mixed cell population in the effusion. Lymphocytic effusion is a pathological finding, particularly when combined with large amount of red blood cells. Differential diagnosis includes tuberculosis and malignancy (including lymphomas). Tuberculous effusion usually includes mature lymphocytes (a) but some follicle centre cells including

plasma cells can be present (b). Mesothelial cells are sparse or absent, reflecting the surface of the pleura being covered with chronic inflammatory exudate. Cell marker studies reveal the majority of the lymphocytes to be of T-cell phenotype, resembling the T/B ratio in peripheral blood. The possibility of a low-grade T-cell lymphoma has to be excluded.

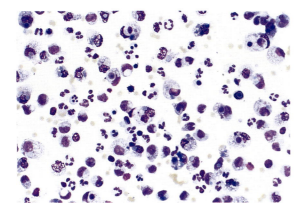

Fig 4.14 Acute inflammatory exudate

MGG ×1160 Pleural effusion

Serous fluids sometimes contain a significant number of polymorphs. These range from relatively few in cases of ascites due to alcoholic liver disease to numerous in cases of empyema and peritonitis. This case illustrates a postpneumonic pleural effusion with polymorphs, lymphocytes and macrophages.

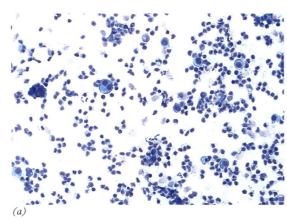

(a)

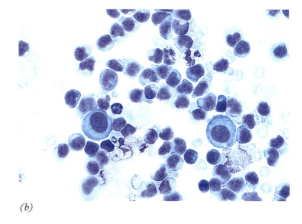

(b)

Fig 4.15 Ascites in alcoholic liver disease

(a) MGG ×420 (b) ×840 Ascitic fluid: liver cirrhosis

Ascites from patients with alcoholic liver disease can be cellular and in addition to mesothelial cells and macrophages also contain inflammatory cells, including polymorphs. Mesothelial cells can be pleomorphic, in clusters of cells with prominent nucleoli and macrophages with irregular chromatin pattern.

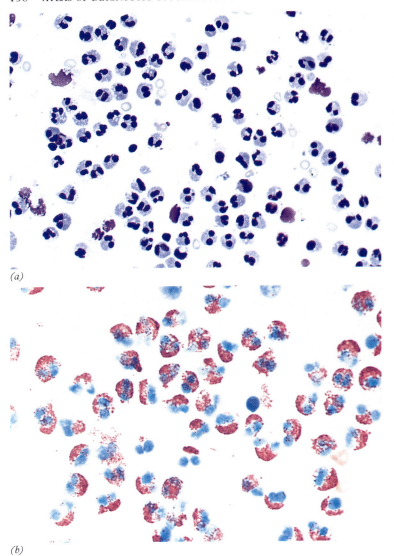

(a)

(b)

Fig. 4.16 Eosinophilic pleural effusion

(a) MGG ×580 (b) Hansel's stain

Eosinophils in the pleural effusion usually signify exposure of the pleura to air; repeated tap and pneumothorax are the commonest. Occasionally, eosinophils are found in young men suffering from idiopathic eosinophilic pleurisy. Other causes are hypersensitivity states, as in the cases illustrated. Case (a) was a drug reaction and (b) a young male with a history of asthma.

If left overnight, fluid with many eosinophils will develop Charcot–Leyden crystals.

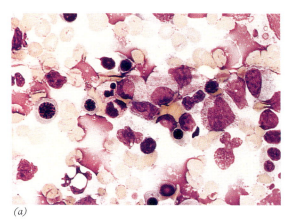

(a)

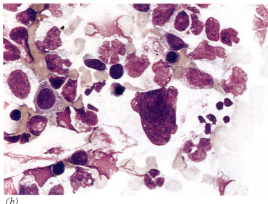

(b)

Fig. 4.17 Myeloid metaplasia

MGG ×525; ascitic fluid (a) normoblasts; myelocyte
(b) megakaryocyte nucleus

A very occasional early neutrophil granulocyte may be present in some effusions, but they and immature blood cells in appreciable numbers are more likely to be present in effusions associated with leukoerythroblastic anaemia. The case illustrated is of a male patient with chronic myelofibrosis, hepatosplenomegaly and ascites. Extramedullary haematopoiesis is an integral part of chronic myelofibrosis. The ascitic fluid (a) contained large numbers of normoblasts in different stages of maturation, a fair number of finely granular myelocytes (a) and one free convoluted megakaryocyte nucleus (b).

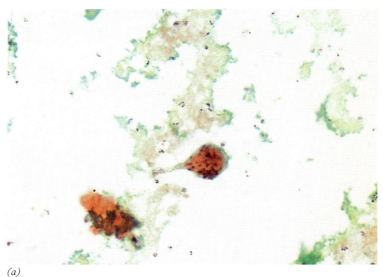

(a)

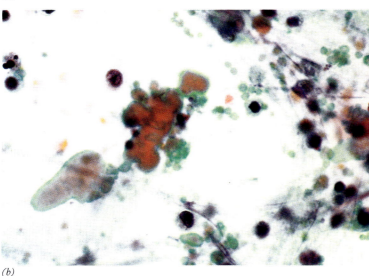

(b)

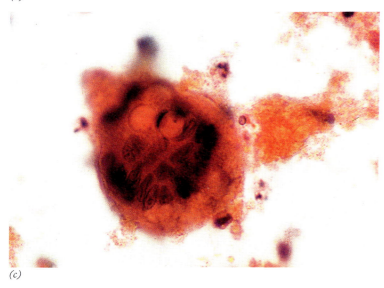

(c)

Inflammatory disease

Fig. 4.18 Rheumatoid effusion

Papanicolaou (a) ×183: pleural fluid (b) ×720; another case (c) ×720: pleural fluid; same case as (a) (d) ×720: pleural fluid; same case as (a) and (c) (e) MGG ×1740: pleural fluid; another case (f) ×720: pleural fluid; same case as (e)

The pulmonary manifestations of rheumatoid disease, a systemic disorder of probable immunological aetiology, include lung nodules and pleuritis, both of which may precede the onset of joint symptoms. The rheumatoid nodule is formed by an initial proliferation of mesenchymal cells, followed by a fibrinoid change in the collagen, which is loosened into simpler products consisting of mucopolysaccharides and glycoproteins; these form the core of the necrobiotic nodule. The cheesy centre is surrounded by a palisade of histiocytic spindle cells and occasional giant cells. This layer is in turn surrounded by fibroblasts, lymphocytes and plasma cells. The rheumatoid lesions of the pleura may be nodular or linear, and may be associated with a serous effusion.

A rheumatoid effusion is an exudate with a low glucose content (1.65 mmol/l, 30 mg%) and high lactic dehydrogenase values. It is usually small and unilateral and may be persistent or recurrent. The cytological appearance may be non-specific, the fluid being predominantly lymphocytic or with an excess of plasma cells, or it may resemble pus.

A rheumatoid nodule occasionally calcifies, and calcium may be seen in the serous fluid. Cholesterol crystals may be formed in an unabsorbed effusion. Often enough, the several components of a rheumatoid nodule are released into the fluid to produce a virtually pathognomonic picture.

A typical rheumatoid effusion contains amorphous debris, epithelioid macrophages and leukocytes. The debris is usually abundant and dominates the picture. Its colour is variable in a Papanicolaou-stained smear. It may be basophilic (a, c) or eosinophilic (d) and may coalesce into large irregular masses which are orange with green edges (b). Consisting as it does of mucopolysaccharides and glycoproteins, it is positive with Alcian blue and PAS after digestion with diastase (see Fig. 12.9c, d).

The epithelioid cells are variable in number, size and shape. The tailed tadpole (a) or fish-shaped (c) epithelioid cell is distinctive to a rheumatoid effusion. It may be small and mononuclear, but usually has more than one nucleus and is often large and multinucleated. Its staining reaction may be similar to that of the orange and green aggregates of debris (a, c). Elongated forms are seldom numerous; generally a greater number of round multinucleated giant forms (d–f) occur. These often contain several well-circumscribed vacuoles (d, e). Fragments of tissue consisting of spindle-shaped fibroblasts intermingled with small and large multinucleated epithelioid cells (f) may be shed into the effusion. The leukocytic infiltrate varies from case to case. In some cases, the majority of leukocytes are polymorphonuclear neutrophils. Most of these show a shift to the right and have four or five lobed nuclei (a, c) which disintegrate into small pyknotic fragments of chromatin (a, c). In other cases, degenerating lymphocytes are more abundant (b, e).

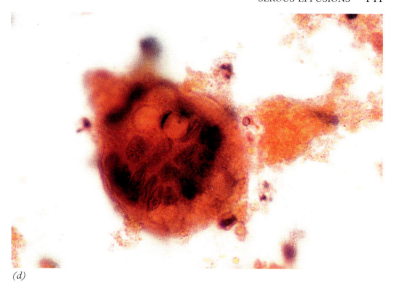

(d)

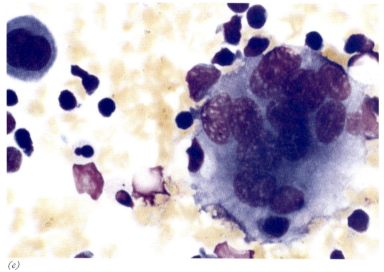

(e)

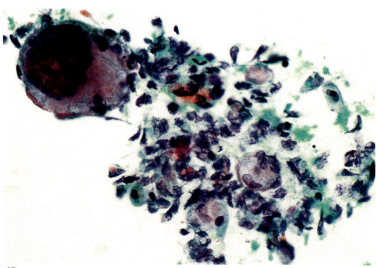

(f)

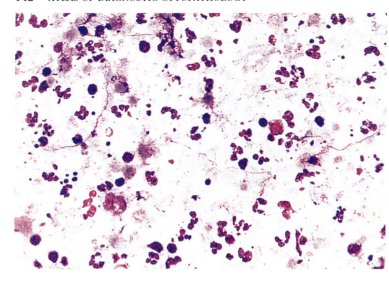

Fig. 4.19 Tuberculous empyema

MGG ×183: pleural fluid

A tuberculous effusion, as described earlier, is characterized by a preponderance of lymphocytes; neutrophils are few in number. With the onset of tuberculous empyema, this ratio is reversed. Degenerate neutrophils showing pyknotic degeneration and frank pus cells dominate the picture. A few macrophages and lymphocytes usually persist.

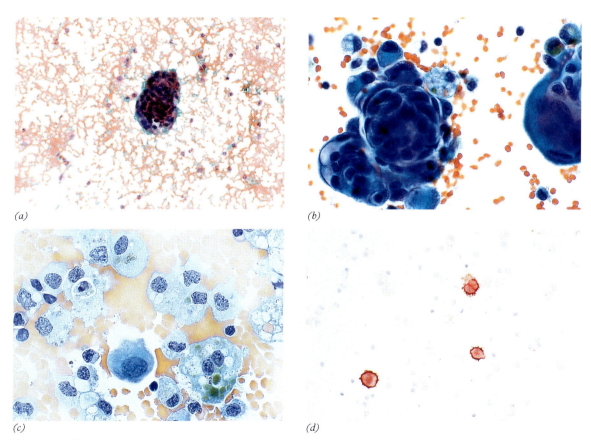

(a)   *(b)*

(c)   *(d)*

Fig. 4.20 Endometriosis of the pleura

(a) Papanicolaou ×840 (b) ×1260 (c) ×1260 (d) BerEP4 APAAP ×1260

This is a case of a young woman with recurrent, cyclical bilateral pleural effusions. She had known pelvic endometriosis. Pleural effusions taken on numerous occasions showed three-dimensional clusters of cells, suggesting epithelium (a). On higher magnification these were forming cell balls. Individual cells were difficult to distinguish from mesothelium; macrophages showed extensive haemosiderin deposition (c). Epithelial markers were repeatedly positive in single cells (d). Biopsy of the pleura was negative. No primary malignant tumour was found. The patient was discharged with a presumed diagnosis of pleural endometriosis.

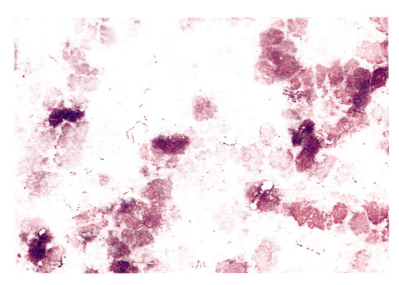

Fig. 4.21 Streptococcal empyema

MGG ×720: pleural fluid

Entry of pyogenic organisms into a serous effusion effects a dramatic change in its appearance and cellular composition. The fluid becomes turbid and may be quite thick. Mesothelial cells quickly disappear. The predominant cell is the pus cell; this is an extremely degenerate neutrophil which has an indistinct cell border and a pale, blurred, virtually amorphous nucleus. It disintegrates easily and the background of a smear of an empyema is covered with cellular and proteinaceous debris. The pathogenic organism may not always be evident. This empyema was due to a haemolytic streptococcus. Short chains of cocci are seen in this field.

METASTATIC TUMOURS

Carcinoma

The commonest cause of a malignant effusion is metastatic adenocarcinoma. This is as might he expected since the majority of human cancers are adenocarcinomas of one sort or another. In cytological smears as in small histological biopsies, there are a few appearances of individual cells, cell formations or distinctive secretory products which can pinpoint the primary. The increasing availability of monoclonal antibodies and application of immunocytochemical methods have extended the scope for a more precise definition of the nature and likely source of a metastatic deposit. In most cases, the primary, whether currently present or in the past, is known and the cytopathologist's immediate concern is to determine whether the effusion does or does not contain malignant cells. This is no idle exercise as an effusion in a cancer patient may be a transudate due to external pressure on blood or lymphatic channels, or hypoproteinaemia of cancer-associated malnutrition or the effusion may be an exudate due to concomitant inflammatory disease.

Identification of tumour cells is usually obvious in 70–80% of malignant effusions and in a substantial proportion of cases is practically a 'spot diagnosis'. Cancer cells are often larger than mesothelial cells and generally display greater pleomorphism. The individual malignant nucleus, except in small-celled tumours, is again usually larger than the nucleus of a mesothelial cell and occupies a disproportionately greater area of the cell. Nucleoli, which are almost always present in mesothelial cells, are not of great significance unless they are exceptionally large. Some cancer cells have macronucleoli and in such cases, the nucleolar-nuclear ratio is valuable in the assessment of malignancy. Biochemical characteristics such as mucin secretion are of considerable diagnostic value if interpreted with care. Both benign hyperplastic and malignant mesothelial cells may synthesize hyaluronic acid, which reacts positively with acid mucin stains such as Alcian blue. Hyaluronic acid is digested by the enzyme hyaluronidase, but not diastase. Mast cells have Alcian blue-positive granules (see Fig. 4.15b).

A useful exercise in a diagnostically difficult case is to compare the morphological features of the suspected malignant cells with typical mesothelial and similar cells. If intermediate forms can be traced, it is safer to assume that all the cells are of mesothelial origin. If, on the other hand, two distinct cell populations are clearly identifiable, it is reasonable to consider that one is native to the serous cavity and the other alien, i.e. metastatic.

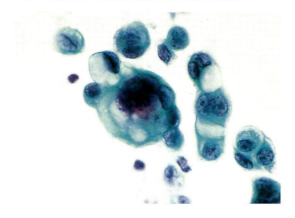

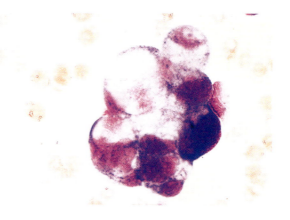

Fig. 4.22 Adenocarcinoma of lung

Papanicolaou ×525: pleural fluid

This micrograph illustrates malignant cells which are identifiable as adenocarcinoma cells, but are non-contributory as to the source of the primary. The tumour cells are larger than the degenerate histiocytoid mesothelial cells in size, the number of nuclei per cell and the nuclear-cytoplasmic ratio. Nucleoli are not remarkable. The cell type is recognized by the presence of clearly bordered mucous vacuoles within some of the tumour cells. The two small cells are lymphocytes.

Fig. 4.23 Adenocarcinoma of lung

MGG ×525: pericardial fluid

A typical example of an adenocarcinoma cluster is shown.

The large cells are aggregated into a three-dimensional cluster with a smooth, scalloped outline. Some cells have virtually no cytoplasm; others are distended with mucin, have peripheral nuclei and have assumed signet-ring forms.

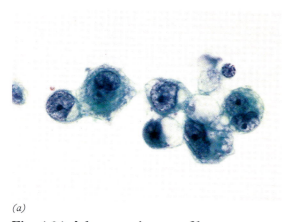

(a)

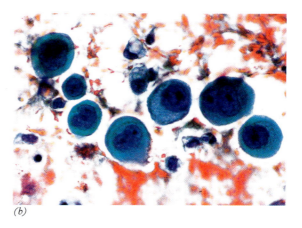

(b)

Fig. 4.24 Adenocarcinoma of lung

Papanicolaou ×525: (a) pleural fluid (b) pericardial fluid

In another example of a mucin-secreting adenocarcinoma of lung, the nuclei are large and variable in size. The cytoplasm is foamy (a). A few intracytoplasmic vacuoles are circumscribed and have the appearance of mucus droplets; most are hazy and are probably hydropic (a). The cells in the pericardial fluid are better preserved, and have a

different appearance. The cell margins are well-defined and the cytoplasm is deeply basophilic. One cell in the centre contains a cobweb of fine vacuoles which may be secretory or may have contained lipid. A few macrophages and leukocytes and many red blood cells are seen in the background.

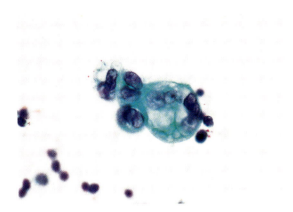

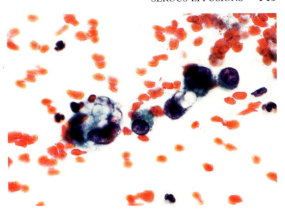

Fig. 4.25 Adenocarcinoma of pancreas

Papanicolaou ×525: ascitic fluid

A group of adenocarcinoma cells from a mucus-secreting carcinoma of pancreas are illustrated. The nuclei are extremely hypochromic and have crenated outlines; both features indicate degenerative changes. The variation in cell size and the arrangement of the cells which contain mucin vacuoles are similar to that seen in Figure 4.23.

Fig. 4.26 Adenocarcinoma of breast

Papanicolaou ×525: pleural fluid

Breast carcinoma is one of the commonest causes of a metastatic malignant effusion. The cells from this case show all the stigmata of malignancy and two cells have vacuolated cytoplasm. They fulfil the cytological criteria of adenocarcinoma cells, but their appearance is not specific to any one organ.

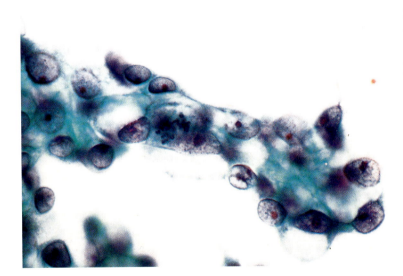

Fig. 4.27 Mucinous cystadenocarcinoma of ovary

Papanicolaou ×720: ascitic fluid

This is another example of an adenocarcinoma which is immediately recognizable as such but is uninformative as to the source of the primary. The ballooning of the cells at the right upper border of the sheet appears to be of a hydropic nature; the sharply bordered vacuole at the lower border is a mucous vacuole. Note that, while all the nuclei are hypochromic, several contain finely stippled chromatin and are not degenerate. One mitotic figure is seen in the centre of the field.

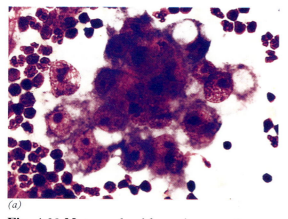

(a)

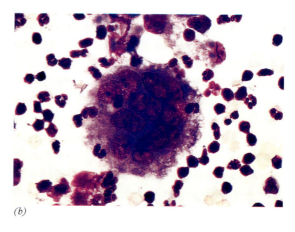

(b)

Fig. 4.28 Mesonephroid carcinoma of ovary

MGG ×525 (a) pleural fluid (b) same smear; another field

The pleural fluid of a woman with a history of mesonephroid carcinoma of ovary contained large adenocarcinoma cells and a few multinucleated carcinoma cells. The feature of note in the obviously malignant cells in (a) is the size of the nucleoli. These are larger than any nucleoli likely to occur in mesothelial cells. Despite the large size of each nucleus, the nucleolar-nuclear ratio in these epithelial cells is abnormal enough to be diagnostic of malignancy. Compare the giant multinucleated malignant cell (b) with the multinucleated mesothelial cell in Figure 4.4; note the difference between the granular chromatin of the malignant nuclei and the evenly reticulated chromatin of the mesothelial cell nuclei.

The nucleoli are similar in both cells.

The peg-like cells which constitute the second cell type in a mesonephroma (see Fig. 3.87) were not evident in this case. The diagnosis of metastatic ovarian carcinoma was based therefore not on the cellular appearance but on clinical assessment. An ovarian tumour may be associated with a pleural effusion in the initial absence of ascites. In the syndrome first described by Meig and named after him, the ovarian tumour was a fibroma and the pleural effusion was benign. The condition in which a malignant ovarian tumour metastasizes to the pleural cavity is sometimes referred to as pseudo-Meig's syndrome.

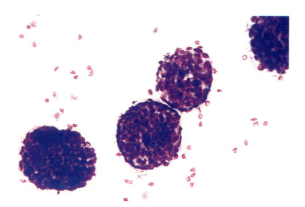

Fig. 4.29 Adenocarcinoma of breast

MGG ×133: pleural fluid

One of the few appearances seen in an effusion which is virtually diagnostic of the causative primary is produced by the type of breast carcinoma that used to be referred to as spheroidal cell carcinoma. The individual tumour cell has less cytoplasm than a mesothelial cell, a similar-sized nucleus and a greater nuclear-cytoplasmic ratio. Single forms are sparse and the typical picture is produced by numerous clusters of hundreds of tightly packed monomorphic cells. The size and shape of the clusters can vary, but the majority are large and spherical.

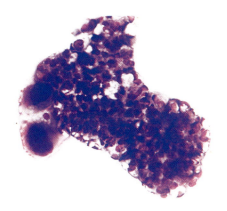

Fig. 4.30 Papillary cystadenocarcinoma of ovary

MGG ×133: ascitic fluid

It is by no means uncommon for a papillary carcinoma of ovary to shed fragments of tissue into an effusion, which acquires a granular turbidity. Microscopically, the fine granules which may be visible to the naked eye are seen as cell aggregates which may be large enough to cover and extend beyond a low-power field. These aggregates differ from the clumps of breast carcinoma cells illustrated in the preceding micrograph in several respects. Individual cells have more cytoplasm which is visible at the edge of the cluster and which results in greater separation of the nuclei. Some cells are finely vacuolated. Fairly often, substantially larger cells with one or several nuclei are seen in juxtaposition to the smaller cells and there may be some clumps composed predominantly of larger cells. The presence of smaller cells and significantly larger cells in an effusion from a female patient is most often seen in cases of ovarian carcinoma. The appearance is therefore suggestive of an ovarian primary but is not diagnostic, as other tumours including the occasional breast carcinoma show a similar pattern (see Fig. 2.29).

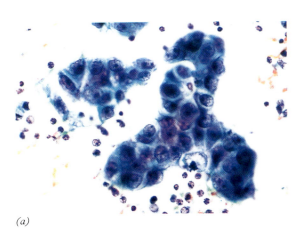

(a)

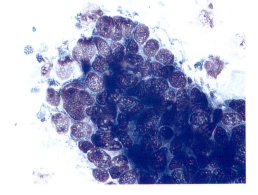

(b)

Fig. 4.31 Papillary adenocarcinoma of gallbladder

(a) Papanicolaou ×333: ascitic fluid (b) MGG ×1260: ascites

A papillary tumour, by definition, forms frond-like projections, each of which has a slender fibrous stalk covered with layers of tumour cells. A true papilla with a central fibrovascular core may be recovered in a needle aspiration but is seldom exfoliated. A papillary tumour may, however, be identified in some cases by a cellular presentation, which suggests that the cells have been shed from the tip of an outgrowth with a free surface. The cells

appear in aggregates which may branch to form finger-like processes. The luminal border has an orderly configuration, the surface cells are palisade and the distal nuclear borders are roughly equidistant from the free edge of the cell aggregate. A papillary carcinoma in this respect shows a cell arrangement which is usually more characteristic of benign glandular cells.

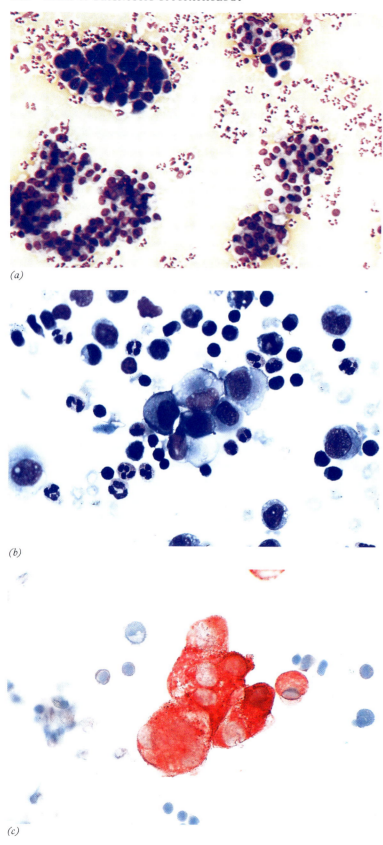

(a)

(b)

(c)

Fig. 4.32 Papillary adenocarcinoma of pancreas

(a) MGG ×183 (b) ×1740 (c) APAAP AUA1: ascites

The non specific appearance of papillary clusters (a) and small bland-looking cells may be misleading. Immunocytochemistry staining for epithelial markers proves the cells to be of epithelial rather than mesothelial origin (c) and confirms metastatic carcinoma.

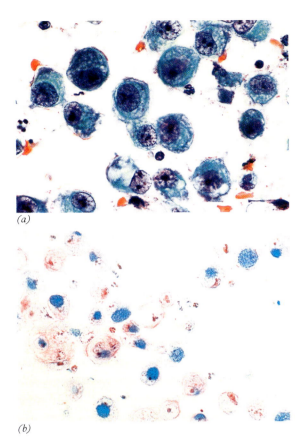

(a)

(b)

Fig. 4.33 Adenocarcinoma of stomach

(a) Papanicolaou ×525: ascitic fluid (b) Alcian blue ×333: same specimen; another smear

Biochemical activity of adenocarcinoma cells may be easily ascertained by the use of special stains. The metastatic stomach carcinoma cells in this micrograph have abundant foamy cytoplasm with the appearance of a large-meshed sieve. Numerous mucin droplets are demonstrated with Alcian blue; some form compact rounded masses, others are more diffusely stained.

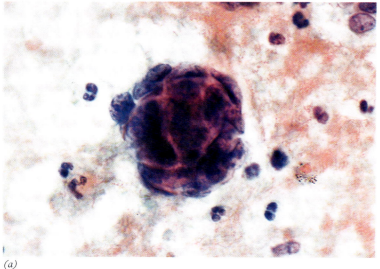

(a)

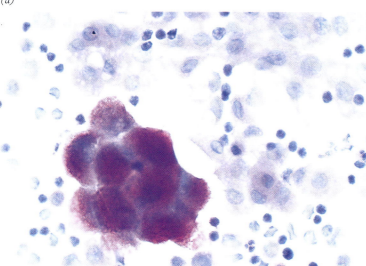

(b)

Fig. 4.34 Adenocarcinoma of colon

(a) Papanicolaou ×720 (b) PAS diastase ×1740

In a very poorly differentiated adenocarcinoma, loss of distinguishing morphological features may be accompanied by loss of function. This micrograph illustrates an example of a poorly differentiated, mucin-depleted carcinoma of colon. The cells are packed together in a tight cluster. The spherical arrangement is suggestive of glandular origin but the scant cytoplasm lacks any morphological or functional feature that may identify the cell type. The malignant nature of the cells is indicated by the nuclei, which practically fill the cells, are variable in size and have disorganized chromatin patterns (a).

PAS diastase stain shows the presence of mucin within the cells, thus confirming their epithelial origin (b).

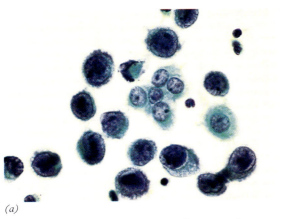

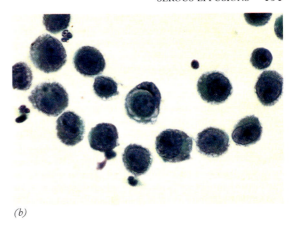

(a)   *(b)*

Fig. 4.35 Adenocarcinoma of stomach

Papanicolaou ×525: (a) ascitic fluid (b) same smear; another field

Reduced cohesiveness is one of the more notable characteristics of malignant cells. In some cases, this is so marked that the malignant effusion contains mainly dissociated cells. The carcinoma cells need to be distinguished from mesothelial cells and from high-grade lymphoma cells.

    Micrograph (a) shows malignant cells from a carcinoma of stomach, one discrete mesothelial cell (opposite 3 o'clock) and a group of five cohesive mesothelial cells in the centre of the field. The two cell types are roughly the same size. The significant differences between the malignant and benign cells are seen in the nuclei. The malignant nuclei are larger, variable and have hyperchromatic chromatin clumps which are irregular in size and distribution. The cell-within-a-cell formation (b), referred to as a bird's-eye appearance, may be seen in a variety of tumours and in some benign cells.

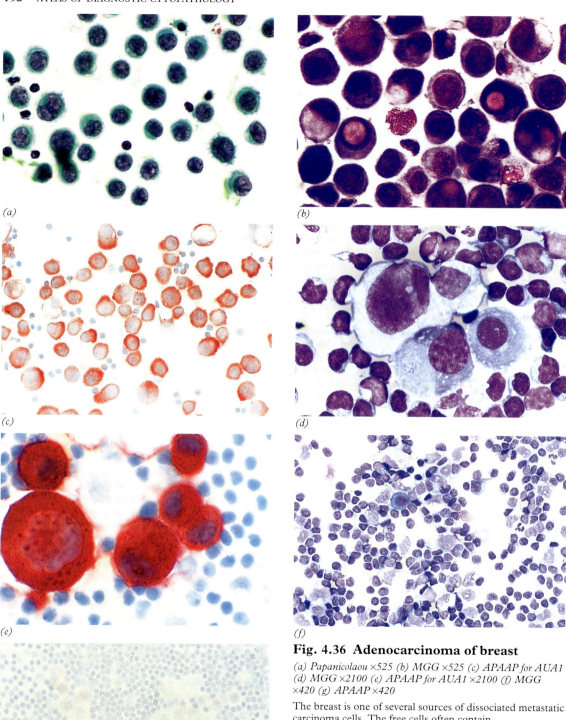

Fig. 4.36 Adenocarcinoma of breast

(a) Papanicolaou ×525 (b) MGG ×525 (c) APAAP for AUA1
(d) MGG ×2100 (e) APAAP for AUA1 ×2100 (f) MGG
×420 (g) APAAP ×420

The breast is one of several sources of dissociated metastatic carcinoma cells. The free cells often contain intracytoplasmic vacuoles (a, b). Immunocytochemistry for epithelial markers helps in establishing their epithelial origin (c, e, g). This is particularly important in lymphocytic effusions with single cells intermixed with inflammatory cells (f). These are highlighted by the special stains (g).

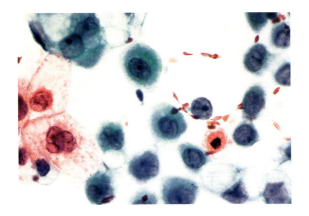

Fig. 4.37 Serous cystadenocarcinoma of ovary

Papanicolaou ×525: ascitic fluid

Another source of cells which either float free or form loose connections is a serous cystadenocarcinoma of the ovary. The cells with this type of presentation closely resemble mesothelial cells in size, shape and staining reaction. All epithelial tumours of the ovary are considered to arise from its serosal covering. Recognition of malignancy may be difficult on occasion; as a rule, the nuclei of the tumour cells are larger and more pleomorphic and the nuclear-cytoplasmic ratio is fairly high. Two additional features which are sometimes met with in a malignant effusion due to a serous cystadenocarcinoma of ovarian origin are seen in this micrograph. A few cells contain mucin vacuoles. A serous tumour of ovary can be heterogeneous and may contain foci of mucous differentiation. The other feature to note is the anomalous eosinophilia of some tumour cells. This is occasionally seen in degenerating cells, benign or malignant, and does not indicate squamous differentiation.

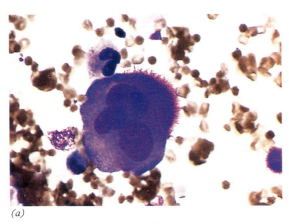

(a)

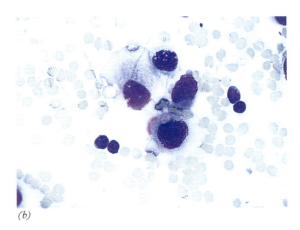

(b)

Fig. 4.38 Serous cystadenocarcinoma

(a) MGG ×525: ascitic fluid (b) ×1260: pleural fluid

Free-floating tumour cells may occasionally have a covering of microvilli. These are generally uneven in length and considerably longer than the microvilli of benign mesothelial cells. The hair-like pseudocilia are usually present at one pole of the cell, but may entirely cover the cell. They may be seen in breast or gastric carcinomas, but are most frequently encountered in serous tumours of the ovary. They are difficult to see in Papanicolaou-stained smears, but are clearly visible in MGG-stained smears.

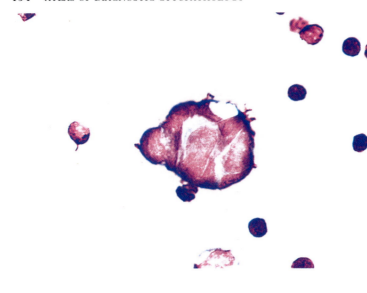

Fig. 4.39 Small cell carcinoma (SCC) of lung

MGG ×720: pleural fluid

The air-dried Romanowsky method of preparation is of particular value in the identification of SCC of lung metastatic to an effusion. The cells form a flat monolayer. The nuclei have a homogeneous, almost smudged appearance and stain a uniform shade of purple, appreciably paler than the accompanying lymphocytes. Adjacent nuclei are separated by a linear cleft which, unlike that in alcohol-fixed smear, is seldom crescentic in shape.

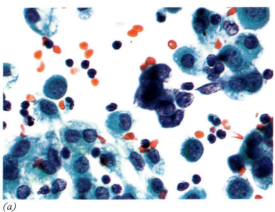

(a)

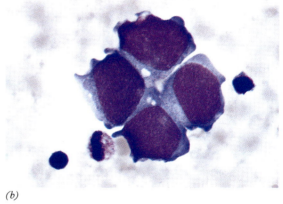

(b)

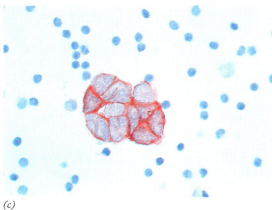

(c)

Fig. 4.40 Small cell carcinoma of lung

(a) Papanicolaou ×525: pleural fluid (b) MGG ×2100 (c) AUAI: pleural fluid

Correct typing of SCC cells and distinction from a poorly differentiated adenocarcinoma may be difficult in a wet-fixed smear (a). Oat cells are said to be a little larger than lymphocytes. The comparison is based on appearances seen in sections. In an effusion, the individual oat cell appears substantially larger and approximates more closely to the mesothelial cell in size. The crescentic line of separation between moulded nuclei may be wider, the cytoplasm more abundant and lacy than in bronchial secretions.

The same cells appear even larger when air-dried (b). Compare the size of oat cell to lymphocytes—it is 8–10 times larger. Immunocytochemistry for epithelial antigens confirms the diagnosis of metastatic carcinoma (c). (See Chapter 3, Fig. 3.53a, b).

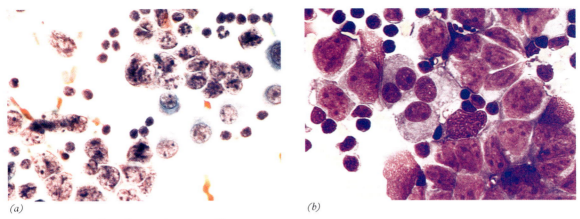

(a)   *(b)*

Fig. 4.41 Small cell carcinoma of lung

(a) Papanicolaou ×525: pleural fluid (b) MGG ×525: same specimen; another smear

The relatively greater size of the metastatic SCC cell in a fluid is even more evident when the tumour is composed of cells at the larger end of the spectrum. In this example (a), the neoplastic cells are moderately pleomorphic and several are larger than mesothelial cells. The nuclear moulding seen here is not usually remarkable in a Papanicolaou-stained fluid.

This specimen was unusual in as much as it contained a great number of carcinoma cells in large aggregates and was partially air-dried.

The features seen in the alcohol-fixed smear are greatly enhanced by air-drying (b). Note the multiple conspicuous nucleoli and the large size of the malignant nuclei.

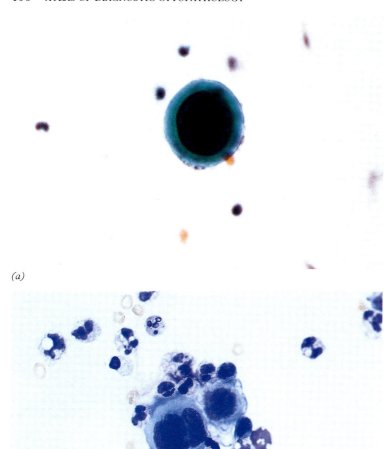

(a)

Fig. 4.42 Malignant squamous cells in fluids

(a) Papanicolaou ×720: pleural fluid (original) (b) MGG ×1740: ascites (c) MGG ×2900: pleural fluid

Malignant squamous cells are not often seen in serous effusions, even from a lung primary. When present, they usually show two features. First, they are rarely keratinized, even when the primary carcinoma is well-differentiated. Second, they appear as single forms or, at most, in very small groups. With the Papanicolaou stain, the cytoplasm is usually basophilic and opaque but may have a paler periphery. The nucleus is hyperchromic and the chromatin coarse (a).

Despite the cytoplasm acquiring a rounded shape, the nuclei of squamous cell carcinoma are irregularly shaped and angular (b). Chromatin is coarse (c).

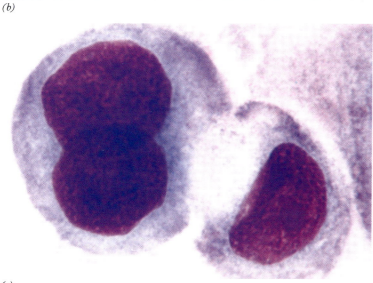

(b)

(c)

Fig. 4.43 Squamous cell carcinoma of lung

MGG ×720: pleural fluid

A cell-within-a-cell formation is shown in this micrograph. The cell is recognized as being of squamous origin by its cytoplasm. In an MGG-stained smear, cytoplasm with some keratin appears colourless or pale blue. The coarse chromatin of the malignant squamous cell is usually arranged in criss-crossing strands.

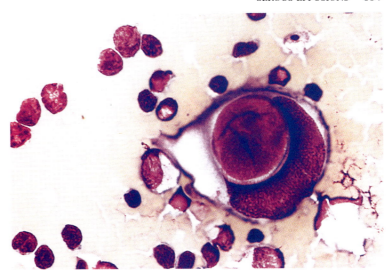

Fig. 4.44 Transitional cell carcinoma

MGG ×720: ascitic fluid

This micrograph shows a large multinucleated malignant cell with copious amphophilic cytoplasm, coarsely stranded chromatin and prominent nucleoli. The appearance was considered to be suggestive of a squamous origin. The cell was present in the ascitic fluid of a patient with a history of transitional cell carcinoma of the prostatic urethra. There was no evidence of another primary and the cell is assumed to be urothelial in type.

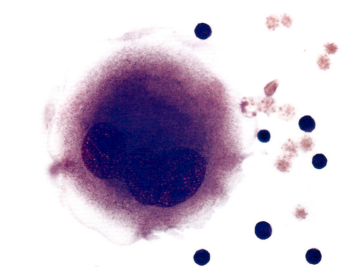

Sarcoma

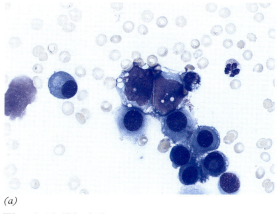

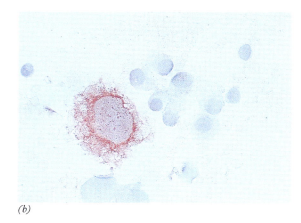

(a)   *(b)*

Fig. 4.45 Rhabdomyosarcoma

(a) MGG ×1260: pleural fluid (b) APAAP for antidesmin ×1260; same case

Effusions caused by metastases of mesenchymal tumours do not differ greatly from those in other malignancies. Cells are usually more pleomorphic than in carcinomas and often are single, with a rounded appearance. Nuclei are frequently large and pleomorphic. A history of sarcoma elsewhere and immunocytochemistry help to confirm the tumour type. The case illustrated is that of a rhabdomyosarcoma with pleural metastases (a). Antidesmin antibody is positive, confirming muscle differentiation of the cell (b).

LYMPHOPROLIFERATIVE AND MYELOPROLIFERATIVE DISORDERS

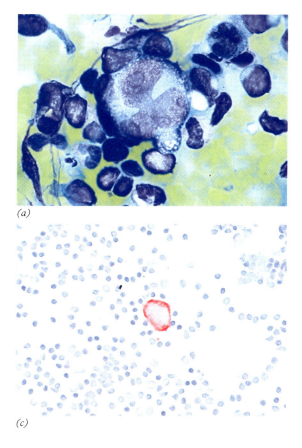

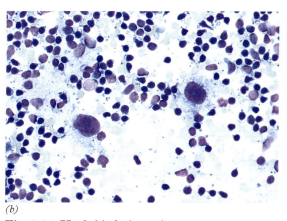

(a)   *(b)*

Fig 4.46 Hodgkin's lymphoma

(a) MGG ×2100 (b) ×840 (c) APAAP CD30: pleural fluid

Effusions in cases of Hodgkin's lymphoma are usually lymphocytic with admixture of macrophages and eosinophils. In order to diagnose Hodgkin's disease in fluid it is essential to find Reed–Sternberg cells. They have features similar to those in the lymph node, polylobated nucleus and prominent nucleoli with a dense nucleolar rim (a, b). Immunocytochemistry (CD5 and CD30) positivity in the appropriate cells confirms the diagnosis (c).

(c)

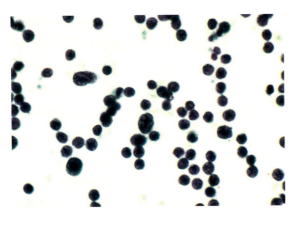

Fig. 4.47 Sézary's syndrome

Papanicolaou ×525: ascitic fluid

The neoplastic cell of Sézary's syndrome, a leukaemic variant of mycosis fungoides, is a malignant T lymphocyte with little cytoplasm and an irregular nucleus characterized by deep convolutions reminiscent of the cerebrum, hence it is referred to as a cerebriform cell. Three typical Sézary cells accompanied by small lymphocytes are illustrated in the ascitic fluid of a man who presented with ascites, lymphadenopathy and erythrodermal lesions which started on the abdominal wall and gradually spread. A few abnormal T cells were noted in the peripheral blood at this stage. The disease progressed with the development of a T-cell leukaemia blood picture.

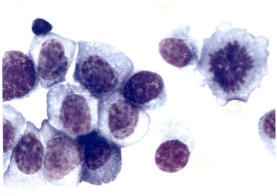

(a)

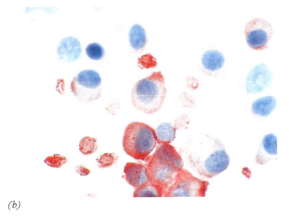

(b)

Fig 4.48 Plasmablastic plasmocytoma

(a) MGG ×2100 (b) APAAP CD45: ascites

These cells originate from the ascitic fluid of a patient with extramedullary plasmacytoma which spread into peritoneal cavity. Cells (a) are large with eccentric nuclei and prominent nucleoli. Some resemble mature plasma cells,

some are blastic and others in mitosis. CD45 staining, usually negative in mature plasma cells, stains the immature plasma cells (b).

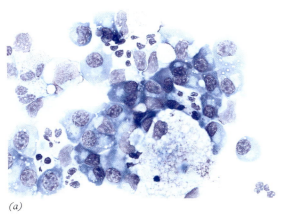

(a)

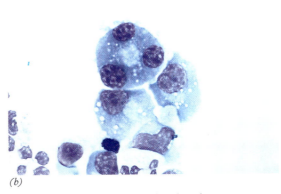

(b)

Fig. 4.49 Low-grade lymphoma of mucosa-associated lymphoid tissue in the thymus

(a) MGG ×1260 (b) ×1260 FNA of the mediastinum

Aspiration of the mediastinum yielded fluid in which, in addition to macrophages and some lymphoid cells, many plasma cells were seen (a, b). The patient was young and, although serum immunoglobulins showed an abnormal pattern, the morphology of plasma cells was normal.

Castleman's disease was suspected on cytological material. After the excision of mediastinal mass, a low-grade lymphoma of mucosa-associated lymphoid tissue, most probably originating in the thymus, was diagnosed.

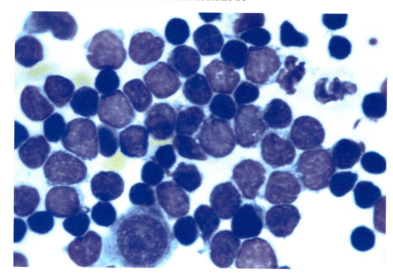

Fig. 4.50 Malignant lymphoma: centrocytic

(a) MGG ×1740: pleural fluid

Medium-sized lymphoid cells dominate the picture. The patient had a history of centrocytic lymphoma so that pleural disease influenced the staging. Care is necessary in grading lymphomas in fluids. Cells often appear larger and more pleomorphic so that there is a temptation to call most lymphomas high-grade.

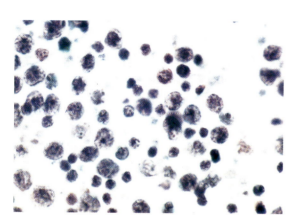

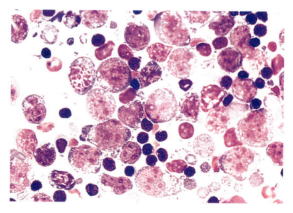

Fig. 4.51 Malignant lymphoma: centroblastic–centrocytic

Papanicolaou ×525: peritoneal dialysis fluid

This micrograph illustrates a typical cellular presentation of a centroblastic–centrocytic lymphoma in a fluid specimen. The fluid contains a virtually pure culture of discrete neoplastic cells; several have nuclear clefts characteristic of follicle centre cells. A continuous spectrum of size from small lymphocyte to large blast forms is seen. Nucleoli are evident in the larger blast cells and are small and inconspicuous in the smaller cells. The diagnosis of centroblastic–centrocytic malignant lymphoma was initially made by cytological examination of peritoneal dialysis fluid, which the patient wisely brought in for examination, as it was milky in colour. Lymph node histology confirmed the diagnosis and demonstrated a follicular pattern.

Fig. 4.52 Malignant lymphoma: centroblastic

MGG ×525: pleural fluid

Centroblastic lymphoma cells are large and, like all marrow-derived cells, are discrete. Their cytoplasm is basophilic, and usually moderately pyroninophilic. It often contains immunoglobulins which are PAS-positive. The nuclei are usually round, although a small dent may be seen in a few. Each nucleus contains several prominent nucleoli of varying sizes; some nucleoli are closely apposed to the nuclear membrane. Note that this specimen contains two distinct cell populations: malignant blast cells and benign mature lymphocytes. Compare this appearance with the centroblastic–centrocytic lymphoma (Fig. 4.51) in which all stages of transition from lymphocyte-like to lymphoblast can be appreciated.

A centroblast with an intensely pyroninophilic cytoplasm and a single large central nucleolus is known as an immunoblast.

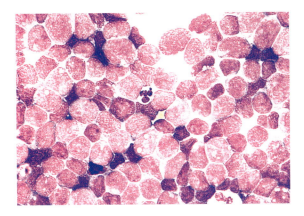

Fig. 4.53 T-cell acute lymphoblastic leukaemia

MGG ×525: pericardial fluid

The blast cells in the pericardial fluid of a 13-year-old girl are medium-sized and moderately monomorphic. The cytoplasm is agranular; the nuclei almost fill the cells and do not show indentation and convolutions; one or two nucleoli are present but are inconspicuous. The cells are similar in size to myeloblasts with which they may be confused; neither can they be distinguished from centroblasts. The T-cell origin of the primitive blast cells was established by appropriate immunocytochemical and histochemical studies.

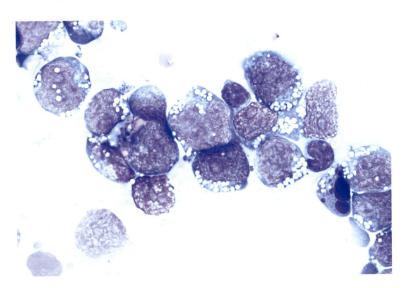

Fig. 4.54 Malignant lymphoma: lymphoblastic, Burkitt like

MGG ×1740: ascites

Ascitic fluid abounds with immature lymphoid cells with nuclear characteristics of blast cells. Cytoplasm has fine vacuolation. Primary disease was in the gastrointestinal tract and was histologically typed as non-Hodgkin's lymphoma, Burkitt like.

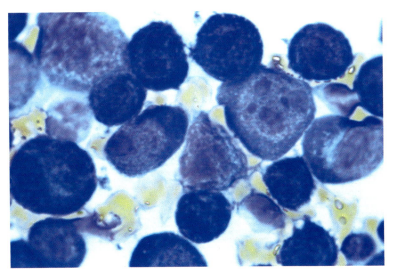

Fig. 4.55 Malignant lymphoma: immunoblastic

MGG ×2900

Immunoblastic lymphoma is not an unusual finding in the ascitic fluid of patients with lymphomas who are human immunodeficiency virus (HIV)-positive. Cells are large, have round eccentric nuclei, prominent single or multiple nucleoli and strikingly basophilic cytoplasm.

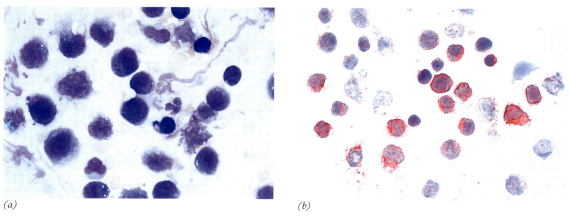

(a)   *(b)*

Fig. 4.56 Malignant lymphoma: HTLV I-associated T-cell lymphoma

(a) MGG ×1260 (b) APAAP for CD3: pericardial fluid

Large pleomorphic single cells which resemble both lymphoid cells and macrophages are indicative of high-grade lymphoma in the pericardial fluid of this HIV-positive patient (a). CD3 staining is patchy but confirms the majority of bizarre cells to be of T-cell origin (b).

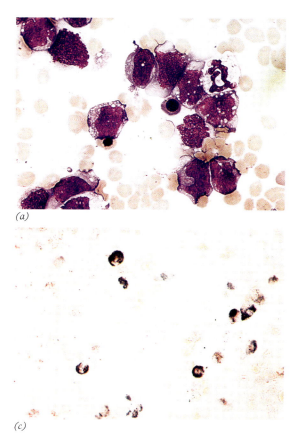

(a)

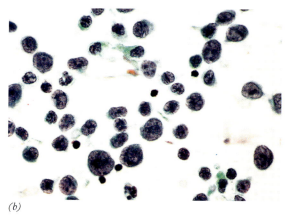

(b)

Fig. 4.57 Acute myeloid leukaemia

(a) MGG ×525: pleural fluid (b) Papanicolaou ×525: pleural fluid; another case (c) Sudan black B ×333: same specimen as (b); another smear

A large population or a pure content of leukaemic cells is seen in an effusion when the serous membrane is infiltrated. Two cases of pleural effusion associated with acute myeloid leukaemia are illustrated. The cells in (a) are large, but lack the basophilia of myeloblasts. The cytoplasm is more ample and in a few cells has a suggestion of fine granular stippling. Four to five nucleoli are discernible. The large cells have the appearance of promyelocytes. Several nuclei have irregular indentations found in cells referred to as parapromyelocytes. The two small acidophilic cells with condensed central nuclei are normoblasts. One degenerate polymorph is seen (upper right).

The primitive variable-sized cells in (b) appear smaller; this is in part due to wet fixation in alcohol. Little or no cytoplasm is evident and the nuclei are indented or grossly convoluted. The appearance is similar to that seen in high-grade T-cell lymphomas. The myeloid origin of the leukaemia cells was established by demonstrating Sudan black B-positive granules (c); these are not present in cells of lymphoid origin.

(c)

MESOTHELIOMA

A primary tumour of the mesothelial lining, known as mesothelioma, may be benign or malignant. The latter is induced by asbestos, usually of the crocidolite group.

A benign mesothelioma develops from the pleura as a localized mass, often pedunculated, and is typically of the fibrous type (fibroma of pleural origin); epithelial and mixed or biphasic forms are uncommon.
A malignant mesothelioma involves the visceral and parietal surfaces of the pleura, is usually diffuse and often encases the lung. The majority have a biphasic structure, although monomorphic forms also occur. The extremely rare peritoneal malignant mesothelioma is also associated with exposure to a cancer-inducing asbestos.

The diagnosis of malignant mesothelioma in a pleural effusion is a particularly difficult one. The fibrous component of the commonest biphasic variety is rarely exfoliated. Well-differentiated epithelial-type tumour cells may be difficult to distinguish from benign reactive mesothelial cells. The more obviously malignant forms often closely resemble metastatic adenocarcinoma cells. The problem is not necessarily resolved by the use of special staining techniques. Both types of cancer cells may be rich in glycogen which stains red with PAS. The presence of diastase-resistant PAS (D-PAS)-positive epithelial mucin distinguishes a mucin-secreting adenocarcinoma but a negative reaction does not discriminate between a mesothelioma and a non-secretory adenocarcinoma.

The use of immunocytochemistry, in particular epithelial markers, as illustrated in the paragraph on carcinomas in fluids, excludes the diagnosis of mesothelioma. As yet, there is not a reliable marker to discriminate between benign and malignant mesothelial cells.

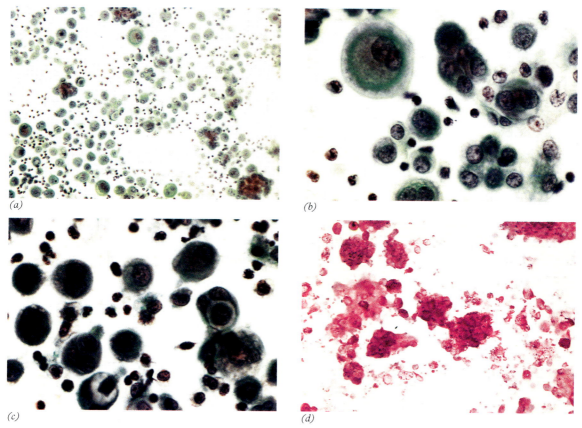

(a)

(b)

(c)

(d)

Fig. 4.58 Malignant mesothelioma

(a) Papanicolaou ×133: pleural fluid (b) ×525: same field (c) ×525: another part of same field (d) PAS ×133: same specimen; another smear

A pleural fluid from a case of malignant mesothelioma often contains abundant epithelial-type cells which occur singly, in small groups and in large mulberry-like clusters (a). The field in (b) shows leukocytes and large cells which clearly belong to one family. They display a wide range in size, and in the number of nuclei. The chromatin is finely stippled in some nuclei and coarsely granular in others. The nucleoli vary in size and some are prominent. Compare the tumour cells with benign mesothelial cells (Fig. 4.3). The similarities of shape and cytoplasmic features suggest a common origin. The two bird's-eye forms seen in (c) are rarely found in benign mesothelial cells. The malignant cells in this effusion contained much glycogen (d) and were negative with D-PAS and Alcian blue.

5. Cerebrospinal fluid

Cerebrospinal fluid (CSF) may be lumbar puncture fluid from the central canal of the spinal cord, fluid from the ventricles of the brain or occasionally from a shunt inserted to relieve hydrocephalus.

The colour and volume of the CSF should be noted and a cell count performed on lumbar CSF. A normal CSF contains up to five mature lymphocytes per cubic millimetre; the cell count is often raised in pathological conditions. Ventricular and shunt fluids may contain fragments of tissue and a cell count is seldom feasible. The cells are concentrated for study in a cytocentrifuge or membrane filter preparation and stained by the Papanicolaou or Romanowsky methods. In smears made from centrifuged deposit, the notch of the lymphocyte may be accentuated and the cell may appear histiocytoid.

Aspiration or imprint smears from the brain may be obtained at operation. The use of these specimens is usually confined to specialist units attached to neurosurgical units.

BENIGN CONDITIONS

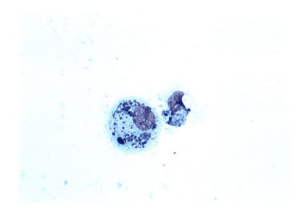

Fig. 5.1 Subarachnoid haemorrhage

MGG ×1260: lumbar puncture, 1-month-old baby

Haemosiderin-laden macrophages are a feature of the CSF in this 1-month-old baby. They originate from the subarachnoidal mesenchyme, measure 15–25 μm in diameter and show various stages of evolution of a macrophage. The presence of haemosiderin confirms subarachnoid haemorrhage of at least 5–6 days' duration.

Erythrophagocytosis is an earlier event occurring approximately 4 h after the haemorrhage and persisting for about 2 weeks. A transient increase in polymorphs can be noted due to meningeal irritation. This lasts 1 week approximately. Pigmentophages can be present in the fluid for more than 6 months.

Red blood cells frequently present in the CSF are usually due to the trauma of the needle rather than spontaneous subarachnoidal haemorrhage. In the presence of red blood cells, the type and quantity of other haemopoietic cells are less reliable.

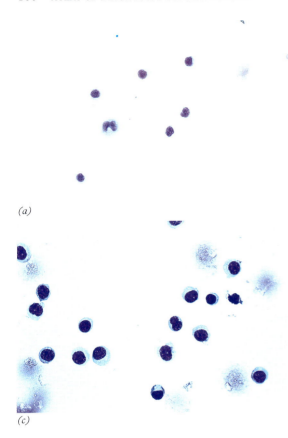

(a)

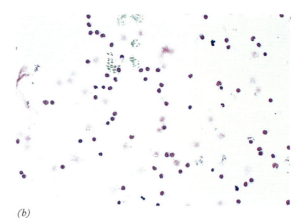

(b)

(c)

Fig. 5.2 Meningitis

(a) MGG ×840 (b) ×420 (c) ×1260: lumbar puncture CSF

A raised number of lymphocytes in the CSF can be due to meningitis or meningoencephalitis, most often without the causative agent being known. The number of lymphocytes is in excess of 30/mm³ and is usually between 100 and 1000/mm³ in viral meningitis. Cells are predominantly mononuclear with mature lymphocytes and some monocytes (a–c). Possible causative agents include polio, ECHO, coxsackie, arbovirus, mumps, myxovirus, Epstein-Barr virus, herpes zoster and others.

Polymorphs are absent from normal CSF. Their number is raised in cases of bacterial meningitis. Cell count varies between 3 and 12 000/mm³. Fluid is usually turbid, opaque or purulent. Common causative agents are meningococci, pneumococci, streptococci, staphylococci and *Haemophilus influenzae*.

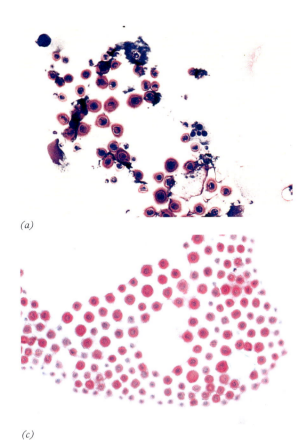

(a)

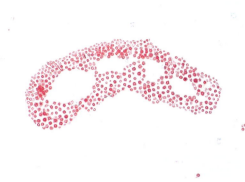

(b)

Fig. 5.3 Mycotic infections. *Cryptococcus neoformans*

(a) MGG ×525: HIV-positive patient (b) mucicarmine ×420 (c) ×1260

CSF of this immunocompromised patient contains numerous *Cryptococcus neoformans* organisms. Their capsule is refractile; they are rounded in shape, approximately the size of mononuclear cells. Capsule stains strongly with mucicarmine but organisms can be recognized on routine staining (c).

(c)

NEOPLASMS

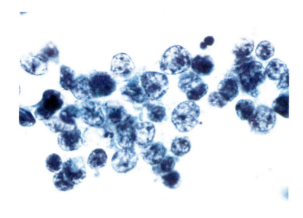

Fig. 5.4 Ependymoma

Papanicolaou ×832: lumbar CSF

The ventricles and the central spinal canal are lined by a single layer of specialized glial cells, referred to as ependymal cells. Tumours derived from these cells are known as ependymomas and constitute one variety of glial tumours or gliomas.

An ependymoma may develop in the brain or in the spinal column, the most common being a papillary tumour of the fourth ventricle. The tumours occur mainly in children and adolescents.

The tumour cells illustrated were recovered in great numbers from the lumbar CSF of a young boy several months after treatment of a histologically proven central ependymoma. The cells are small and have little cytoplasm. The nuclei are round, monomorphic and finely granular. The cells are loosely attached to each other and arranged around small spaces in a pseudoacinar manner.

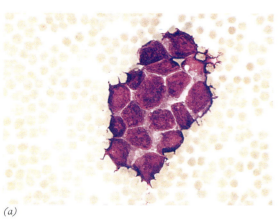
(a)

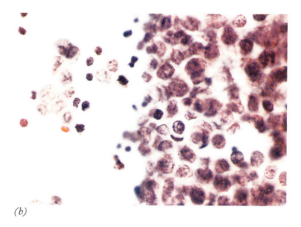
(b)

Fig. 5.5 Pinealoma

(a) MGG ×525: lumbar CSF (b) Papanicolaou ×525: lumbar CSF; another specimen from the same case

Another tumour of children, adolescents and young adults arises from the pineal gland (a specialized endocrine gland), the function of which is not fully understood. Histological variants include germinomas and teratomas. The case illustrated is the poorly differentiated small-celled variety and occurred in a young boy. Micrograph (a) illustrates a group of cohesive cells with variable-sized nuclei and little cytoplasm. Small multiple nucleoli are faintly discernible. Another specimen of fluid obtained some months after treatment contained similar cells (b). These appear smaller because they have been fixed in alcohol. The cell size approximates to that of lymphoblasts. The granularity of the nuclei is better appreciated in the Papanicolaou preparation.

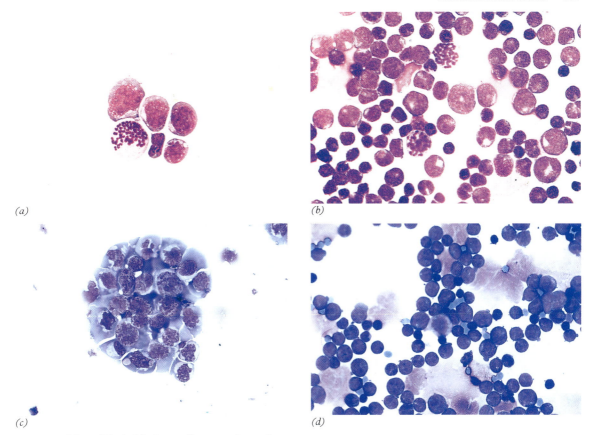

Fig. 5.6 Non-Hodgkin's malignant lymphoma

MGG ×525 Lumbar CSF (a) postnasal lyphoma (b) lymphoblastic lymphoma (c) MGG ×1260: immunoblastic lymphoma (d) ×1260: high-grade non-Hodgkin's lymphoma

Involvement of the central nervous system by disseminated lymphoma is not uncommon and CSF cytology is often performed as part of the initial staging and subsequent assessment procedures. Distinction between benign reactive lymphocytes and a low-grade lymphoma can be difficult; high-grade tumours are more easily identifiable and CSF cytology plays an important and generally, primary, role in establishing central involvement.

The cell count is always raised in these cases and may be very high. Two cases of high-grade lymphoma are illustrated in these micrographs. The cells in (a) are primitive and large.

Anisocytosis and anisonucleosis are marked. Multiple macronucleoli are seen in the top left nucleus; below it is an abnormal mitotic figure. A mixed population of small lymphocytes and poorly differentiated large lymphoma cells are seen in (b). Several of the large nuclei are convoluted. Note the two abnormal mitoses. Occasionally cells of high-grade lymphomas show marked convolutions, as in the case of B-cell immunoblastic lymphoma in a patient with acquired immunodeficiency syndrome (AIDS; c). The morphology of lymphoid blasts is otherwise similar to those elsewhere.

In cases in which the distinction between discrete carcinoma cells, lymphoma cells or tumour cells of glial origin is not clear, the problem may be resolved by immunocytochemical typing of the cells.

Fig. 5.7 Metastatic carcinoma

MGG ×720 (a) squamous cell carcinoma of the lung (b) adenocarcinoma of the breast (c) MGG ×1740 (d) ×1740: APAAP for epithelial marker (AUA1)

Metastatic disease of the central nervous system is said to be more common than primary tumours. The commonest source of secondary deposits is a bronchogenic carcinoma, the breast being the second most frequently encountered site. Lumbar CSF may contain numerous tumour cells when the meninges are involved (carcinomatous meningitis). Micrograph (a) illustrates poorly differentiated malignant squamous cells from a lung primary. Unlike glial tissue, the four cells seen are clearly demarcated from each other and appear to be of epithelial origin. Adenocarcinoma cells with smooth borders, high nuclear-cytoplasmic ratios and prominent nucleoli seen in (b) were recovered from the lumbar CSF of a woman with disseminated breast carcinoma. The cohesive cluster of large vacuolated carcinoma cells with eccentric nuclei are characteristic of a mucus-secreting adenocarcinoma (c). The patient presented with symptoms of a space-occupying lesion in the cranium and a diagnosis of metastatic adenocarcinoma was established by lumbar CSF cytology. The primary was not established, but was suspected to be of colonic origin.

In cases where the epithelial origin of the cells has to be established, the use of immunocytochemistry, in particular epithelial markers (d), is very helpful.

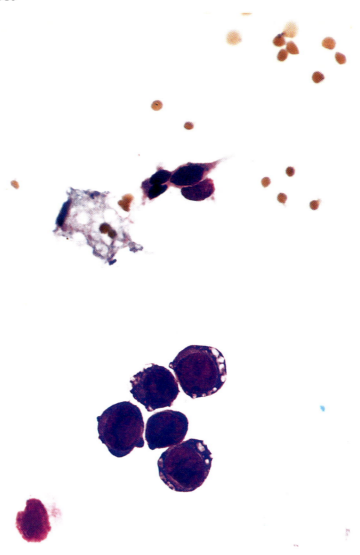

(a)

(b)

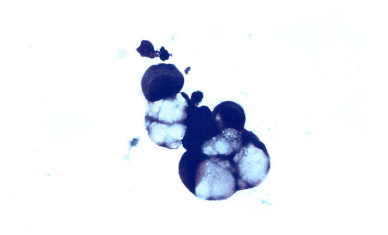

(c)

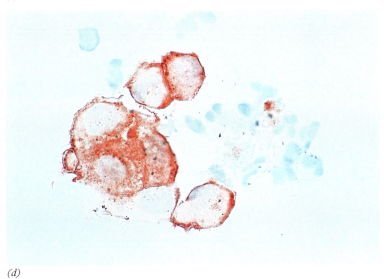

(d)

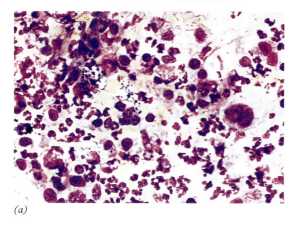

(a)

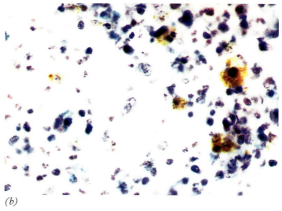

(b)

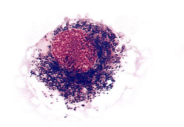

(c)

Fig. 5.8 Melanoma

(a) MGG ×525: ventricular CSF (b) Papanicolaou ×525: same specimen; another smear (c) MGG ×2100

Discrete tumour cells are seen interspersed between inflammatory cells in these micrographs. The neoplastic cells are variable in size and nuclear-cytoplasmic ratio, and a large convoluted nucleus is seen opposite 3 o'clock in (a). Abundant intracellular pigment, blue-black in the MGG preparation (a, c) and golden-brown in the Papanicolaou smear (b), is seen. The differential diagnosis lies between iron pigment and melanin. The latter was demonstrated by the Masson–Fontana stain and the tumour identified as a melanotic melanoma.

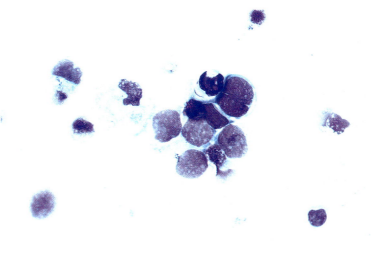

Fig. 5.9 Rhabdomyosarcoma

MGG ×2900: CSF child

Malignant cells from rhabdomyosarcoma mimic lymphoid blasts and vice versa. Immunocytochemistry for muscle-specific antigens, including desmin, should confirm rhabdomyosarcoma. In cases where staining is negative for both leukocyte and muscle antigens, a repeat immunocytochemistry with wider panel of haemopoietic markers is advised.

6. Oesophagogastrointestinal tract

The role of cytopathology in the field of gastroenterology has been extended in the last decade by the introduction of the flexible fibreoptic endoscope. It is now possible to visualize the entire gastrointestinal tract and acquire permanent documentation of the lesion under investigation by the use of a camera attachment.

The instruments have single or double channels through which diagnostic material may be obtained for biopsy histology and brush cytology and it is customary to obtain both types of specimens. The diagnostic rate for oesophageal and colonic carcinomas is high and equal by both methods. Biopsy histology is more successful than brush cytology in the diagnosis of gastric carcinoma of the fundus and the body. The cardia and the antrum beyond the incisura are not easily reached by the biopsy forceps but are generally accessible to the brush. The overall diagnostic rate for gastric carcinoma is improved by the combined use of cytology and histology.

Opinion varies as to the optimal sequence of collection of the specimens. In some centres brush specimens are collected prior to biopsy as it is considered that the bleeding caused by the biopsy forceps has an adverse effect on the smear. As against that, a brush rolled over an ulcer crater covered with slough or over an infiltrating carcinoma may not contain diagnostic cells, whereas a specimen obtained after prior biopsy has removed the slough or breached the surface over an infiltrating carcinoma may be more informative. The brush specimens illustrated in this section were obtained as a matter of policy, after biopsies which generally numbered four to six, and the blood was not found to interfere with the quality of the preparation or the interpretation.

A Romanowsky stain is not suitable for a gastrointestinal brush specimen on account of the mucin present. To avoid dehydration, which damages morphology in an alcohol-fixed, Papanicolaou-stained smear, it is essential to spread and fix the smears one at a time. It is generally possible to make three or four good smears from a brush.

The technique of endoscopic retrograde cholangiopancreatography (ERCP) is used to visualize the pancreatic duct system by fluoroscopy after injection of contrast medium. The endoscope is introduced into the pancreatic duct through the ampulla of Vater and pancreatic juice obtained prior to injection of the dye may be used for cytological and biochemical analysis.

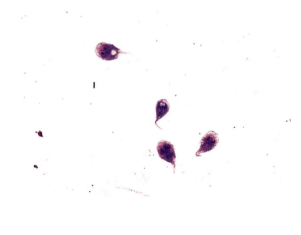

Fig. 6.1 *Giardia lamblia*

MGG ×525: pancreatic juice; ERCP

The gastrointestinal tract is a potential portal of entry for a wide variety of pathogens—viral, bacterial and parasitic. *Giardia lamblia*, an actively motile, multiflagellated, unicellular protozoon, parasitizes the duodenum and the jejunum where it divides by simple binary fission. Infection is acquired by ingestion of water contaminated with faeces containing the ovoid cystic forms. The trophozoite released in the human intestine is pear-shaped with two nuclei and a central parabasal body, and resembles a human face.

G. lamblia is endemic in the tropics and in some parts of the USA and infects mainly children who suffer from a watery diarrhoea. In heavy chronic infestation, the jejunal mucosa may be covered with a host of parasites and malabsorption may occur. In recent years, giardiasis has emerged as a significant cause of traveller's diarrhoea. This is seldom acute and some subjects may remain asymptomatic for long periods.

The trophozoites illustrated were recovered from pancreatic juice collected in the course of ERCP, and are likely to be from the duodenum traversed by the endoscope.

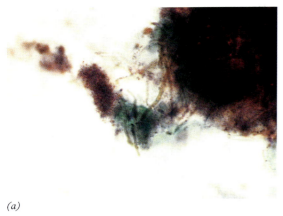

(a)

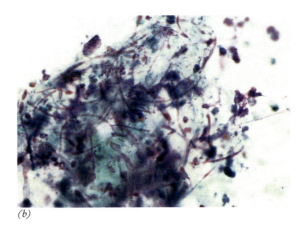

(b)

Fig. 6.2 Bacteria: *Candida* spp.

Papanicolaou ×525 (a) oesophageal brush (b) gastric brush

Candida may be present in an oesophageal brush specimen in immunocompromised subjects and patients on antibiotic therapy, and bacteria and the fungus may be seen in cases of oesophagitis, ulcer or carcinoma.

The acidity of the normal stomach inhibits bacterial growth and a healthy stomach is sterile. In hypochlorhydria and achlorhydria, the stomach may be colonized by the opportunistic *Candida albicans*, and a chronic ulcer may show a polymicrobial invasion. Both *Candida* and bacteria are most frequently seen in association with gastric carcinoma.

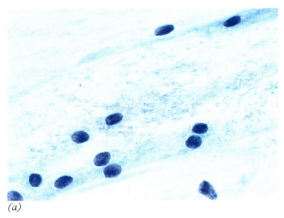

(a)

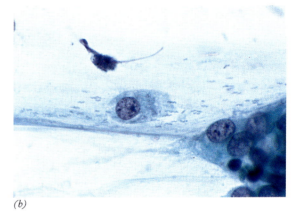

(b)

Fig. 6.3 *Helicobacter pylori*

(a) Papanicolaou ×2100: gastric brushing (b) ×2100

These bacteria are associated with gastric ulcers. Cytologically they can be seen in routinely stained preparations, best in the mucus next to the gastric epithelium or amidst the bare nuclei (a, b). They are often present in large numbers and can be recognized under high magnification. They are described as 'seagulls in flight', having a wavy rod-like appearance.

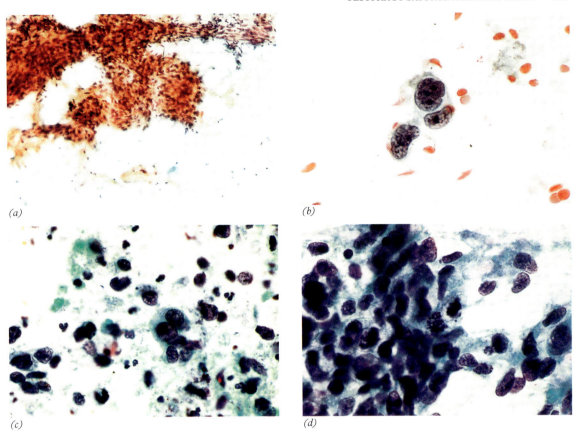

(a)

(b)

(c)

(d)

Fig. 6.4 Squamous cell carcinoma

Papanicolaou: oesophageal brush (a) ×133: well-differentiated (b) ×525: another case; moderately differentiated (c) ×525: another case; poorly differentiated (d) ×525: another case; anaplastic

The oesophagus is lined by stratified squamous epithelium which changes abruptly to gastric mucosa at the cardio-oesophageal junction. The lower third may contain ectopic foci of gastric mucosa. The majority of oesophageal malignant tumours are of the squamous cell type. The well-differentiated squamous cell carcinoma contains round or bizarre-shaped cells identical in appearance to the keratinized carcinoma cells of the genital tract or bronchogenic squamous cell carcinoma. Micrograph (a) shows a well-differentiated malignant cell in the lower half of the field and a sheet of cohesive, flattened tumour cells in the upper half. The moderately differentiated carcinoma cells in (b) are free of keratin. The nuclei are variable in size and markedly variable in shape. The nuclear chromatin is aggregated into small and coarse granules and is irregular in distribution; the chromatin pattern is different in each of the

four nuclei. The nucleoli are prominent to the same degree as in moderately differentiated squamous cell carcinomas in other organs. The cells in (c) are poorly differentiated and display a greater degree of anisocytosis. Although distinctive cytoplasmic features of squamous cells are lacking, the lack of cell cohesion, the irregularity of cell shape, the absence of depth of focus or of intracellular mucin and the coarseness of the nuclei favour a presumptive diagnosis of a squamous cell origin. Note the scattered necrotic tumour cells. Total anaplasia is evident in the sheet of cells in (d). The nuclei vary in size and in shape from round to fusiform. The scant cytoplasm lacks recognizable limiting membranes and nucleoli are inconspicuous. The four mitotic figures present in one high-power field are indicative of a rapid rate of cell proliferation.

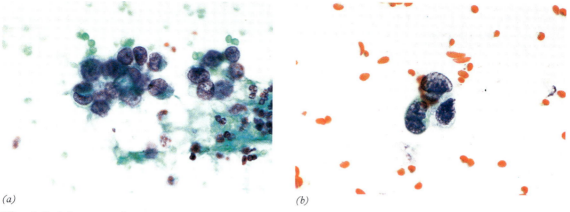

(a)   *(b)*

Fig. 6.5 Adenocarcinoma

(a) Alcian blue ×525: oesophageal brush (b) Papanicolaou ×525: gastro-oesophageal anastomosis brush; another case

Adenocarcinoma of the oesophagus is rare, and usually occurs in the lower third in an ectopic focus of gastric mucosa. More commonly it is an upward extension of a gastric primary.

Micrograph (a) of a brush smear from the lower third of the oesophagus illustrates adenocarcinoma cells. The cluster to the right shows an acinar arrangement. One cell in the cluster to the left contains a sharply delineated mucous vacuole; the mucin in the other cells is diffuse. The patient presented with symptoms due to an oesophageal stricture. In view of the rarity of adenocarcinoma in this area, a suggestive appearance of an adenocarcinoma can be altered to a definitive diagnosis by the use of appropriate special stains to demonstrate mucin. The primary tumour in this case originated in and involved the stomach. The adenocarcinoma cells in (b) were recovered from a recurrence of a gastric carcinoma at the site of anastomosis 23 years after a gastrectomy.

STOMACH

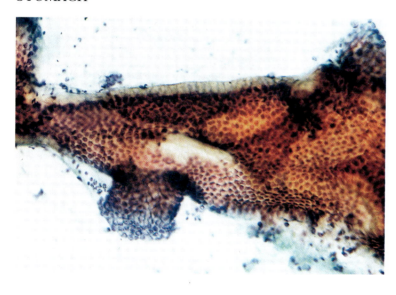

Fig. 6.6 Normal gastric mucosa

Papanicolaou ×183: gastric brush

This micrograph illustrates a fragment of normal gastric mucosa. The surface cells form a regular palisade and have abundant pale-staining cytoplasm with basally located nuclei. The same cells are seen deeper down lining the gastric pits or fovea. Foveal cells contain neutral mucin which stains strongly with periodic acid-Schiff (PAS), but reacts weakly with Alcian blue. The other cells that make up the gastric mucosa, the hydrochloric acid-secreting parietal or oxyntic cells and the pepsinogen-secreting peptic or chief cells, are not easily discriminated in a Papanicolaou-stained smear.

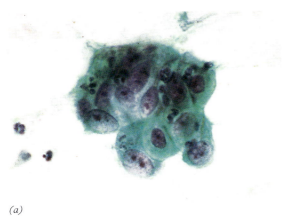

(a)

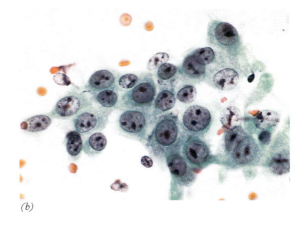

(b)

Fig. 6.7 Regenerating gastric mucosa

Papanicolaou ×525: gastric brush (a) a case of chronic gastritis (b) another case

One of the major diagnostic problems met with in gastric cytopathology is presented by regenerating mucosal cells. These are seen particularly in hypersecretory chronic gastritis which is not a significant precursor of gastric carcinoma. The regenerating cells usually appear in sheets, have deeply basophilic cytoplasm, display some anisonucleosis and invariably contain prominent nucleoli which may be multiple and are often polymorphic. An occasional mitotic figure may be present. The features that aid in the correct identification of the benign proliferating cells are the relative flatness of the cell aggregate which is two-dimensional in the manner of lining cells, and, despite the anisocytosis, an overall impression of a more or less comparable nuclear-cytoplasmic ratio. In addition, the nuclei are vesicular and the chromatin pattern is not disorganized.

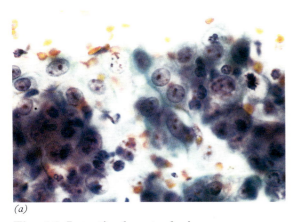

(a)

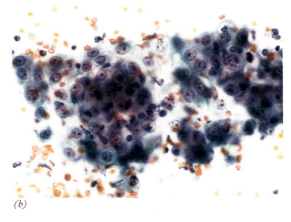

(b)

Fig. 6.8 Intestinal metaplasia

Papanicolaou (a) ×525: gastric brush (b) ×333: gastric brush

Chronic gastritis due to environmental causes is prevalent in populations at high risk of developing gastric carcinoma, as in Japan, but occurs in sporadic cases in other parts of the world. The condition may result in atrophy of the gastric mucosa which is replaced by metaplastic epithelium of the intestinal type. The metaplasia may be complete and contain all the cell types seen in the small intestine or be incomplete and more closely resemble colonic metaplasia. Paneth and argentaffin cells are not identifiable in routine cytological smears and require special staining procedures for their demonstration. At a simple level, intestinalized gastric mucosa is seen to consist of goblet cells and absorptive cells. The goblet cell is larger, has a paler cytoplasm and contains mucous vacuoles; its distal border is often fuzzy and fine tags of cytoplasm extend beyond the luminal surface. The absorptive cell is smaller, has a deeper and more uniformly stained cytoplasm and does not contain intracytoplasmic secretory vacuoles. It is covered with fine, short microvilli and the line of attachment of the microvilli, although not as broad as the terminal bar of the ciliated cell, is sharp and imparts a clear definition to the luminal surface of the cell. Areas of intestinal metaplasia may also contain mitoses and a mitotic figure is seen opposite 1 o'clock (a). The cell arrangement is more disorganized than is the case with regenerating gastric mucosa cells. The benign nature of the cells is indicated by the extreme regularity of the nuclei, the uniformly low nuclear-cytoplasmic ratio and the blandness of the nuclei (a). The relative flatness of the clusters is better appreciated at a lower magnification (b).

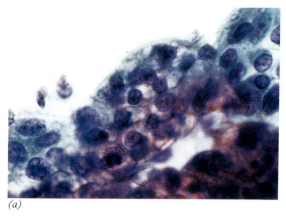

(a)

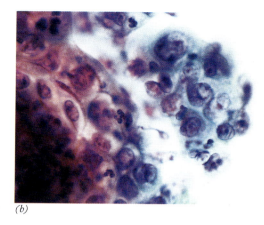

(b)

Fig. 6.9 A case of pernicious anaemia

Papanicolaou ×525: gastric brush (a) intestinal metaplasia (b) dysplasia

The chronic gastritis associated with the pernicious anaemia syndrome is the result of injury to the intrinsic factor and the parietal cells by autoantibodies. Like gastritis due to environmental causes, it leads to atrophy and subsequent intestinal metaplasia and is a significant precursor of gastric carcinoma. A sheet of benign intestinal metaplasia cells is illustrated in (a). An absorptive cell with a clear narrow end-plate is seen interposed between two mucin-containing cells at the free edge of the sheet; the majority of the cells are of the goblet type. The cells are approximately the same size; the nuclei are regular and small.

Intestinal metaplasia may show cellular atypia and become dysplastic. The cells illustrated in (b) were seen in the same smear. They are larger and more variable in size. The nuclei show considerable variation in size and the nuclear-cytoplasmic ratio is high. The chromatin content is increased and there is some disorganization of the chromatin pattern. The nucleoli are larger and more prominent. The cellular atypia is consistent with mild dysplasia.

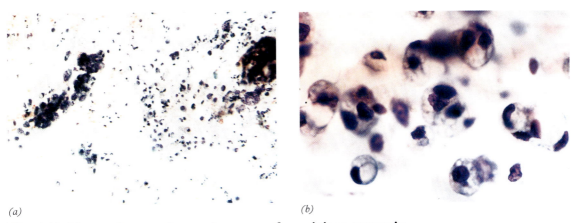

(a)

(b)

Fig. 6.10 Signet-ring carcinoma in a case of pernicious anaemia

Papanicolaou gastric brush (a) ×133 (b) ×525: another field

A large number of neoplastic cells, some discrete, others in cohesive sheets, are seen against a background of pale pink free mucin (a). At high magnification (b) the cells are seen to be distended with mucin. In some cells the mucous vacuoles are small and multiple; in others, the nucleus is pushed to one pole by a single, large secretory globule and the cell has acquired a signet-ring appearance. The nuclear-cytoplasmic ratio is low and the nuclei compressed by mucin are small and intensely hyperchromic. Sparse, scattered, signet-ring carcinoma cells are easily overlooked or mistaken for histiocytes. High-power examination of cells caught in amorphous material is advisable to avoid a false-negative report. If required, the acidic mucin in the cells may be confirmed with mucicarmine or Alcian blue.

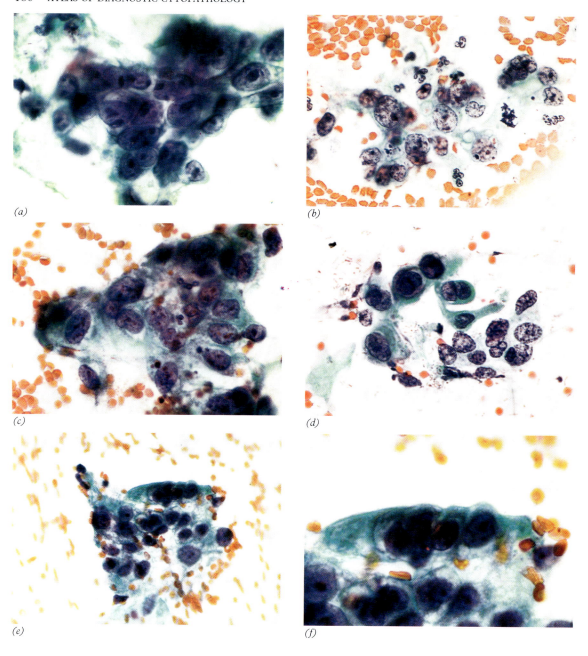

(a)

(b)

(c)

(d)

(e)

(f)

Fig. 6.11 Adenocarcinoma of the stomach

Papanicolaou: gastric brush (a) ×525 (b) ×525: another case (c) ×525: another case (d) ×525: another case (e) ×333: another case (f) ×832: same field as (e)

The common cytological features of malignancy met with in endoscopic gastric brush cytology are illustrated in these micrographs by five cases. The first point to note is that, although all the cases are of adenocarcinoma, the three-dimensional globular clusters characteristic of spontaneously exfoliated glandular cells are not a feature of a brush smear. The cell arrangement in clusters and sheets with uneven ragged borders is similar to that seen in bronchial brush and lung aspirate smears. The familiar appearance of rounded adenocarcinoma cells is an artefact as much of the type of specimen as of the nature of the cell and should not be sought in a brush smear of an adenocarcinoma.

The malignant cells in these micrographs are pleomorphic, the variation in shape and size being most evident in the nuclei and the nuclear-cytoplasmic ratio. Reasonably well-preserved nuclei, freshly obtained from a tumour by brush or aspiration, are not remarkable for hyperchromasia; they may be moderately hyperchromic (a), normochromic (b) or hypochromic (c). Nucleoli are usually present in gastric carcinoma cells, but vary in size and prominence from case to case. In (a) they are a dominant

feature, like a dilated pupil in the cornea. In (b) and (c) they are appreciably smaller and less conspicuous than in benign regenerating cells (Fig. 6.7). The staining reaction of the nucleoli is as variable in malignant cells as in benign cells. As a rule, the nucleolus in a hypochromic nucleus is more likely to be eosinophilic (c).

The cytoplasm also varies from case to case. It is intensely basophilic in (a), paler and more fragile in (b) and (c). Cytoplasmic vacuolization is not an outstanding feature of these cases, but at least one cell in (a), (b) and (c) contains a mucous vacuole. A centrally located eosinophilic dot of condensed mucin within a clear vacuole and an abnormal mitotic figure are present in (b).

The cells in (d) evince advanced degenerative changes, as indicated by the many stripped malignant nuclei, and the perinuclear vacuolization of the binucleate cell.

In most cases, carcinoma cells in a brush smear do not exhibit any kind of architectural organization. On occasion, a strip of luminal neoplastic cells may be recovered along with deeper cells (e). The luminal cells are aligned in a palisade and their polarity is maintained. The distal surface is neat and covered with a microvillous brush border (f).

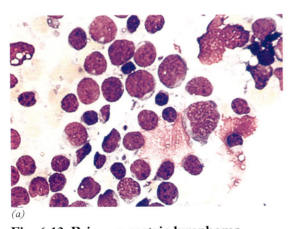

(a)

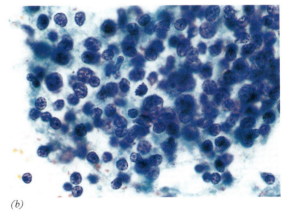

(b)

Fig. 6.12 Primary gastric lymphoma

(a) MGG ×525: gastric brush (b) Papanicolaou ×525: gastric brush; another case

These micrographs illustrate two cases in which a cytological diagnosis of non-Hodgkin's lymphoma was confirmed by histology; a full diagnosis of B-cell lymphoma was established by immunocytochemical study on the case shown in (b). The smears show a mixed population of discrete cells which include a few small lymphocytes with hyperchromic condensed nuclei and numerous immature lymphoid cells which show a progressive gradation in size (a, b). Some of the nuclei are notched and several contain small multiple nucleoli.

A presumptive cytodiagnosis of primary gastric

lymphoma can be of value as this tumour is eminently treatable, may occur in the younger age groups and may present with the symptoms and appearance of a benign ulcer. Since, however, lymphocytes and plasma cells may occur in small numbers in a normal upper gastrointestinal brush smear, or in abundance in chronic gastritis, a cytological diagnosis of malignant lymphoma calls for careful morphological assessment and should always be confirmed by appropriate histological and immunological studies.

Fig. 6.13 Leiomyoma of stomach

Papanicolaou ×525: gastric brush

Another non-epithelial neoplasm of the stomach is a smooth-muscle tumour which may be benign or malignant. Initially submucous, it may project into the gastric cavity as a polypoid mass and erode the surface mucosa. Tumour tissue may be obtained in a brush smear at this stage. In the example of a leiomyoma illustrated, numerous smooth-muscle cells are seen. The plump, fusiform nuclei are more or less alike in shape and size and mitoses are not evident (see Fig. 14.8a, b). The nuclei of a poorly differentiated leiomyosarcoma are generally bizarre and pleomorphic and the diagnosis is self-evident. A well-differentiated leiomyosarcoma shows relatively little nuclear deviation and the diagnosis of malignancy may have to be based on the number of mitotic figures seen per microscopic field in a histological specimen.

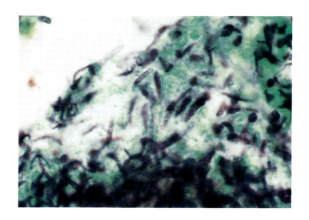

COLON

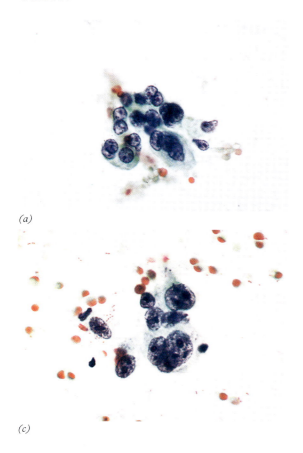

(a)

(c)

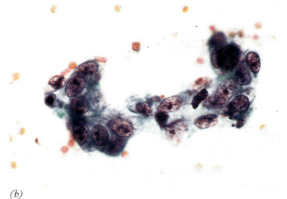

(b)

Fig. 6.14 Adenocarcinoma of the colon

Papanicolaou ×525: colonic brush (a) carcinoma of the caecum (b) carcinoma of the sigmoid colon; another case (c) carcinoma of the rectosigmoid colon; another case

Brush samples are obtainable from the entire colon up to the ileocaecal valve. The majority of the primary colon carcinomas occur in the descending part. The tumours are adenocarcinomas and cytologically similar to gastric carcinomas. A well-differentiated adenocarcinoma originating in the caecum is illustrated in micrograph (a). The cells are small, intercellular borders are well-defined and nuclear variation is of a low degree; the nucleoli are small. A moderately differentiated carcinoma of the sigmoid colon has yielded cells which have more cytoplasm; the limiting membrane of the cells, however, is less well-defined. The nuclei and nucleoli are larger than in (a). In a poorly differentiated tumour of the rectosigmoid, intercytoplasmic membranes are still less distinct, and the cytoplasm appears to form a syncytium. Anisonucleosis is marked and the nucleoli are prominent and variable in number and shape. Note the perinucleolar condensation of chromatin round the nucleoli in (c).

Fig. 6.15 Polyp with surface dysplasia

Papanicolaou (a) ×720: colonic brush
(b) ×183: colonic brush; same field as (a)
(c) ×720: colonic brush; same case;
another field

Interest has centred in recent years on the early recognition and grading of dysplastic changes that occur in some lesions of the colon such as a villous adenoma, familial polyposis coli and long-standing ulcerative colitis known to carry a high potential of malignant transformation. Whilst the high sensitivity of cytology in identifying dysplasia is universally acknowledged, distinction between severely dysplastic cells and cells brushed from the surface of an infiltrating lesion remains problematical. This may be achieved if an adequate amount of tissue is present.

These micrographs illustrate a polypoid lesion of the sigmoid colon with severe dysplasia. The cells in (a) bear stigmata of malignancy; the nuclei are pleomorphic, the nuclear chromatin is stippled and the nuclear-cytoplasmic ratio is high. At a lower magnification (b), they are seen to form the surface of a non-malignant fragment of colonic tissue. A milder degree of dysplasia in hyperplastic mucosa is seen in (c). The cells are enlarged and nucleoli are prominent but the arrangement is orderly and polarity is maintained. Note the microvilli and the narrow end-plate of the luminal absorptive cells.

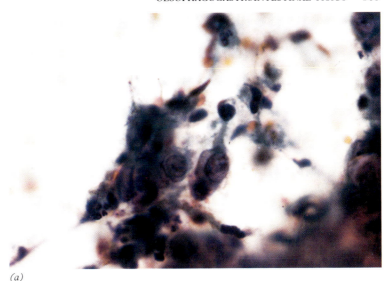

(a)

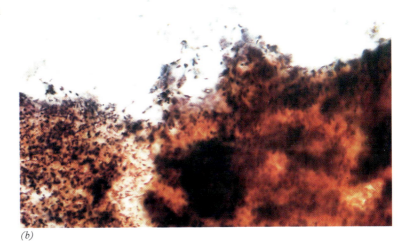

(b)

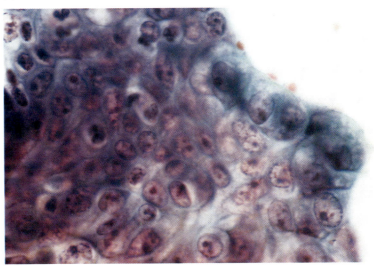

(c)

7. Pancreas, liver and extrahepatic bile ducts

The main aim of diagnostic cytology in this area is to establish the presence or absence of a neoplasm. For this reason a number of techniques in a variety of settings have been developed to obtain cells for diagnosis. With the development of imaging techniques, the favoured methods are preoperative fine-needle aspiration (FNA) cytology, intraoperative FNA cytology and endoscopic retrograde brush cytology (ERBC). Cytology of the pancreatic juice and cytology of bile are used less frequently. All of these methods can, singly or combined with radiological investigations, establish the diagnosis, thus avoiding surgery in many cases. Cytological methods carry a less than 1% risk of serious complications. They can be performed as an outpatient procedure. Preoperative pathological diagnosis diminishes the need for hospitalization associated with diagnostic laparotomy and has a major impact on the economics of treating the patient with pancreatic carcinoma. When compared with other diagnostic methods (sonography, computed tomography, endoscopic retrograde cholangiopancreatography, roentgenography and angiography), cytology gives a higher proportion of positive results.

Cytology of malignant epithelial neoplasms of the pancreas is as difficult as it is important in terms of clinical management. In terms of surgical management, only 30% of pancreatic carcinomas are resectable at the time of diagnosis and they are confined to the head. There is hardly any other area of the body, apart perhaps from the central nervous system, which is more difficult to access in terms of sampling and yet where cells show a relatively limited spectrum of morphological changes. At the same time, cytological opinion given on the basis of these cell changes should be sufficiently clear as to enable surgical decision-making. In the case of pancreatic cancer this decision almost invariably carries a grave prognosis for the patient. Given the responsibility that lies with the cytopathologist in terms of accuracy and clarity of reporting, it is our view that only those lesions which show clear cytological criteria of malignancy should be reported as carcinoma. Any other abnormalities of doubtful cytological significance should be referred for tissue biopsy. This approach will ensure that the error rate is kept to a minimum and will sharpen our resolve to achieve accurate definitive diagnosis.

Cytological criteria for the diagnosis of pancreatic carcinoma do not greatly differ from those encountered in other organs. However, in cases of pancreatic carcinoma some of these features are more important than others. These features, listed in order of priority are: presence of disoriented or crowded cells in three-dimensional groups, extreme nuclear enlargement with nuclear contour irregularity, unevenly distributed chromatin, anisonucleosis and prominent nucleoli. Nuclear hyperchromasia and coarse chromatin pattern are not helpful diagnostic criteria of malignancy in cases of pancreatic carcinoma.

Although the cytopathologist is aware of the histological classification of pancreatic carcinoma, the nature of the cytological sample often enables only the assessment of nature (i.e. benign or malignant) rather than the type of the tumour. Some histological subtypes of pancreatic carcinoma have their equivalent in cytological preparations. *Duct adenocarcinoma* constitutes more than 90% of all forms of pancreatic neoplasms and the morphological features described thus far apply mainly to duct carcinoma. It is important to distinguish papillary carcinoma of the bile duct from pancreatic duct carcinoma because of their different anatomical and biological behaviour. Cytologically, papillary carcinoma of the bile duct has round to polyhedral cells arranged in papillary-like pattern. This distinction is not so easy in cases of moderately to poorly differentiated papillary bile duct carcinomas. Similarly, distinction is difficult in cases of *papillary and cystic* (solid and cystic) carcinoma of the pancreas. *Giant cell carcinoma* is a rare pancreatic tumour (incidence 2.1–6.5% of all non-endocrine neoplasms). Cytologically it is characterized by the presence of bizarre tumour giant cells and abundant mitoses. Tumour giant cells have to be distinguished from benign 'osteoclast like' giant cells. These can be seen in granulomatous diseases such as tuberculosis and sarcoidosis, vasculitis (Wegener's granulomatosis) and other conditions, including fat necrosis. Giant cell carcinoma of the pancreas can be diagnosed by a combination of clinical history, imaging findings and FNA biopsy. Because of its morphological similarity to sarcoma, the differential diagnosis includes soft-tissue tumours, e.g. rhabdomyosarcoma, malignant fibrous histiocytoma and liposarcoma. Ultrastructural features reveal an undifferentiated malignant tumour lacking specific features found in the mesenchymal tumours, which it might resemble morphologically. The prognosis of these tumours is very poor, with a short survival of 2–3 months. Giant cell carcinoma occasionally contains benign osteoclast-like giant cells in addition to pleomorphic cells. Immunocytochemically these tumours stain for vimentin, actin, α_1-antitrypsin, α_1-antichymotripsin, synaptophysin and neuron-specific enolase (NSE) but not for epithelial markers. *Mucinous cystadenocarcinoma* is cytologically characterized by papillary clusters of mucin-secreting cells in an inflammatory necrotic and cystic background (Fig. 7.9f–h). *Adenosquamous carcinoma* cytologically shows two types of cells. One is distinctly of squamoid type with polyhedral cells forming flat sheets and having keratinized cytoplasm. The other cells appear to be from a poorly differentiated tumour with pseudoglandular features. Necrotic background is often present. Differential diagnosis includes a rare mucoepidermoid carcinoma of the bile ducts which has to be excluded by radiological investigations.

Cytological features of *acinar cell carcinoma* have only recently been reported. They include cellularity with acinar and occasional glandular structures. The neoplastic cells are about twice the size of normal acinar cells, arranged in sheets with mild overlapping. They have eccentrically located, round or oval hyperchromatic nuclei. Nuclear membrane often shows foldings and appears irregular under high-power magnification. The diagnosis is made on cytoplasm which contains granules but no mucin. Mitoses are frequent. Ultrastructurally, cytoplasm of tumour cells contains electron-dense granules, but no neuroendocrine or mucoid granules. Immunocytochemistry shows positive staining for α_1-antitrypsin, lipase, trypsinogen, chymotripsinogen and antielastase (except α_1-amylase) and fails to stain with antisera against carcinoembryonic antigen, CA 19-9, NSE and pancreatic endocrine hormones. *Papillary cystic carcinoma* shows features of malignancy including pleomorphism and prominent nucleoli. Cells are arranged in papillary clusters. Other features occasionally seen in cytological preparations of pancreatic carcinoma are: pseudostratification, mucinous metaplasia, phagocytosis, intranuclear vacuoles, signet-ring cells and neuroendocrine-type cells. The relevance of various morphological subtypes has yet to be established. Until such time, the main object of cytological investigation is finding reliable morphological criteria for establishing the presence of cancer.

Diagnostic accuracy of the cytological examination is high in cases with representative aspirates. The experience of the radiologist in localizing and puncturing of the lesion can significantly influence the correct cytological diagnosis. The overall sensitivity of the preoperative FNA for detection of pancreatic neoplasms ranges between 48 and 97%. Specificity ranges between 78 and 100%. The false-negative rate is largely due to a non-representative sample and ranges between less than 10 and 24%. The false-positive rate is reported infrequently and is low.

Cytology of the *endocrine neoplasms* is more difficult than the cytology of non-endocrine tumours. The features of islet cell tumours, particularly when they are composed of a monotonous proliferation of single cells, are often sufficient to suggest the diagnosis. Additional techniques, including immunocytochemistry and electron microscopy, are necessary to confirm the diagnosis. Despite this, cytological diagnosis of these tumours remains difficult. Recognition of diagnostic limitations of cytology in diagnosing neuroendocrine tumours is essential if these clinically indolent tumours are to be managed according to the FNA reports alone.

PANCREAS

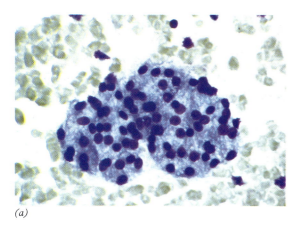

(a)

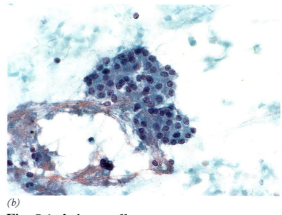

(b)

Fig. 7.1 Acinar cells

(a) MGG ×840: FNA pancreas (b) Papanicolaou ×420 (c) ×840

Acinar cells of the pancreas show these characteristic features: round, cohesive, complex aggregates with no central lumen. The nucleus is round, eccentrically placed and shows a slight variation in size, with a conspicuous nucleolus and coarsely granular chromatin condensed beneath the nuclear membrane. It often shows degenerate changes due to autolysis or fixation. Cytoplasm is abundant and granular, not clearly outlined, defined by acinar arrangement and containing intracytoplasmic zymogen granules (periodic acid-Schiff (PAS) trichrome: bright orange).

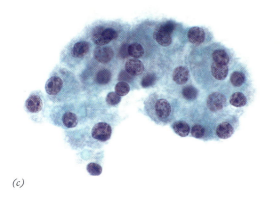

(c)

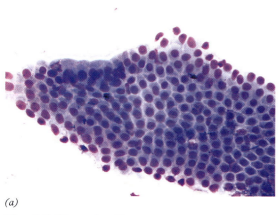

(a)

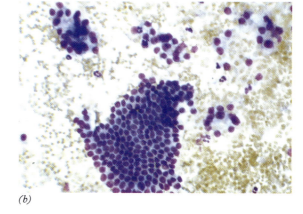

(b)

Fig. 7.2 Ductal cells

FNA pancreas: (a) ductal cells: MGG ×840 (b) ductal and acinar cells: MGG ×420

Ductal epithelium presents in FNA as large monolayered sheets with uniformly spaced oval nuclei, showing minimal or no overlapping and small inconspicuous nucleoli. These are surrounded by a moderate amount of ill-defined cytoplasm luminal border without visible microvilli.

In benign conditions, anisonucleosis is not more than double in size; nucleoli can be prominent but multinucleation is consistently absent.

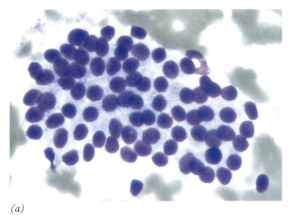

(a)

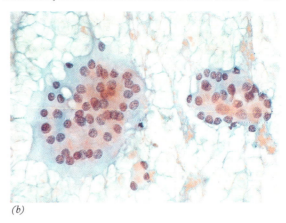

(b)

Fig.7.3 Islet cells

FNA pancreas: (a) MGG ×840 (b) Papanicolaou ×840

Pancreatic islet cells are difficult to distinguish from acinar cells. They are usually present in flat rounded aggregates, have more distinct cytoplasmic outline than acinar cells with centrally placed nucleus and inconspicuous nucleolus. Granules in the cytoplasm (alcohol-fixed preparations) can be confirmed with PAS-trichrome stains: β cells are pale yellow-green with yellow-orange granules, δ cells exhibit translucent green cytoplasm, α cells have a deep orange cytoplasm. They stain with chromogranin similar to acinar cells.

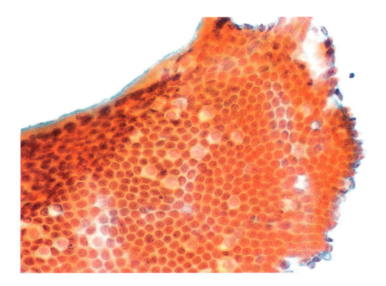

Fig. 7.4 Duodenal cells

FNA pancreas: Papanicolaou ×580

These are present particularly in the brushings performed at ERCP but also in FNA preparations. They differ from pancreatic and biliary duct cells in that they have a more prominent brush border. When present in large flat sheets, they are usually interspersed with numerous goblet cells.

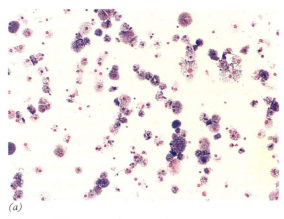

(a)

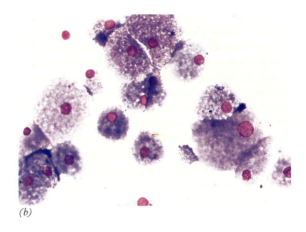

(b)

Fig. 7.5 Pancreatic pseudocyst

FNA pancreas: (a) MGG ×840 (b) ×2100

Pancreatic pseudocyst contains numerous macrophages, often containing haemosiderin. No epithelium is present.

Aspirates from pseudocysts should be differentiated from simple congenital cysts in patients with von Hippel-Lindau disease. These contain very few cells. They are mostly normal epithelial cells in monolayers mimicking the reparative process. Most of the cells have a single nucleus; a few have two or more nuclei and may be found in association with mononuclear cells or as solitary cells. Cytoplasm of these cells is abundant and delicate. Nuclei have fine, evenly distributed chromatin and frequently multiple nucleoli. Other cystic lesions of the pancreas include: retention cysts, adenomas, papillary and cystic neoplasm, mucinous cystadenoma, mucinous cystadenocarcinoma, cystic acinar adenocarcinoma and solid neoplasms with cystic degeneration.

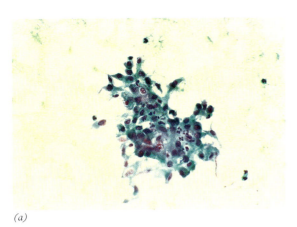

(a)

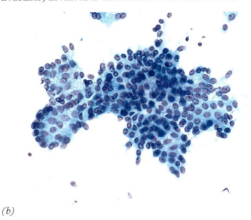

(b)

Fig. 7.6 Pancreatitis

(a) Papanicolaou ×840 (b) ×840

FNA of chronic pancreatitis (a, b) can vary in cellularity depending on the degree of scarring. In cases of marked fibrosis, fibrocytes and other mesenchymal elements can be seen. Chronic inflammatory cells including lymphocytes and plasma cells are frequently present. Acinar and ductal epithelium, when present in the aspirate, can show marked regenerative and degenerative changes (b). Acinar cells can have enlarged nuclei, increased nuclear-cytoplasmic ratio and prominent nucleoli. Ductal cells can show marked anisonucleosis and nuclear enlargement. They are present in sheets but can show some overlapping and nuclear atypia. When pronounced, epithelial atypia in chronic pancreatitis is difficult to distinguish from the well-differentiated adenocarcinoma. Under inflammatory conditions endothelial cells of small blood vessels may appear pleomorphic and bizarre-looking but are still arranged in a single-layered sheet, unlike malignant cells. Similarly, irritated mesothelial cells may show prominent nucleoli and coarse chromatin clumping but still remain in a monolayer.

Pancreatitis with its epithelial atypia is the most frequent cause of false-suspicious cytology reports. Cytological differentiation between chronic pancreatitis and a well-differentiated adenocarcinoma is difficult. The usual criteria of malignancy—nucleoli, nuclear contour irregularity, nuclear hyperchromasia, coarse chromatin and elevated nuclear-cytoplasmic ratio alone—can be found in most cases of both chronic pancreatitis and well-differentiated carcinoma. Nuclear contour irregularity of cells in benign conditions consists of angularity and notching, not the smoother deep convolutions of malignant cells. The cells with nuclear irregularity in cases of benign disease often present in monolayers, showing cell degeneration whilst preserving a honeycomb arrangement. Marked nuclear enlargement (five times and more), together with nuclear overlapping, irregular nuclear contour and three-dimensional cell arrangement are the best single criteria of malignancy.

FNA of acute pancreatitis contains tightly packed clusters of necrotic acinar cells with pyknotic nuclei. The background of the smear contains necrotic debris and inflammatory exudate with pus cells. Degenerate ductal cells are also seen. Lipid-laden macrophages and calcium deposits can be detected with special stains.

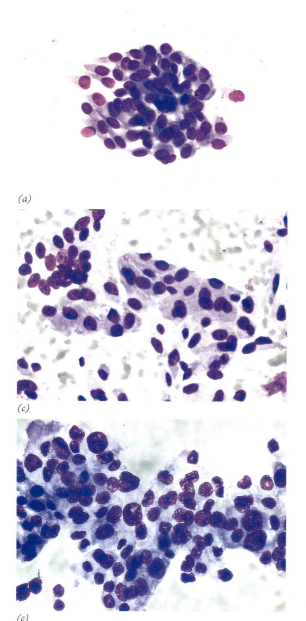

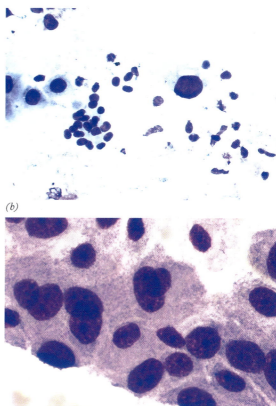

(a)

(b)

(c)

(d)

Fig. 7.7 Carcinoma of the pancreas

FNA pancreas: (a) MGG ×840 (b) ×840 (c) ×840 (d) ×2100 (e) ×840

Cytological criteria of pancreatic carcinoma listed in order of priority are: extreme nuclear enlargement with nuclear contour irregularity, disoriented or crowded cells in three-dimensional groups, unevenly distributed chromatin, anisonucleosis, elevated nuclear-cytoplasmic ratio and prominent nucleoli.

Cells from a well-differentiated adenocarcinoma may show very few of the classical features of malignancy. Instead, criteria listed above seem to be most appropriate for the diagnosis of malignancy. Of these, nuclear crowding (a), extreme nuclear enlargement compared to benign duct cells (b) and disorientation of nuclei with overlapping (c, d) are the most helpful. Poorly differentiated adenocarcinoma (e) can be diagnosed relatively easily due to the usual pleomorphism of malignancy.

(e)

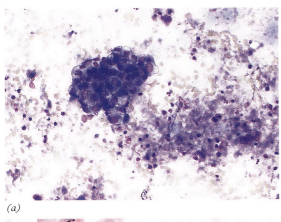

(a)

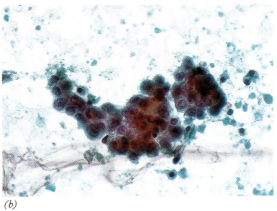

(b)

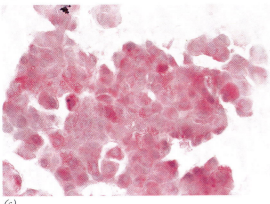

(c)

Fig. 7.8 Mucinous cystadenocarcinoma

(a) ×420 (b) Papanicolaou ×840 (c) PAS diastase ×840

Mucinous adenocarcinoma is characterized by papillary clusters of mucin-secreting cells in an inflammatory necrotic and cystic background.

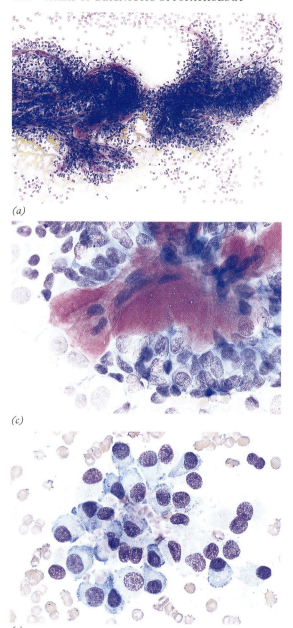

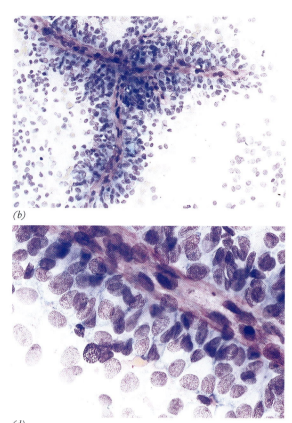

Fig. 7.9 Papillary and solid neoplasm

(a) MGG ×210 (b) ×420 (c) ×1260 (d) ×1260 (e) ×1260 (courtesy of Dr I Kardum-Skelin)

This is a distinctive uncommon tumour of low-grade malignancy which primarily occurs in girls and young women. Histologically it is predominantly a solid tumour with numerous thin-walled blood vessels, but dystrophic changes and haemorrhage yield pseudocystic areas filled with blood, and papilla-like structures.

Material obtained by FNA shows high cellularity with numerous papillary fronds (a) composed of fibrovascular stalks (b) with narrow capillaries surrounded by hyalinized rims (c) and lined with one or more layers of cuboidal cells with variably abundant cytoplasm which frequently contains PAS diastase-resistant eosinophilic inclusions (d). The cells are round or oval with euchromatic nuclei with a monotonous appearance and a smooth contour (e). One or two inconspicuous nucleoli and nuclear folds can be seen. Foamy cells, blood and cellular debris are also present. Immunoperoxidase shows positive staining for vimentin, NSE, very weak cytokeratin staining and focal positive staining for α_1-antichymotripsin. There is no staining for chromogranin or hormonal markers.

Preoperative diagnosis is fundamental in view of the low potential for local invasion and metastases.

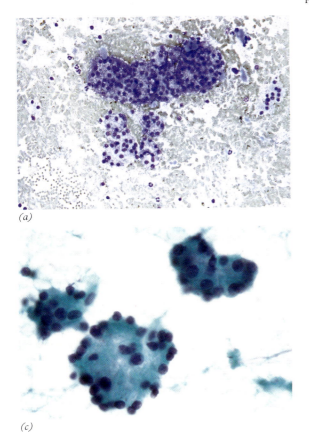

(a)

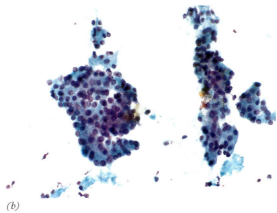

(b)

Fig. 7.10 Islet cell tumour

FNA pancreas: (a) MGG ×420 (b) Papanicolaou ×420 (c) ×840

Cytology of islet cell tumours is characterized by monotonous proliferation of cells with rounded nuclei and a moderate amount of well-outlined, sometimes granular, cytoplasm. They are arranged in small cell aggregates or singly (a, b). Nuclei are often eccentrically placed and plasmacytoid and usually contain a small nucleolus (c). Mitotic figures are infrequent. The background is usually 'clean' with no necrosis. The uniformity of cell features and the cellularity of the specimen are the most striking features. Despite this, it is often difficult to distinguish islet cell tumours from normal cellular constituents of the pancreas, well-differentiated adenocarcinoma and lymphoma. Normal pancreatic acinar cells have abundant granular cytoplasm but are frequently present in clusters whereas the islet cell tumours often present singly, although there are exceptions to this, as in our case. Well-differentiated adenocarcinoma of the pancreas usually has a coarser chromatin structure and an irregular nuclear outline and is also mostly present in aggregates. Lymphomas can usually be recognized by the fact that the cells are always single and do not have the uniformity or the amount of cytoplasm that islet cells have.

Whenever possible, immunocytochemistry should be performed on direct smears or deposits of a cell suspension to confirm the diagnosis. Chromogranin appears to be the most useful of the currently available markers for islet cell tumours.

(c)

BILIARY TRACT

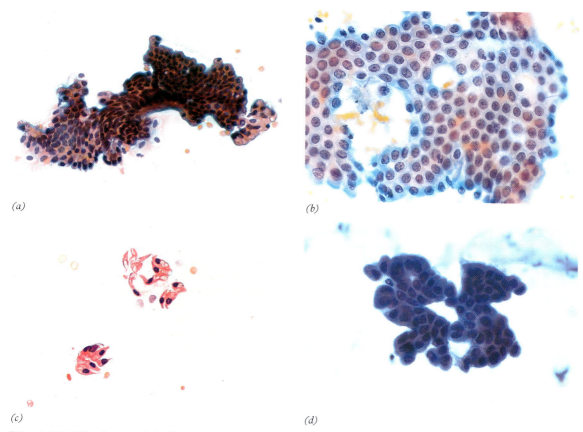

(a)

(b)

(c)

(d)

Fig. 7.11 Bile duct epithelium

Bile duct brushings: (a) Papanicolaou ×420 (b) ×1260 (c) ×840 (d) ×840

Cells from the periampullary region and bile ducts are mainly found in pancreatic juice obtained at endoscopic retrograde cholangiopancreatography (ERCP), in the bile or the endoscopic brushings performed at ERCP. Differentiation between bile duct and pancreatic duct cells is not always possible.

Bile duct cells have a rounded appearance and mainly represent uniform low columnar epithelial cells arranged in sheets that form a honeycomb pattern when viewed on end (a, b). Because of their columnar shape with bulging terminal nuclei and basal cytoplasmic process, they are known as 'matchstick' cells (c). The background of bile duct brushings sometimes contains granular bile pigment. Sheets of bile duct epithelium can frequently show architectural patterns with loops and branching cords in cytological smears.

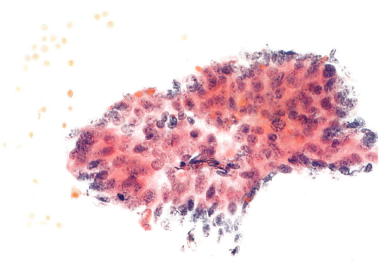

Fig. 7.12 Villous adenoma

Bile duct brushing: Papanicolaou ×1160

ERCP investigation of bile duct obstruction occasionally reveals tumour in or around Vater's papilla. Cytological smears are composed of numerous clusters of hypercrowded columnar cells with irregular feathered edges and somewhat coarser chromatin than the surrounding 'normal' bile duct and intestinal epithelium. Distinction from malignant tumours from this area is important because of the possibility of cure of such a lesion by means of surgical resection.

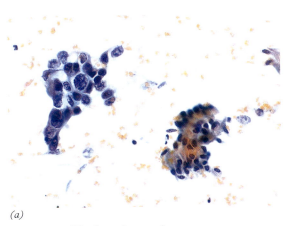

(a)

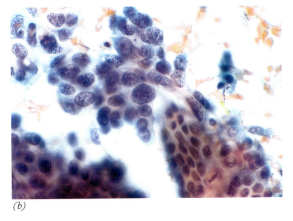

(b)

Fig. 7.13 Cholangiocarcinoma

Bile duct brushing: (a) Papanicolaou ×840 (b) ×1260

Cells with features of malignancy can be contrasted with benign epithelium (a, b). Malignant cells are larger and show crowding, overlapping and anisonucleosis.

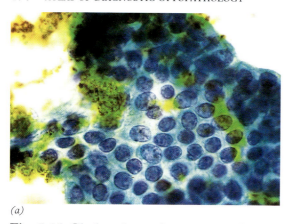

(a)

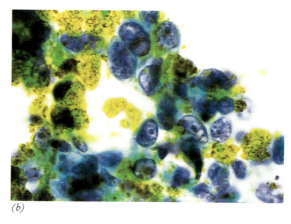

(b)

Fig. 7.14 Cholangiocarcinoma, extrahepatic

Papanicolaou ×525: bile (a) benign ductal cells (b) malignant ductal cells

Percutancous transhepatic cholangiography is a diagnostic procedure used to examine the extrahepatic biliary system. A needle introduced through the skin is guided into an intrahepatic bile duct under fluoroscopic control, dye is injected and the biliary system examined radiologically. An indwelling catheter may be used to drain a dilated biliary tree into the duodenum or percutaneously and to relieve obstructive jaundice. The bile drained externally may be examined for the presence of neoplastic cells. It should however be reasonably fresh as cells left in bile deteriorate rapidly.

These micrographs illustrate cells in bile drained through a catheter. Abundant yellow bile pigment is seen in both micrographs. The cells in (a) are benign ductal cells in a sheet. The nuclei are evenly spaced, monomorphic and normochromic; the nuclear chromatin is sparse. The carcinoma cells in (b) are appreciably larger; the nuclei vary in size and shape and the nuclear-cytoplasmic ratio is high. The nuclear chromatin is increased in quantity and disorganized in arrangement.

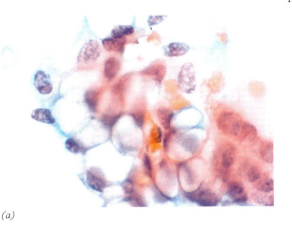

(a)

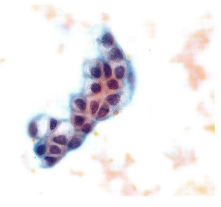

(b)

Fig. 7.15 Mucinous cystadenoma/ cystadenocarcinoma of bile ducts

(a) Papanicolaou ×1260 (b) ×840 (c) ×1260

Biliary cystadenoma tends to occur in women. It has a well-known tendency for malignant transformation. It is composed of columnar or cuboidal mucin-secreting epithelium which is mostly uniform (a, b). In mucinous cystadenocarcinoma (c) cells differ in size, nuclei show a coarse chromatin pattern and haphazard arrangement (c).

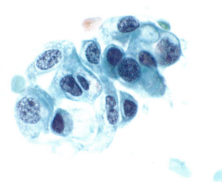

(c)

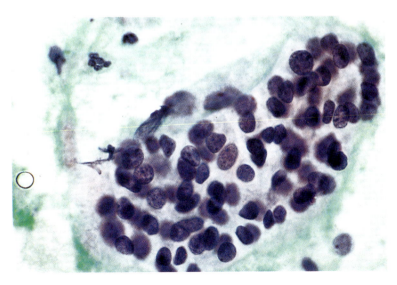

Fig. 7.16 Cholangiocytes

Papanicolaou ×720: FNA; liver

The liver synthesizes bile which is secreted into a system of fine canaliculi which drain into intrahepatic bile ducts, whence it is transported to the duodenum via the common bile duct. The lining cells of intrahepatic bile ducts, known as cholangiocytes, vary from cuboidal in the small ducts to low columnar in the larger ducts.

The cytoplasm of cholangiocytes is cyanophilic and sparse. The nuclei, about the size of a neutrophil, are round or oval, hyperchromic and granular. The nuclear-cytoplasmic ratio is high and a small nucleolus may be present. Cholangiocytes usually occur in groups and sheets and the monomorphism of the nuclei is a striking feature.

LIVER

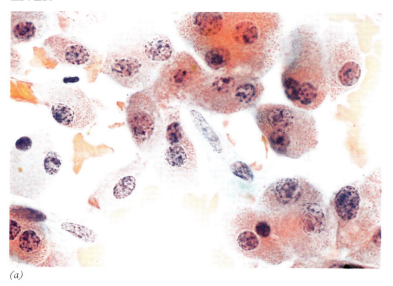

(a)

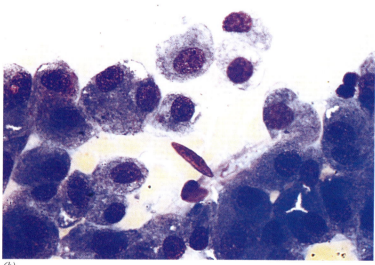

(b)

Fig. 7.17 Hepatocytes: Kupffer cells: bile pigment

(a) Papanicolaou ×720: FNA; liver (b) MGG ×720: same specimen; another smear (c) Papanicolaou ×720: FNA; liver; another case

The parenchymal liver cell or hepatocyte is a large polyhedral cell with abundant cytoplasm. This is eosinophilic with the Papanicolaou stain (a) and violet with MGG (b); however, the intensity of cytoplasmic staining varies with the metabolic state of the cell and may not be uniform throughout. The healthy liver cell is rich in organelles and glycogen, and at times lipid, and the cytoplasm may appear finely granular. The nucleus of the hepatocyte is round with evenly dispersed chromatin and the nuclear-cytoplasmic ratio is low on account of the large volume of cytoplasm. One or more prominent nucleoli are always present. The normal liver often contains a fair proportion of cells with double or quadruple the diploid complement of chromosomes. The tetraploid and polyploid cells may have large nuclei; in consequence, anisonucleosis is a frequently encountered feature of liver aspirates. Binucleate forms are often present (a, b) and the occasional cell may contain three (a) or more nuclei. Variation in the size and number of liver cell nuclei is without any diagnostic significance. Bile may be seen in the form of yellow or light brown intracytoplasmic granules of variable size (c). The sinusoids between plates of liver cells are lined by flattened slender cells with scant pale cytoplasm and elongated nuclei (a, b). These cells have a phagocytic function and are referred to as Kupffer cells.

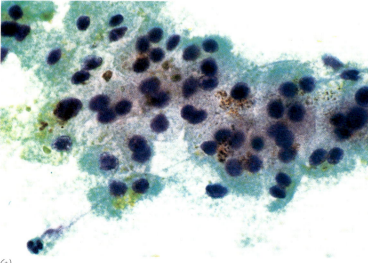

(c)

Fig. 7.18 Cirrhosis

FNA liver: Papanicolaou ×1160

Diagnosis of cirrhosis cannot be made on cytological material. Prominent anisonucleosis, inflammatory cells including polymorphs and stromal fragments are suggestive of this condition.

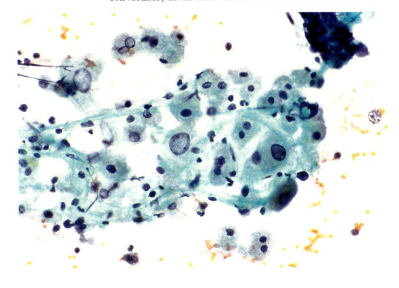

Fig. 7.19 Abscess

FNA liver: Papanicolaou ×580

FNA of liver in cases of known abscess is usually avoided. Cytological material showing abscess usually comes in the laboratory as a result from investigation of a 'cystic' lesion of unknown nature. In that context, the cytologist can helpfully diagnose abscess and exclude malignancy. Occasionally organisms, in particular amoebae, can be seen. For hydatid cyst fluid morphology see Chapter 3, Figure 3.32.

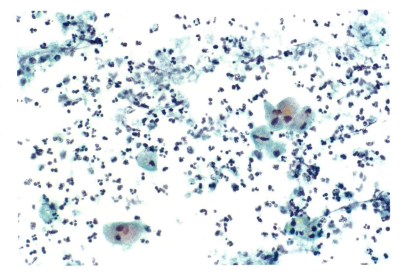

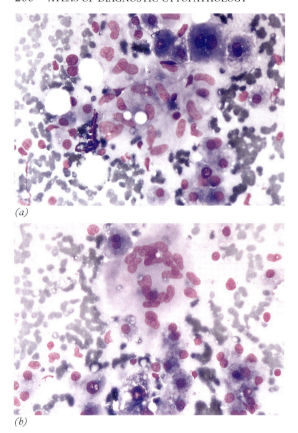

(a)

(b)

Fig. 7.20 Granuloma

FNA liver: (a) MGG ×840 (b) ×840 (courtesy of Dr Couchand Priollet)

The presence of epithelioid cells in combination with or without multinucleate giant cells suggests liver granulomas. Granulomas are associated with a variety of liver diseases and the cause needs detailed clinical and radiological investigation.

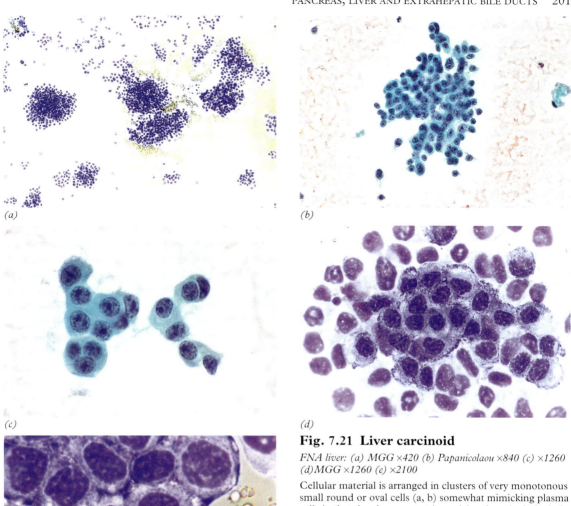

(a)

(b)

(c)

(d)

(e)

Fig. 7.21 Liver carcinoid

FNA liver: (a) MGG ×420 (b) Papanicolaou ×840 (c) ×1260 (d)MGG ×1260 (e) ×2100

Cellular material is arranged in clusters of very monotonous small round or oval cells (a, b) somewhat mimicking plasma cells in that they have eccentric nuclei and particularly dark basophilic cytoplasm on MGG stain (c–e). Careful examination reveals one or more small nucleoli (c, e) Immunocytochemistry to confirm neuroendocrine origin of the tumour (chromogranin) is helpful.

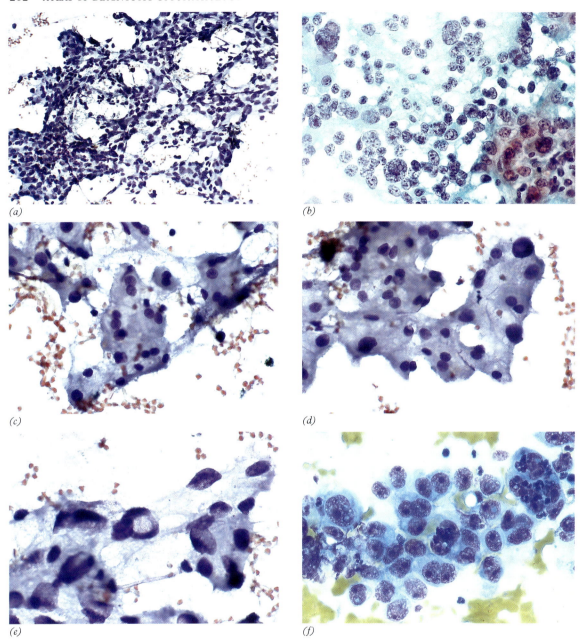

(a)

(b)

(c)

(d)

(e)

(f)

Fig. 7.22 Hepatocellular carcinoma

FNA liver: (a)Papanicolaou ×210 (b) ×840 (c) ×1260 (d) ×1260 (e) ×1260 (f) MGG ×1260 (g) AFP ×840

Primary liver cell carcinoma is a common cancer in some African countries but is relatively rare in the west. It often develops in pre-existing cirrhosis. Cells of well-differentiated hepatocellular carcinoma contain a nearly homogeneous population of morphologically normal hepatocytes, sometimes arranged in trabeculae or papillary-like clusters and often single (a, b). In some cases these are difficult to distinguish from regenerative liver epithelium (c, d). In these cases, extreme anisonucleosis, prominent nucleolus, presence of intranuclear vacuoles, transgressing endothelium (see Fig 7.23a, b), necrosis or intracellular bile granules may help to diagnose malignancy (e, f). Some authors emphasize the importance of atypical hepatocytic 'naked' nuclei for the diagnosis of hepatocellular carcinoma (b). These are not found in liver regeneration, nodular hyperplasia or other liver tumours. Staining of malignant hepatocytes for α-fetoprotein confirms their differentiation (g).

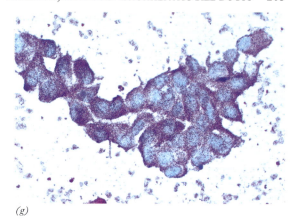

(g)

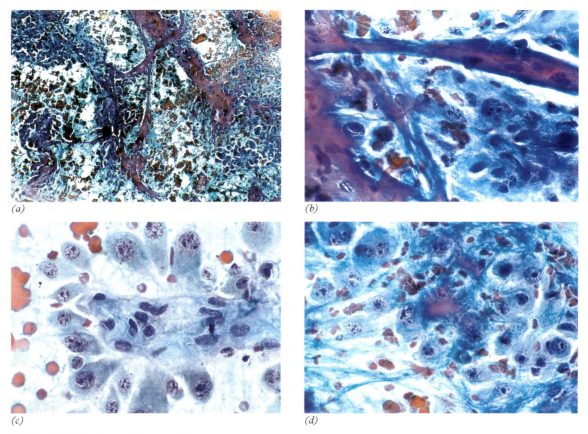

(a)   *(b)*

(c)   *(d)*

Fig 7.23 Fibrolamellar carcinoma

FNA liver, Pap stain: (a): ×420 (b) ×1260 (c) ×1260 (d) ×840 (courtesy of Dr Schroff, India)

This is biologically and morphologically a different tumour from all other hepatocellular carcinomas. It occurs in young adults (under 35) and arises in non-cirrhotic liver. Most of the patients have tumour confined to the liver at the time of diagnosis. Patients seldom have elevated serum AFP levels. They may resemble focal nodular hyperplasia in that they usually present as a single mass. Histologically, the tumour has thick collagen bands separating oxyphilic tumour cells.

Aspirates from this tumour are often scanty due to prominent fibrosis. Classically, they may contain collagen bundles and transgressing endothelium (a, b) surrounding dishesive oxyphilic cells (c) with frankly malignant, pleomorphic, hyperchromatic nuclei; macronucleoli; and abundant granular cytoplasm. Often, the smear contains only a few naked nuclei and oxyphilic cells with characteristic hyaline intracytoplasmic inclusions (d) and intranuclear pseudoinclusions.

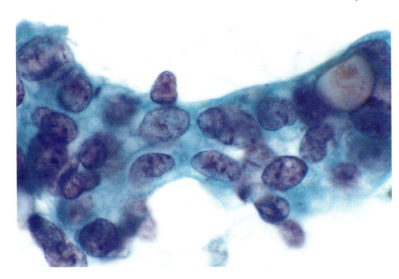

Fig. 7.24 Intrahepatic cholangiocarcinoma

FNA liver: Papanicolaou ×1160

Primary carcinoma of intrahepatic bile ducts is even more uncommon than primary liver carcinoma. Malignant cholangiocytes are larger than benign duct lining cells and the appearance and arrangement of the cells are that of an adenocarcinoma. Occasionally, as illustrated, intracellular bile is noted. Most cholangiocarcinomas are mucin-producing, which distinguishes them from hepatocellular carcinoma but not from a metastatic mucin-producing adenocarcinoma.

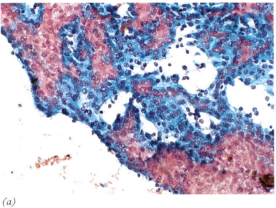

(a)

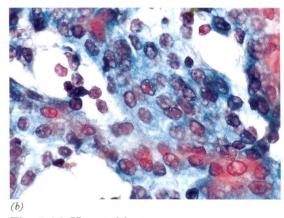

(b)

Fig. 7.25 Hepatoblastoma

FNA liver, child: Pap stain (a) ×200 (b) ×600 (c) ×600 (courtesy of Dr Schroff, India)

Hepatoblastoma is the most common primary liver tumour in children. Histologically, tumour types are subdivided into: epithelial; mixed epithelial and mesenchymal; and anaplastic or small cell undifferentiated, the epithelial type having the best prognosis after surgical resection.

Aspirates of *epithelial* type are very cellular and contain flat sheets and trabeculae of small round, crowded abnormal hepatocytes (a). Cells have a high nuclear-cytoplasmic ratio, prominent nucleoli and vacuolated or granular cytoplasm (b,c). Cells may form acini but transgressing epithelium has not been described.

Mixed, epithelial and mesenchymal type contains a mesenchymal component and shows more pleomorphism of epithelium. Small cell undifferentiated type is similar to other small cell tumours of childhood and relies on special techniques for definitive diagnosis (EM, immunocytochemistry).

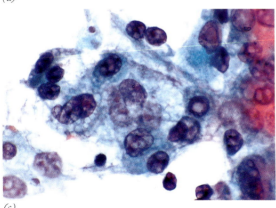

(c)

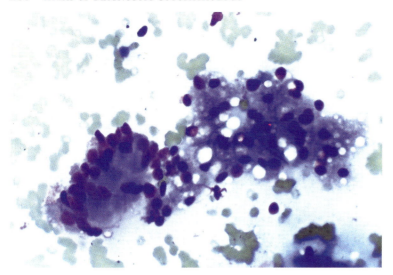

Fig. 7.26 Metastatic adenocarcinoma

FNA liver; MGG ×580

FNA cytology is relatively commonly used for confirmation of radiological suspicion of metastatic tumours. Sometimes, as in the case illustrated, it is possible to suggest that the tall columnar pseudostratified malignant cells probably originate from colonic carcinoma. Note the benign liver epithelium.

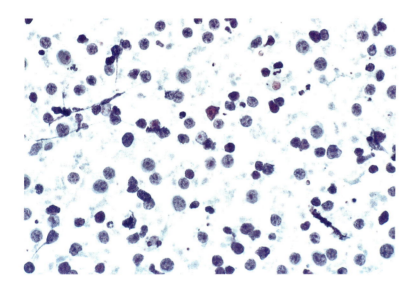

Fig. 7.27 Lymphoma

FNA liver; Papanicolaou ×1160

Liver FNA cytology is occasionally performed as part of the staging of patients with known non-Hodgkin's lymphomas. Only rarely is this the initial finding of the disease. Our case illustrates a high-grade B-cell non-Hodgkin's lymphoma composed of a uniform population of lymphoid blast cells. The immunocytochemistry panel of lymphoid and epithelial markers is helpful in distinguishing this from any other small-cell tumour, although the lack of cell cohesion and typical morphology and speckled chromatin pattern of lymphoid cells should cause no problems for diagnosis.

8. Urinary system

The role of cytopathology in this field is mainly limited to the diagnosis of malignant disease, a few benign disorders and a few parasitic infestations such as schistosomiasis and the occasional trichomoniasis of the male urethra may also be identified. The variety of inflammatory and autoimmune disorders, particularly of the kidney, is outside the scope of cytology.

SAMPLING TECHNIQUES

The different types of specimens that may be obtained and examined are normally voided and catheter specimens of urine, bladder washings, endoscopic brush and fine-needle aspiration (FNA) samples.

An early-morning specimen of urine, formerly recommended, is unsuitable as the cells in the highly concentrated urine are too degenerate to be assessable. A fresh specimen voided at any time may be used; a mid-morning specimen passed preferably 30–60 min after a drink such as tea or coffee is often convenient for the patient and the laboratory. The specimen should be despatched to the laboratory without delay as cell deterioration can be fairly rapid.

Urine and bladder washings are centrifuged and smears made from the deposit. As urine is often hypocellular, it is desirable to concentrate the cells by using part of the specimen to make a millipore filter preparation. Crystals which form *in vitro* may render a urine cloudy and mask the cells in the smear; phosphates may be removed by the addition of 1% acetic acid and urates by gentle heating.

Brush and aspiration smears are prepared and processed as for other organ systems. Smears from all types of specimens listed above may be stained by the Papanicolaou and Romanowsky methods.

URINARY TRACT

Fig. 8.1 Transitional cells

Papanicolaou ×720: ureteric urine

The urinary tract is lined with transitional epithelium, also referred to as urothelium. The morphology of normal transitional cells is illustrated in a fresh specimen of urine obtained through a ureteric ureter, as cells in bladder urine tend to be sparse and degenerate. The cells to the lower right are fairly small and vary little in size. They have a moderate amount of cytoplasm and round or oval nuclei with scanty chromatin and micronucleoli. The shape varies: cuboidal, pyramidal and cylindrical forms are seen. The variation in shape is an artefact created by the spread of the smear. Substantially larger cells with abundant cytoplasm are seen to the top left of the field. The nuclei of these cells are identical in shape, staining reaction and chromatin content with the nuclei of the smaller cells but number from one to three per cell. The larger cells are derived from the surface layer of the urothelium, extend across two or three smaller subjacent cells and are known as umbrella cells.

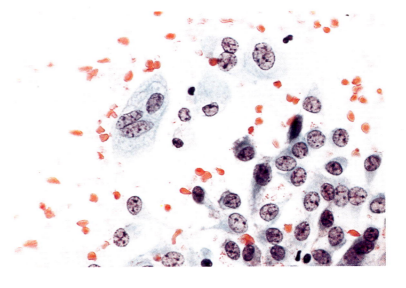

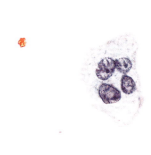

Fig. 8.2 Umbrella cell

Papanicolaou ×525: voided urine

An umbrella cell with four nuclei is illustrated in this micrograph. Apart from the larger size, the distinctive feature of these surface urothelial cells is the exceptional thickness of their distal plasma membrane. The thick membranes render the epithelium impermeable to urine and protect it from the toxic effects of what is essentially a hypertonic toxic solution. The cytoplasm of the umbrella cell is slightly foamy.

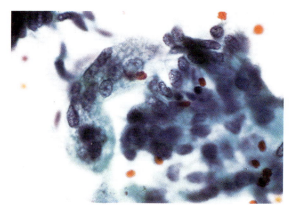

Fig. 8.3 Transitional cells

Papanicolaou ×525: ureteric brush

Diagnostic material may be obtained from the upper urinary tract with a fine endoscopic brush guided at cystoscopy into the ureter as far as the renal pelvis. Cells obtained by this method usually appear in sheets. Normal transitional cells are illustrated in this micrograph. The small overlapping cells in the right lower corner are deeper urothelial cells and two multinucleated umbrella cells are seen to the left.

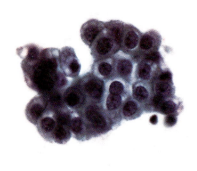

(a)

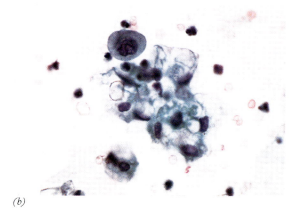

(b)

Fig. 8.4 Reactive transitional cells

Papanicolaou ×525 (a) voided urine (b) voided urine; other case

The cells illustrated in these micrographs were recovered from urine from two patients with large stones in the renal pelvis. The irritation to the renal pelvis epithelium caused by constant friction may induce reactive hyperplastic changes and abnormally excessive exfoliation. The cells in (a) are arranged in a honeycomb pattern. They are uniform in size, have round and regular nuclei and contain perinuclear haloes. The chromatin content is greater than in normal transitional cells and the cytoplasm beyond the vacuoles is dense and basophilic. The appearance is of

hyperplastic cells overtaken by degenerative changes. These are more advanced in (b). Excepting one cell, the cytoplasm is filled with hydropic vacuoles. The nuclei are structureless, crenated and are pushed to the periphery of the cells, which appear signet-ring-shaped.

Changes produced in transitional epithelium by a renal stone may prove misleading and be a potential source of an incorrect interpretation of malignancy, particularly an adenocarcinoma.

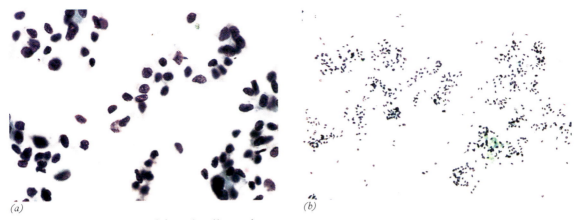

(a)   *(b)*

Fig. 8.5 Papillary transitional cell carcinoma

Papanicolaou (a) ×525: voided urine (b) ×133: same field; pattern of spontaneous exfoliation

The sensitivity of urinary cytology in the diagnosis of urothelial malignancy varies directly with the histological grade and type of tumour and is notoriously poor for low-grade papillary carcinoma. The cells that cover the finger-like projections of these tumours are extremely well-differentiated and virtually indistinguishable from benign transitional cells. Tumour cells from a grade 1 papillary carcinoma of the bladder mucosa are illustrated in micrograph (a). In shape, they resemble benign transitional cells (Fig. 8.1) and in size, are, if anything, smaller on account of the degenerative changes. The hyperchromasia of the nuclei is due to pyknotic degeneration and a cytodiagnostic assessment of nuclear pleomorphism and

disorganized chromatin pattern is inapplicable.

The one significant feature seen here (b) is the degree and pattern of cell exfoliation. Urine, which is normally hypocellular, may in some cases of low-grade papillary tumours contain showers of more or less normal-looking cells. The majority of cells are discrete, but a few cell aggregates or microbiopsies are present. This appearance can be the basis of a correct diagnosis in the absence of cystitis or lithiasis. The criterion, however, is applicable only to normally voided urine and has no relevance to cases in which a significantly large population of normal-looking cells is dislodged by iatrogenic causes such as catheterization or surgical exploration.

Fig. 8.6 Transitional cell carcinoma

MGG ×720: voided urine

Exfoliative urine cytology is of greater value in the diagnosis of higher grades of urothelial carcinomas when the standard criteria of malignancy can be applied. The cells in this case of a grade 3 carcinoma are large. The nuclei and the nuclear-cytoplasmic ratio are significantly variable and nuclear pleomorphism is a notable feature. The degree and pattern of exfoliation are not relevant when frankly malignant cells are seen, and the number of neoplastic cells exfoliated is often small.

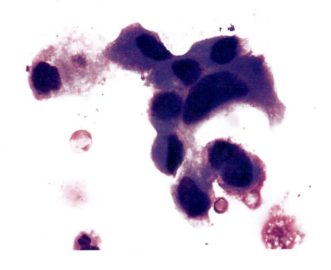

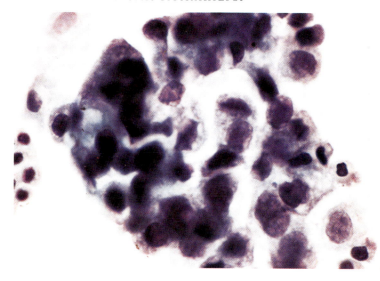

Fig. 8.7 Transitional cell carcinoma

Papanicolaou ×720: bladder washings

The yield of tumour cells may be increased by washing out the bladder with normal saline: this procedure is usually carried out at cystoscopy. Bladder washings contain numerous cells which are often aggregated in large sheets. In this example the cells and nuclei are large and there is significant variation in the size of the nuclei and the nuclear-cytoplasmic ratio.

Bladder washings collected at check cystoscopy are of particular value in patients being followed up after a treated transitional cell carcinoma. Neoplastic transformation of the urothelium occurs in subjects exposed to industrial toxins and is usually multifocal. A transitional cell carcinoma may remain *in situ* for a long period and this and some deeply infiltrating tumours may not be identifiable at cystoscopy or by retrograde urography. Washing out the bladder dislodges many cells, some of which may be informative and form the basis for further management.

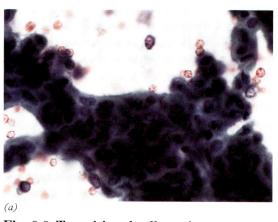

(a)

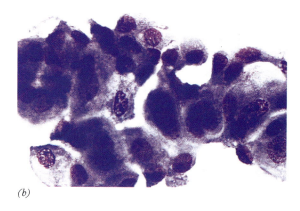

(b)

Fig. 8.8 Transitional cell carcinoma

(a) Papanicolaou ×525: renal pelvis brush (b) MGG ×525: renal pelvis brush; another case

Tumours in the upper part of the urinary tract may be sampled with a brush which removes large numbers of cohesive cells. These micrographs illustrate two cases of grade 2 carcinoma of the renal pelvis. The cells in (a) are small, but the nuclei are disproportionately large and crowded together. A moderate degree of anisonucleosis is seen. The cells in (b), being air-dried, appear larger and variations in nuclear size and nuclear-cytoplasmic ratio are more obvious. Small but distinct nucleoli are seen.

Fig. 8.9 Transitional cell carcinoma

MGG ×720: FNA; renal pelvis

Another useful approach to a tumour in the renal pelvis is by percutaneous fine aspiration. A case of grade 2 transitional cell carcinoma sampled by this method is illustrated in this micrograph. An important point to bear in mind in the assessment of brush and aspiration specimens is that the cells obtained by these methods differ in appearance from cells exfoliated in urine. The arrangement of the cells may resemble that of adenocarcinoma cells and distinction between a urothelial and a renal cell carcinoma may on occasion be difficult.

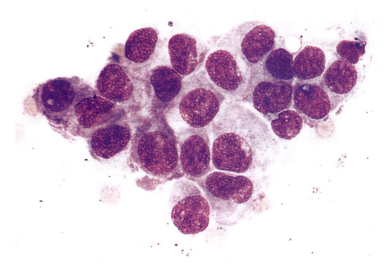

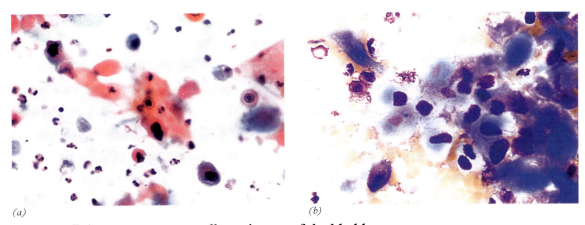

(a)   *(b)*

Fig. 8.10 Primary squamous cell carcinoma of the bladder

(a) Papanicolaou ×525: voided urine (b) MGG ×525: same specimen, another smear

Squamous cell carcinoma of the bladder usually develops in a pre-existing metaplastic squamous epithelium which is formed in response to chronic irritation such as a stone or a parasitic infestation. It is the commonest type of bladder carcinoma in geographical regions in which schistosomiasis is endemic; elsewhere it constitutes less than 5% of urinary tract neoplasms. The male urethra contains foci of squamous epithelium which may, very rarely, become neoplastic.

The case illustrated in this micrograph, of an English woman without renal tract lithiasis, a normal genital tract and no history of exposure to a provocative parasite, is a sporadic one. The malignant cells in the urine are well-differentiated and bizarre-shaped, have cytoplasmic bulbous expansions and India ink nuclei (a). The pale or azure staining of the cytoplasm with May–Grünwald–Giemsa (MGG) is often seen in a keratinized cell.

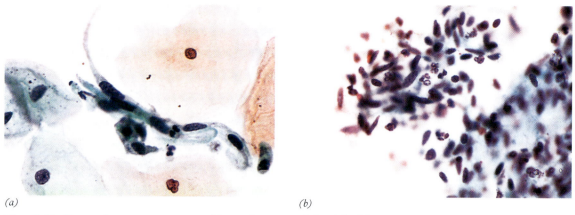

(a)   *(b)*

Fig. 8.11 Secondary squamous cell carcinoma of the bladder

Papanicolaou (a) ×525: catheter urine (b) ×333: catheter urine; another case

Squamous carcinoma of the bladder in the female is more likely to be an extension of a primary genital tract tumour and investigation should include vaginal and/or cervical cytology. Two examples of secondary involvement of the bladder are illustrated in these micrographs. The poorly differentiated, fibre-shaped malignant squamous cells in (a) were recovered from a catheter specimen of urine. Biopsy histology of a puckered ulcerated area on the posterior wall

of the bladder confirmed infiltration by a genital tract squamous carcinoma. The patient had a history of CIN and VAIN and subsequent invasive carcinoma of the vagina. The sheet of poorly differentiated, spindle-shaped malignant squamous cells in (b) is from a woman with stage 4 carcinoma of the cervix and a vesicovaginal fistula. To ensure against vaginal contamination, urine cytology in such a case should be done on a catheter specimen.

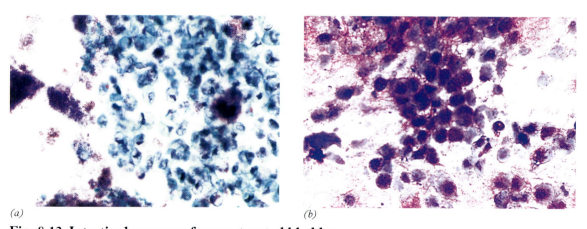

(a)   *(b)*

Fig. 8.12 Intestinal mucosa of reconstructed bladder

Papanicolaou ×525: voided urine; caecocystoplasty (b) MGG ×525: voided urine; ileal bladder, another case

Two examples of urine cytology of patients with bladders reconstructed from the intestine following total cystectomy are illustrated. The cells are of glandular origin and markedly degenerate. In (a) they have signet-ring shapes

and in (b) they are arranged in a honeycomb against a background of homogeneous material. Mucin secreted by the intestinal mucosa cells is often present in these specimens. Neoplastic transformation may occur.

Fig. 8.13 Viral cytopathia

Papanicolaou (a) ×720: voided urine
(b) ×720: voided urine; another case

Urothelial cells may show cytopathic effects in a number of viral infections. The variable appearances illustrated in these micrographs have been attributed to polyomaviruses. The cells in (a) were seen in the urine of a 5-year-old boy with a febrile illness of short duration, abdominal lymphadenopathy and a high erythrocyte sedimentation rate. Mononuclear and multinucleated forms are seen; the size of the cell being proportional with the number of nuclei. These are uniformly pale and homogeneous and are ringed by a narrow band of chromatin on the nuclear membrane. The cells in (b) from the urine of a 3-year-old boy, also with a febrile illness but no lymphadenopathy, contain intranuclear inclusions which are punctate in the cell on the left and large and dense in the cell to the right.

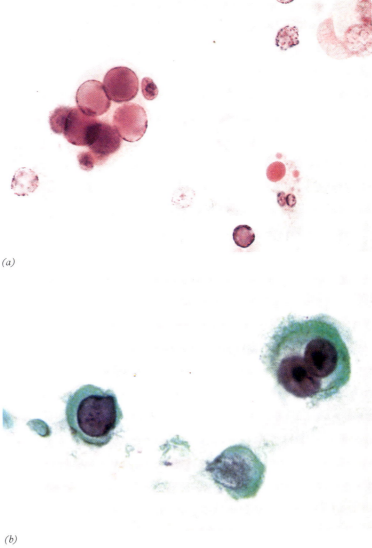

(a)

(b)

Fig. 8.14 Histiocyte with inclusion

Papanicolaou ×720: voided urine

The urine may occasionally have small structures which seem to be peculiar to it, and virtually identify the specimen. These are probably histiocytes and are characterized by the presence of smooth contoured eosinophilic or orange inclusions. The identity of these inclusions is not known and, as far as can be determined, these bodies do not have pathological significance. Compare with viral changes in the preceding micrograph.

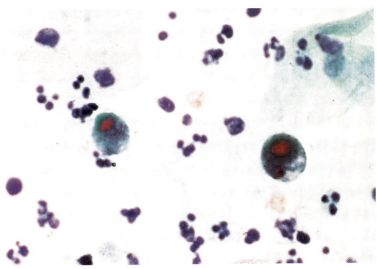

Fig. 8.15 Pollen

Papanicolaou ×525: voided urine

A contaminant which bears a superficial resemblance to a schistosome (see Fig. 8. 16) but is, in fact, a pollen grain, may be seen in urine. It is distinguished from an ovum by its smaller size, the bipolar angular terminations of its capsule and its generalized granularity.

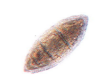

Fig. 8.16 *Schistosoma haematobium*

(a) Papanicolaou ×333: voided urine; ovum (b) MGG ×333: voided urine; ovum; another case (c) Papanicolaou ×333: same smear as (a); another field; miracidium

Schistosomiasis or bilharziasis is caused by three closely related trematodes, whose definitive host is a fresh-water snail. Infection is acquired when cercarial larvae released by the snail into water penetrate the skin of the human host. The larvae enter the venous capillaries and make their way into the systemic circulation by a circuitous route through the right side of the heart, the pulmonary circulatory system, into the left ventricle.

From the mesenteric blood vessels, they enter the portal venous system where the adult worms reach maturity. *S. japonicum* and *S. mansoni* preferentially infest the digestive tract. *S. haematobium* travels to the capillaries of the bladder where the female deposits her eggs. These are embedded in the bladder mucosa which becomes inflamed and eventually responds by undergoing squamous metaplasia. The eggs may rupture through the mucosa and be passed in urine. The ova of the three species are distinguished by their size and the position of the spine. The ovum of *S. haematobium* is large and has a terminal spine (a, b) at one pole. An embryo is faintly discernible in (a). Aggregates of inflammatory cells may accompany the ovum (b). On contact with fresh water, the embryo in the egg hatches into a miracidium, the surface of which is covered with numerous cilia (c). The miracidium penetrates the specific snail host and the life cycle is repeated. The miracidium illustrated in (c) was one of several in a voided specimen of urine; dilution with fresh water is assumed to have occurred at some stage.

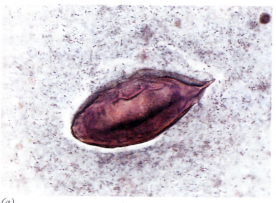

(a)

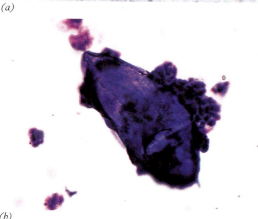

(b)

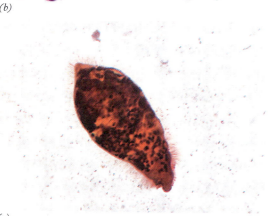

(c)

KIDNEY

Fig. 8.17 Benign renal cyst

Papanicolaou ×133: FNA; kidney

Fluid from a benign renal cyst is generally straw-coloured or, on occasion, slightly tinged with blood. The cell content varies in quantity and consists mainly of large foam cells with degenerate nuclei. Iron-laden macrophages or histiocytic cells with autofluorescent, yellow-green granules of lipofuscin (known as the ageing pigment) may also be seen. The appearance is non-specific and identical to the cellular presentation of some cases of duct ectasia of the breast (Fig. 2.7) or an inclusion cyst of the ovary (Fig. 1.48).

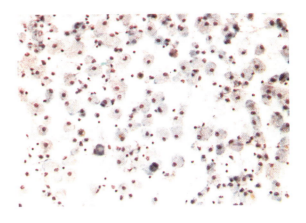

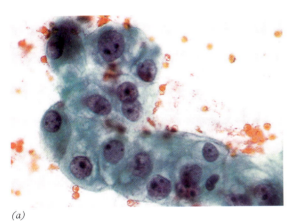

(a)

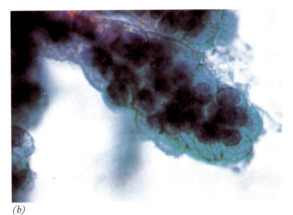

(b)

Fig. 8.18 Renal cell carcinoma

Papanicolaou (a) ×525: FNA; kidney (b) ×832: FNA; kidney; another case (c) same smear as (b); another field

Renal cell carcinoma, also referred to as hypernephroma or clear cell carcinoma, is an adenocarcinoma of the renal tubule epithelium. The tumour cells are large and polygonal in shape (a, b). The cytoplasm is abundant, and vacuolated (a) and may be foamy (b). The nuclei are generally round and may be hypochromic (a); the chromatin content may be small and the nuclear-cytoplasmic ratio low (a, b). In some cases or in some areas of a renal cell carcinoma, the nuclei may appear deceptively bland (a). The diagnosis may prove difficult unless these features are taken into account. Smaller cells with non-vacuolated, uniformly staining cytoplasm and a relatively high nuclear-cytoplasmic ratio (c) may be additionally present or constitute the main or sole population of another histological variant. Large prominent nucleoli are always present in both types of cells.

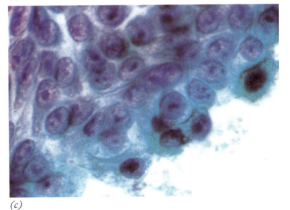

(c)

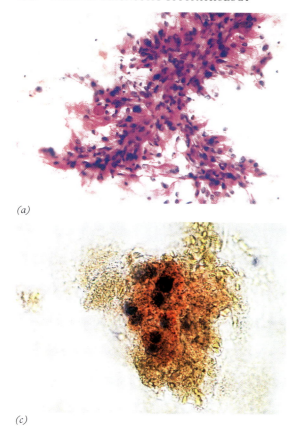

(a)

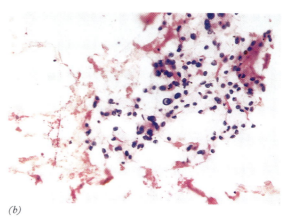

(b)

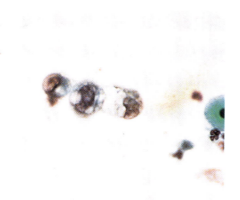

(c)

Fig. 8.19 Renal cell carcinoma

(a) PAS ×133: FNA; kidney (b) D-PAS ×133: same specimen; another smear (c) Sudan III (oil scarlet) ×333: same smear; another smear

The clear or foamy appearance of the cytoplasm of malignant renal cells is due to accumulation of glycogen and lipid; mucin is not secreted by these cells. It is advisable to confirm these biochemical characteristics in a suspected renal cell carcinoma for three reasons. First, a needle aspiration may not contain ancillary evidence by which the target organ can be identified; second, the specimen may be contaminated by benign intestinal mucosa, even when the approach is from the flank; third, a renal cell carcinoma may appear deceptively bland on account of its low nuclear-cytoplasmic ratio and hypochromic nuclei. Micrograph (a) demonstrates the positivity with periodic acid-Schiff (PAS) of both the cells and the connective tissue in which they are embedded in an aspirate of a renal cell carcinoma. Prior digestion with diastase has removed the glycogen from the cells but not the mucopolysaccharides from the connective tissue (b). Abundant intra- and extracellular lipid droplets are confirmed by a fat stain in (c).

Fig. 8.20 Renal cell carcinoma

Papanicolaou ×525: voided urine

Malignant renal cells may be seen in urine when the tumour has ruptured through the renal pelvis. The cells in this micrograph are copiously vacuolated, have smooth outlines and the arrangement of adenocarcinoma cells. The nuclei are variable in size and a nucleolus is seen in the cell to the left. As will be seen, the cells and particularly the nuclei are extremely degenerate. This is usually the case with exfoliated malignant renal cells and a urine cytology diagnosis of a renal primary is, in most cases, tentative.

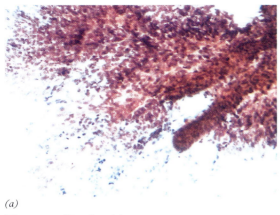

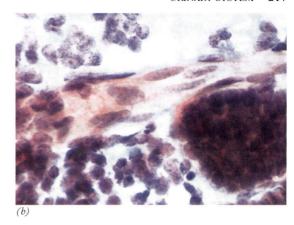

(a)   *(b)*

Fig. 8.21 Nephroblastoma

Papanicolaou (a) ×133: FNA; kidney (b) ×525: same smear; another field

This embryonal tumour, also known as Wilms tumour, is one of the most aggressive and important tumours of early childhood. The neoplastic transformation is believed to occur in embryonic renal blastema in the prenatal period and the tumour contains both sarcomatous and carcinomatous elements (a). Cellular detail is seen in (b). The sarcomatous element consists of pleomorphic plump and slender fusiform or spindle-shaped nuclei in a pink-staining matrix. This is flanked above and below by small, round, undifferentiated cells with virtually no cytoplasm and finely granular nuclei. The epithelial element, seen in the lower right corner, also consists of small round cells which are organized into a tubular structure.

Wilms tumour can be identified in an FNA specimen without difficulty when all the components of the tumour are present. In the absence of a sarcomatous element, the differential diagnosis would include neuroblastoma. In the absence of tubular structures, an undifferentiated rhabdomyosarcoma and a high-grade lymphoma need to be taken into account.

Wilms tumour may occasionally develop in renal tissue rests outside the kidney.

Fig. 8.22 Metastatic squamous cell carcinoma

Papanicolaou ×720: FNA; kidney

The kidney is not infrequently involved in malignant lymphoma and may be the site of a metastatic carcinoma. In considering the latter, care needs to be taken to confirm that the secondary deposit is not in the adrenal, which is a commoner site of metastatic disease. This may not be possible by ultrasound or cytology when the upper pole of kidney appears to be involved. In the case illustrated in the micrograph, extremely well-differentiated malignant squamous cells were aspirated from a mass circumscribed within the kidney. The patient was a known case of squamous cell carcinoma of the lung.

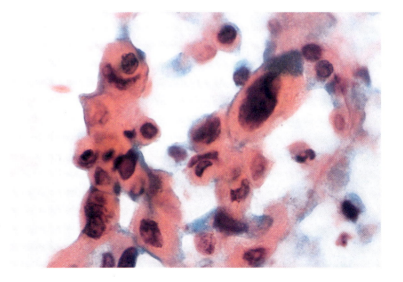

9. Male genital system

The widest application of cytopathology of the male genital system is in fine-needle aspiration (FNA) of the prostate. Testicular tumours are only occasionally sampled for cytology as the complexity of their structure and prognostic assessment require detailed examination of greater amounts of tissue than are obtained with a fine needle. The presence of tumour markers and their focal variation are also better assessed in sections. A specimen commonly submitted for cytology is hydrocoele or spermatocoele fluid.

An important practical point for consideration is that spermatozoa do not adhere firmly to a glass slide, even an albuminized one, and are likely to float off on to other slides processed in the same batch. This may be avoided by using separate jars of fixative and stains for smears of fluid from the scrotal sac.

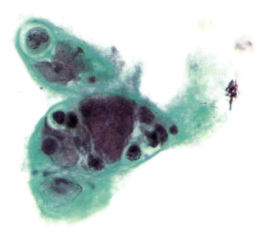

Fig. 9.1 Herpes simplex virus (HSV)

Papanicolaou ×720: penile scrape

A herpetic lesion on the penis, usually caused by the sexually transmitted HSV type 2 may be easily and rapidly diagnosed by cytology. An intact vesicle is ruptured and the droplet of fluid and a scrape of the floor of the vesicle used to make a single smear. Squamous cells with characteristic cytopathic effects, described in Chapter 1, are observed. A secondarily infected herpetic lesion is unsuitable for study.

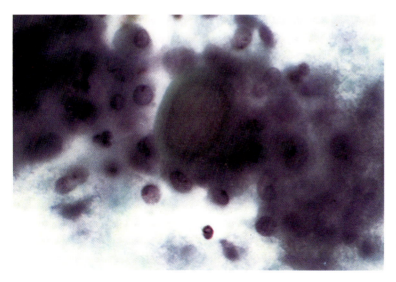

Fig. 9.2 Corpora amylacea

Papanicolaou ×720: voided urine; millipore filter

The elliptical organized structure with concentric rings seen in the centre of the field is a corpora amylacea and is the form in which prostatic secretion is stored. These structures may be seen in the prostate gland of the adult male, and increase in number with advancing years, and may become calcified. The structure illustrated was seen in the urine of a 65-year-old male with benign nodular hyperplasia of the prostate and urinary frequency. Exfoliation of corpora amylacea in urine is uncommon, does not denote a papillary tumour and is without diagnostic significance.

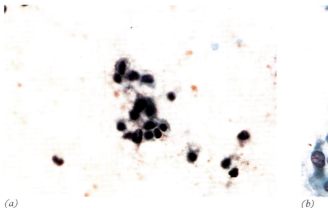

(a)

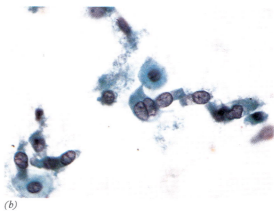

(b)

Fig. 9.3 Prostatic cells

Papanicolaou ×525 (a) prostate fluid (b) prostate fluid: another case

Prostatic epithelial cells are usually present in a needle aspirate. FNA is better avoided in a case of suspected prostatitis and material may be obtained via the urethra after prostatic massage. The appearance of the cells varies with the degree of secretory activity, which is under the influence of androgenic hormones. Inactive prostatic epithelial cells are small, cuboidal and have darkly staining condensed nuclei (a). The active cells are larger and columnar in shape, the cytoplasm may be finely vacuolated; the basally situated nuclei are vesicular (b).

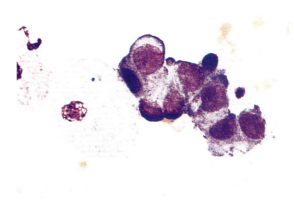

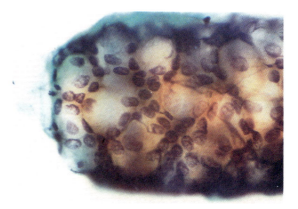

Fig. 9.4 Adenocarcinoma of the prostate

MGG ×525: Franzen needle aspirate; prostate

This micrograph illustrates malignant cells from a well-differentiated adenocarcinoma of the prostate. The cells are large and display anisocytosis and anisonucleosis. Most of the nuclei are eccentric in position and some lie on the outer contour of the cell; nucleoli are often large in prostatic carcinoma and are seen in three nuclei.

The cohesiveness of the cells varies with the degree of differentiation and diminishes with increasing anaplasia.

Fig. 9.5 Rectal mucosa

Papanicolaou ×525: Franzen needle aspirate; prostate

The Franzen needle used for aspiration biopsy of the prostate is introduced per rectum and it is quite common to see benign rectal mucosa in a prostatic aspiration smear. It is important to distinguish it from prostatic tissue and thereby avoid an incorrect diagnosis of a mucin-secreting adenocarcinoma. The colonic mucosa is often arranged in acini and may be identified by the large goblet cells with distended vacuolated cytoplasm and small nuclei.

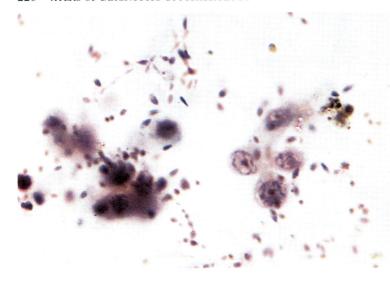

Fig. 9.6 Carcinoma of the prostate

Papanicolaou ×720: voided urine

The adenocarcinoma cells in this micrograph were seen in the urine of a patient with a known carcinoma of the prostate. These tumours may release cells into the urethra, but this occurrence is relatively uncommon. Compare these cells with the exfoliated renal cell carcinoma cells in Figure 8.20 and note the resemblance. Distinction between a prostatic carcinoma, a primary adenocarcinoma of the bladder and a renal cell carcinoma is seldom possible by exfoliative cytology and the presumptive diagnosis should be correlated with the clinical, radiological and biochemical findings. Note the spermatozoa and the fungal pseudohyphae—the latter are contaminants.

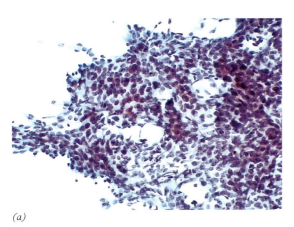

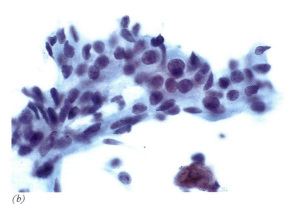

(a)   *(b)*

Fig. 9.7 Carcinoma of prostate

(a) Papanicolaou ×420 (b) ×1260 FNA of prostate

Aspirates of prostatic carcinoma are cellular: cells are arranged in three-dimensional clusters rather than sheets. They often form acini and this microacinar pattern (a) often precedes obvious features of malignancy (b). Malignant cells in less differentiated carcinomas are often more dispersed and show anisonucleosis, overlapping of nuclei and crowding. Nucleoli are small and inconspicuous in well-differentiated carcinoma and prominent, multiple and often angular in poorly differentiated carcinomas.

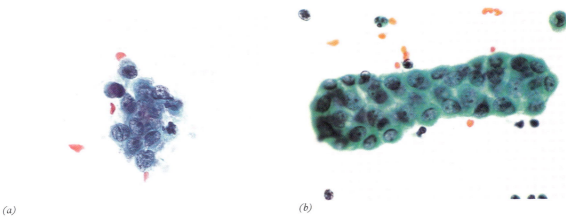

(a)   *(b)*

Fig. 9.8 Hydrocoele

Papanicolaou ×525: (a) FNA: scrotum (b) FNA: scrotum; another case

Aspiration of a fluid from a hydrocoele, which is an accumulation of fluid in the scrotal sac, serves a double function, being both diagnostic and therapeutic. The scrotal sac, an extension of the peritoneum, is lined with mesothelium. The cellular presentation of a hydrocoele is variable. In some cases, all the cells show hydropic degeneration and are foamy; in others, better preserved mesothelial cells are also present. Less commonly, the mesothelial cells are hyperplastic and arranged in acinar (a) or tubular (b) structures. This cytological appearance may be associated with papillary excrescences on the inner surface of the mesothelial lining.

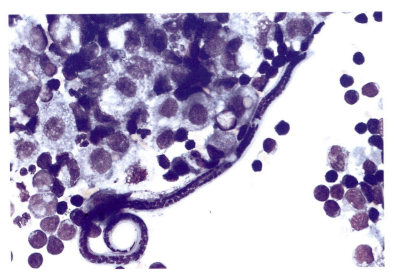

Fig. 9.9 Microfilaria

MGG ×1740

Hydrocoele fluid contains numerous inflammatory cells and microfilarial parasites of the *Onchocerca* species.

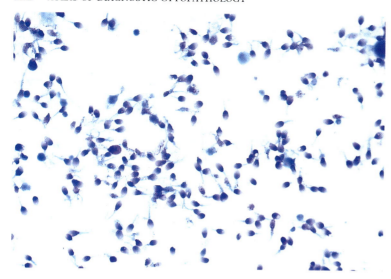

Fig. 9.10 Spermatocoele

MGG ×1740

Fluid within the testicular membranes caused by the occlusion of one of the efferent ducts of the epididymis contains numerous spermatozoa. These can be admixed with precursors of spermatogenesis which appear as darker 'normoblast'-like cells. Mesothelial cells can be present.

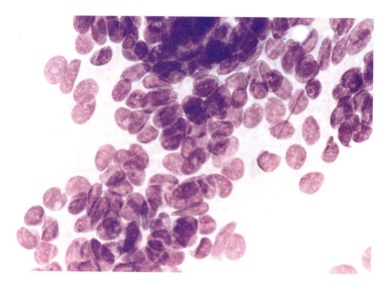

Fig. 9.11 Sertoli cell tumour

MGG ×1740 FNA testis (courtesy of Dr K Trutin Ostovic)

This is a rare tumour, accounting for 1% of testicular neoplasms. Differentiation of this tumour from reactive Sertoli-cell hyperplasia in chromosomal abnormalities and cryptorchidism and predominance of Sertoli cells in testicular atrophy is important. Aspirates of Sertoli-cell tumour contain uniform, lipid-rich Sertoli cells with oval nuclei lying in cohesive aggregates occasionally forming rosettes and tubules.

The large cell calcifying variant of Sertoli cell tumour contains polygonal cells with prominent nucleoli. Calcium and bone formation may be reflected in the aspirates.

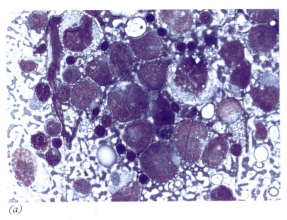

(a)

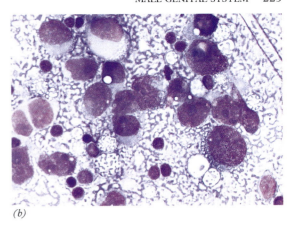

(b)

Fig. 9.12 Seminoma

(a) MGG ×840 (b) 840 imprint of tumour

Seminomas classically present in cytology preparations as loose aggregates and single cells with oval or irregular nuclei, prominent central nucleoli, fine chromatin pattern and vacuolated cytoplasm. There is often an admixture of lymphocytes. A lace-like 'tigroid' background is typical of seminoma.

Spermatocytic and anaplastic variants of seminoma are rare. The former contains an admixture of spermatocytes; the latter is often indistinguishable from testicular teratomas.

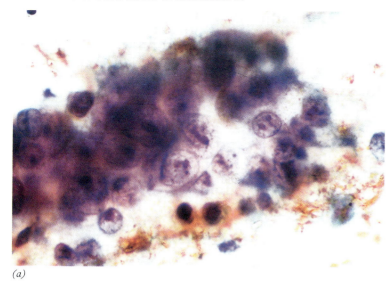

(a)

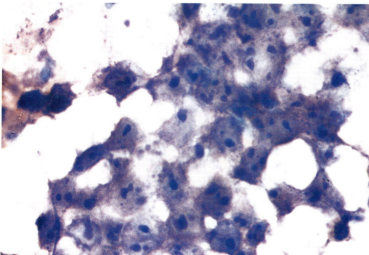

(b)

Fig. 9.13 Malignant teratoma undifferentiated of the testis

(a) Papanicolaou ×720: FNA; testis
(b) MGG ×720: same specimen; another smear

Malignant tumours of the testis include seminomas and teratomas or a combination of the two. The teratomas are thought to be derived from multipotent cells. Many histological variants have been classified. A well-differentiated teratoma may contain an assortment of recognizable adult tissue, whereas an undifferentiated tumour may be totally anaplastic. The tumours occur in younger age groups, and a case of a malignant teratoma in a 35-year-old man is illustrated in these micrographs. The cells are seen in a solid sheet and are poorly differentiated. The large nuclei are surrounded by a narrow rim of cytoplasm and contain polymorphic macronucleoli. The malignant nature of the cells is obvious but it must be appreciated that cytology does not contribute much more than the recognition of malignancy.

Immunocytochemical studies for human chorionic gonadotrophin and α-fetoprotein are possible but interpretation may be rendered difficult by the blood and cell necrosis that is often seen. The diagnosis of malignant teratoma undifferentiated was established by histological examination of the orchidectomy specimen.

10. Lymph nodes and thymus

INTRODUCTION

Role of FNA cytology in diagnosis of lymph node and thymic conditions

Fine-needle aspiration cytology (FNAC) has its application in lymph node pathology in three major clinical settings: primary diagnosis, staging of disease and follow-up.

Primary diagnosis made on FNAC in a patient with lymphadenopathy may be requested for:

1. Anatomical purposes (e.g. confirming that the nodule at the angle of mandible is a hyperplastic lymph node, and not a salivary gland lesion).

2. Confirmation of a suspected clinical condition (e.g. metastatic carcinoma).

3. First-line investigation in a patient with lymphadenopathy of unknown cause.

FNAC report should classify a lesion into one of three main categories:

1. Hyperplastic lymph node (infection/granuloma).

2. Metastatic tumour (or absence of it).

3. Lymphoma (Hodgkin's and non-Hodgkin's).

Staging of disease is usually undertaken in patients with known primary tumour (e.g. lymphoma) to establish the extent of the disease (e.g. subdiaphragmatic).

Follow-up of patients with a history of malignancy (e.g. carcinoma of the breast) provides accurate confirmation of recurrence.

Histological confirmation should be sought by the reporting cytopathologist in all instances where:

1. FNAC contains inadequate material.

2. There is persistent lymphadenopathy in a patient with FNAC report of lymph node hyperplasia.

3. There is a primary diagnosis of lymphoma on FNAC (either Hodgkin's or non-Hodgkin's).

By including this management recommendation as part of the FNAC report, the cytopathologist will avoid the inevitable question from clinicians: "should we biopsy it?"

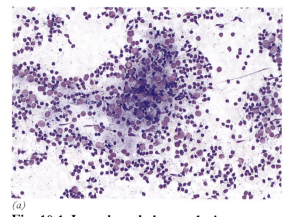

(a)

Fig. 10.1 Lymph node hyperplasia

(a) MGG ×420, (b) same case ×1260 (c) ×1260 (d) ×1260 (e) ×1260

Lymph node aspirate yields numerous lymphoid cells. Low power reveals aggregates of lymphocytes and follicle centre cells, within which bare nuclei of dendritic reticulum cells are seen (a). Their nuclei are oval in shape and often have prominent nucleoli. Cytoplasm is barely visible, poorly outlined and engulfs most of the follicle centre cells (b, c). Apart from small lymphocytes, these include centrocytes, centroblasts and plasma cells (d). Sometimes, tight aggregates of small lymphocytes can also be seen. These are not to be confused with aggregates of metastatic small cell tumours. In cases of acute lymph node reaction, e.g. infectious mononucleosis, numerous centroblasts dominate cytological appearances (d). The presence of follicle centres should point to the condition as reactive and serology often confirms the diagnosis.

Dermatopathic lymphadenopathy often requires a clinical history of skin disease. It is a brisk reactive lymph node hyperplasia with prominence of eosinophils and tingible body macrophages (e). In cases of cutaneous T-cell lymphoma it is probably wise to avoid making a decision about the possible regional lymph node involvement and to suggest biopsy for T-cell receptor gene rearrangement study as an aid to diagnosis in cases of doubt.

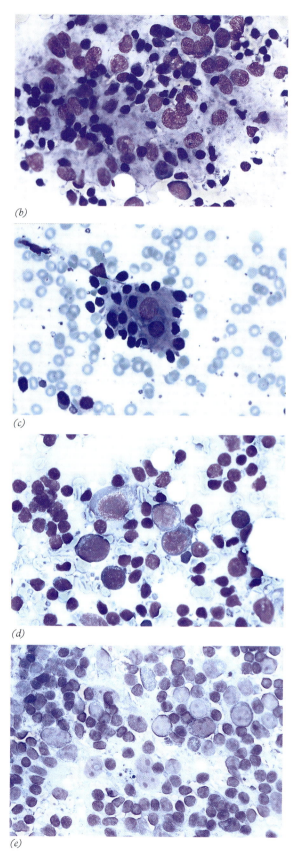

(b)

(c)

(d)

(e)

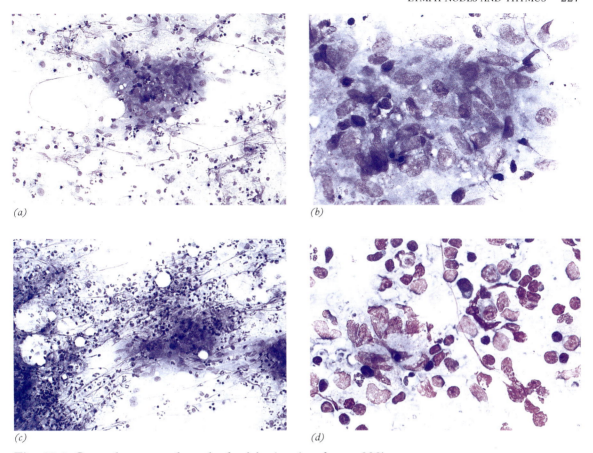

(a)

(b)

(c)

(d)

Fig. 10.2 Granulomatous lymphadenitis *(continued on p. 228)*

(a) MGG ×420 (b) ×1260 (c) different case ×420 (d) ×1260 (e) different case ×420 (f) ×840 (g) ×1260 (h) APAAP for antitoxoplasma ×1260 (i) MGG ×420 (j) ZN ×1260

Aggregates of histiocytes, epithelioid cells with or without giant cells and necrosis make for cytological appearances of a granuloma. The most commonly encountered granulomatous lymphadenitis with necrosis is tuberculous.

Tuberculous lymphadenitis contains aggregates of epithelioid cells, multinucleate giant cells against a necrotic 'dirty' background (a, b). The FNA procedure should include sending material for culture. Ziehl–Neelsen stain shows sparse acid-fast bacilli, particularly within necrotic areas.

Cat-scratch disease often presents as a rapidly developing swelling which is particularly alarming when it presents in a preauricular area of children: the clinical differential diagnosis in that area is rhabdomyosarcoma. FNA reveals a 'dirty' aspirate composed of a mixture of lymphocytes, plasma cells, eosinophils and numerous polymorphs in a necrotic background. Aggregates of epithelioid and/or giant cells can be seen (c, d). It is clearly a non-neoplastic condition and the child is spared a biopsy. Warthin-Starry stain can be attempted to demonstrate causative bacteria.

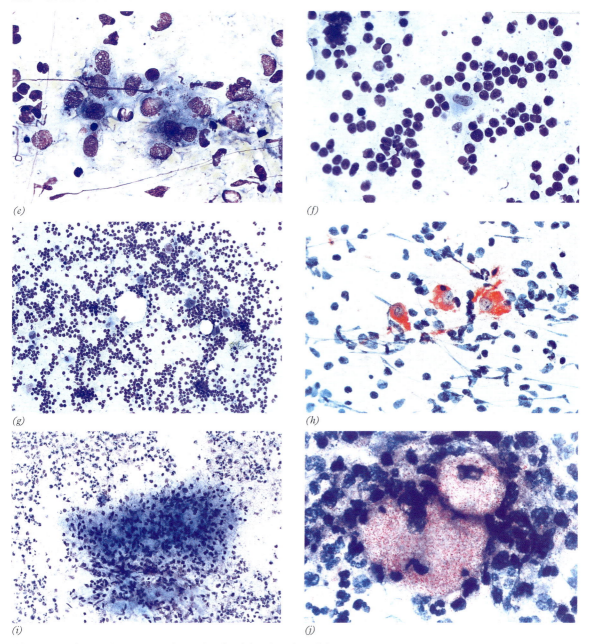

Fig. 10.2 Granulomatous lymphadenitis *(continued from p. 227)*

Toxoplasma lymphadenopathy can in its chronic stage appear very monomorphic, composed predominantly of small lymphocytes (e). Occasional epithelioid cells and multinucleate giant cells point to granulomatous lymphadenitis (f, g). Antitoxoplasma antibodies applied to unstained slides confirm the diagnosis (h). Otherwise, serological tests are advised before a biopsy is required.

Human immunodeficiency virus (HIV)-associated granulomatous lymphadenopathy often contains much necrosis and many pale blue macrophages in which colonies of organisms, usually *Mycobacterium avium-intracellulare*, are demonstrated (i, j).

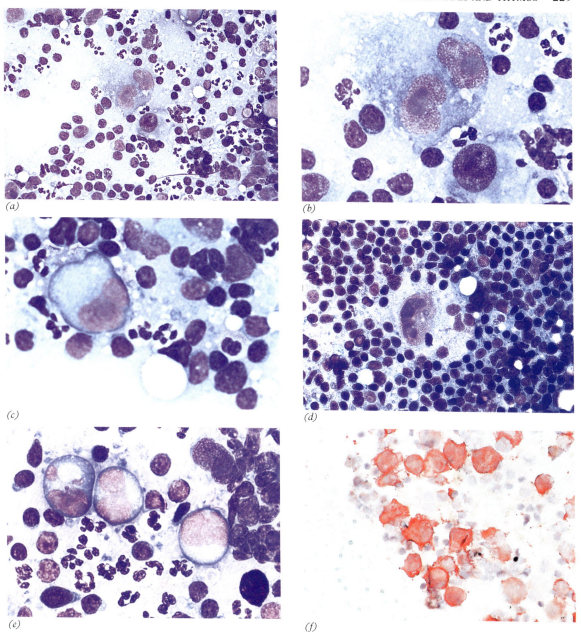

Fig. 10.3 Hodgkin's disease

(a) MGG ×840 (b) ×2100 (oil) (c) ×2100 (d) ×1260 (e) ×1260 (f) APAAP ×1260

FNA reveals a mixed lymphoid cell population in which there are atypical mononuclear and multinuclear Hodgkin and Reed–Sternberg cells respectively (a). These cells have large irregularly shaped nuclei with fine reticular chromatin and prominent, often multiple nucleoli, which are an important feature for diagnosis (b). Cytoplasm is relatively ample with peripheral basophilia in May–Grünwald–Giemsa (MGG) stain (c). Diagnostic cells appear hypochromic compared to the surrounding lymphoid cells (d). Many polymorphs, including eosinophils, may be a helpful feature (e). Hodgkin and Reed–Sternberg cells are CD30-positive, confirming the diagnosis (f). In the previously undiagnosed cases, biopsy is mandatory to establish histological type.

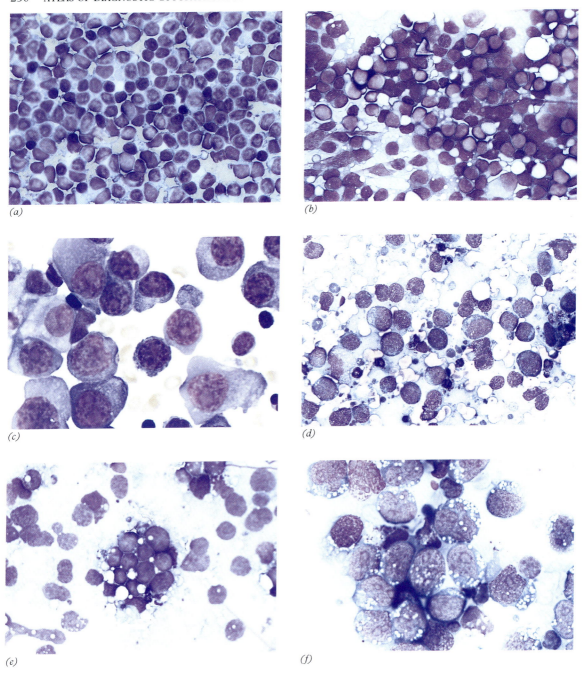

(a)

(b)

(c)

(d)

(e)

(f)

Fig. 10.4 Non-Hodgkin's lymphoma

(illustrations opposite and this page)

a–i MGG ×1260

FNA cytology is usually able to diagnose non-Hodgkin's lymphoma from a lymph node aspirate and in cases of B-cell lymphoma offers a cytological grade and subtype following the Kiel classification.

Low-grade non-Hodgkin's lymphomas yield a monotonous population of small lymphocytes (*chronic lymphocytic leukaemia-type*; a), lymphocytes with plasmacytoid or plasma cell differentiation (*lymphoplasmacytoid type, plasmacytoma*; b, c) or centrocytes (*centrocytic lymphoma*) and centroblasts (*centroblastic/centrocytic lymphoma*; d).

High-grade B-cell lymphomas show a monotonous population of centroblasts (*centroblastic non-Hodgkin's lymphoma*; e), lymphoblasts (*lymphoblastic, including Burkitt's*; f) or immunoblasts (*immunoblastic non-Hodgkin's lymphoma*; g).

T-cell lymphomas are usually diagnosed after immunocytochemistry confirms the cell of origin. Of interest is human T-lymphotropic virus type I (HTLV I)-associated cutaneous T-cell lymphoma. FNA smears contain a population of small lymphocytes, eosinophils, small convoluted blasts and plasma cells (h). Pleomorphic high-grade T-cell lymphomas must be distinguished from anaplastic carcinoma and Ki I lymphoma by means of immunocytochemistry.

Mucosa-associated lymphoid tissue (MALT) lymphomas are described in chapters relating to mucosa-associated pathology (see Fig. 11.6). Illustrated here is the case of a cystic MALT lymphoma of the mediastinum. FNA material showed numerous macrophages and morphologically benign plasma cells. Excision confirmed the diagnosis of MALT lymphoma of the mediastinum.

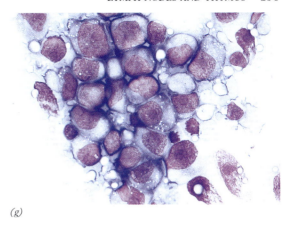

(g)

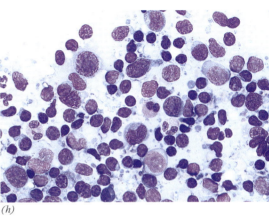

(h)

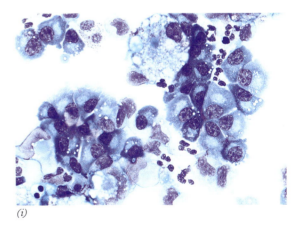

(i)

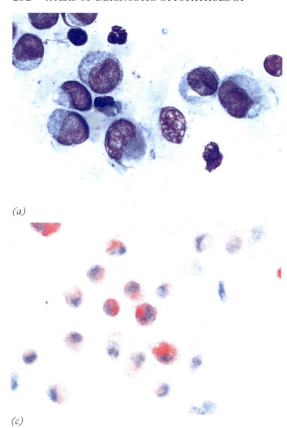

(a)

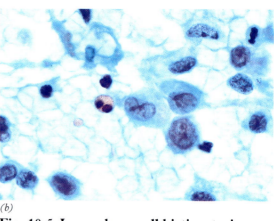

(b)

Fig. 10.5 Langerhans cell histiocytosis

(a) MGG ×1260 (b) PAP ×1260 (c) APAAP ×1260

This is characterized by the presence of typical grooved histiocyte in the background of lymphoid cells, giant cells and eosinophils (a, b). FNA may originate from the bone lesion or from lymph node. Langerhans cells show strong S100-positivity (c) (see also Fig. 14.28).

(c)

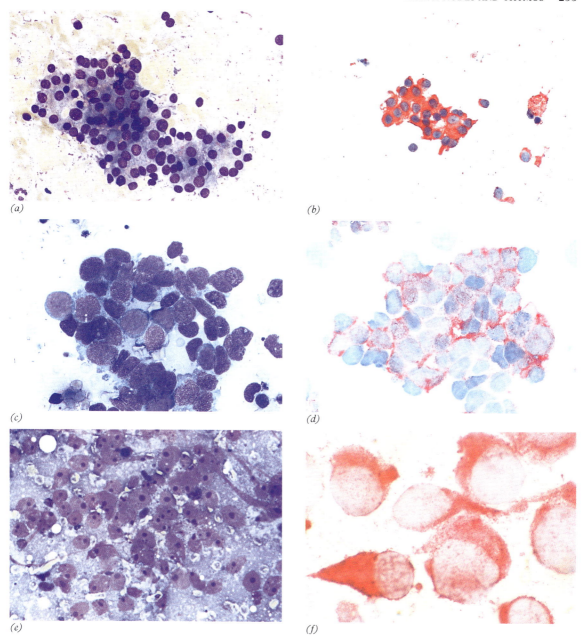

Fig. 10.6 Metastatic disease *(continued on p. 234)*

(a) MGG ×1260 (b) APAAP thyroglobulin ×1260: papillary carcinoma of thyroid (c) MGG ×1260 (d) APAAP UJ 13A ×1260: small cell anaplastic carcinoma (e) MGG ×1260 (f) APAAP CAM 5.2 ×2100: nasopharyngeal carcinoma (g) MGG ×840 (h) APAAP HCG ×840: malignant teratoma (i) ×1260 (j) APAAP CD34 ×2100: Kaposi's sarcoma (k) MGG ×1260 (l) APAAP for HMB 450 ×1260: malignant melanoma.

Lymph nodes are frequent sites of metastases. Some of these, e.g. *carcinoma of thyroid* (a), can be traced to their tumour of origin by means of immunocytochemistry (b). Others, e.g. *small cell anaplastic carcinoma of the lung*, are often morphologically sufficiently characteristic with typical granular reticular chromatin, moulding and scant cytoplasm (c) that immunocytochemistry only confirms its epithelial and neuroendocrine origin (d). *Nasopharyngeal carcinoma* has typical appearance of large nuclei, poorly defined cytoplasm and very prominent nucleoli. Lymphocytes are seen associated with the tumour cells (e). Neoplasms are often so anaplastic that only broad categories (e.g. lymphoma or, in the case illustrated, *carcinoma*) based on immunocytochemistry can be given (f).

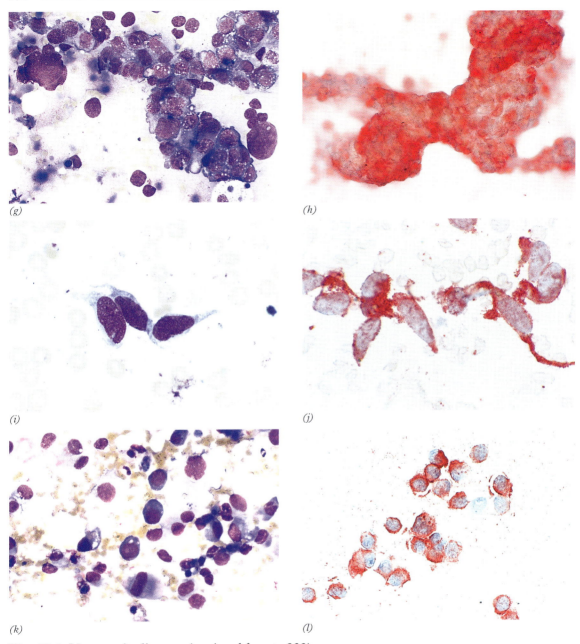

(g)

(h)

(i)

(j)

(k)

(l)

Fig. 10.6 Metastatic disease *(continued from p. 233)*

Germ cell tumours often show bizarre cytological features and have foamy, relatively abundant cytoplasm. Their origin can be confirmed with one or more of the germ-cell tumour markers (β-human chorionic gonadotrophin, α-fetoprotein, placental alkaline phosphatase; (g, h). Positivity for epithelial markers can be useful in distinguishing between seminoma (negative) and other germ-cell tumours (teratomas are positive). *Mesenchymal tumours* can affect lymph nodes and as such are usually detected on the basis of clinical history and tumour markers, e.g. Kaposi's sarcoma in the regional lymph node (i), confirmed by endothelial marker positivity in the atypical spindle cells

with vacuolated cytoplasm (j). *Malignant melanoma* can mimic any tumour and has to form part of the differential diagnosis of any unknown primary. Cytological features are those of mainly single, usually round but also spindle cells with eccentric, often multiple nuclei, very prominent nucleoli and abundant pale cytoplasm with peripheral basophilia on MGG stain (k). Pigment is seen only rarely in metastatic tumours. This is usually fine granules, better seen under high-power/oil immersion. Immunocytochemistry (S100 and other markers) confirms the diagnosis (l).

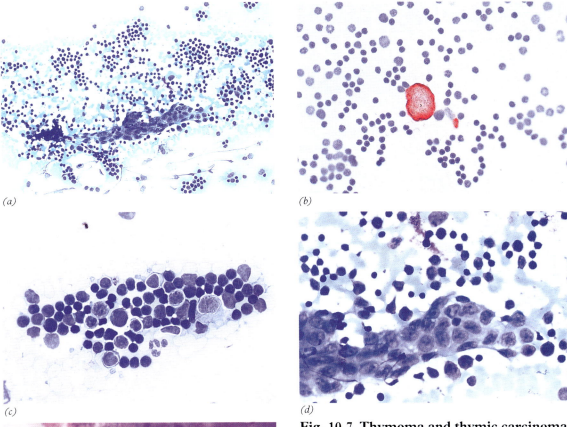

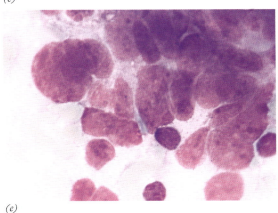

Fig. 10.7 Thymoma and thymic carcinoma

(a) MGG ×420 (b) ×1260 (c) ×1260 (d) APAAP for epithelial antigen ×1260 (e) ×2100

FNAs reflect the dual lymphoid and epithelial cell population of these tumours (a, b). The dominant lymphocytic population is a mixture of small and large, predominantly T-cell lymphocytes and larger dendritic reticulum cells (c). The epithelial component is easily recognizable (b) and can be confirmed by immunocytochemistry (d). Malignant thymomas are usually diagnosed on excised specimens, except in cases where cell anaplasia permits the cytological diagnosis of thymic carcinoma (e). Distinction from germ cell tumours and lymphomas is important and can be made on cytological material.

11. Cytology of salivary glands

Fine-needle aspiration (FNA) cytology of salivary glands is practised more and more widely despite the persistently held minority view among some surgeons that all salivary gland neoplasms require adequate excision and that the choice of surgery depends on the extent of the tumour and not on the histological (or cytological) findings. Most centres using salivary gland FNA do so selectively, in an attempt to obtain a preoperative diagnosis in order to distinguish between neoplasms and non-neoplastic conditions (e.g. sialosis, sarcoid) and thus avoid surgery in conditions which clinically mimic neoplasm.

The above aim—namely distinguishing between neoplastic and non-neoplastic conditions—will be reflected in our general approach to salivary gland cytomorphology.

Diagnostic accuracy varies between centres, reaching 96.4% with 93% sensitivity and 99% specificity in some of the larger series. False-negative and false-positive rates reach up to 5.0%. It is important for clinicians to be aware of the diagnostic difficulties associated with both sampling and the diverse morphology of salivary gland tumours and for the pathologist to be aware of the clinical relevance of the diagnosis.

The safety of the FNA procedure must be promoted, particularly amongst surgeons, who often worry about the needle tract seeding and consequent tumour recurrence following the FNA. Many studies looking specifically at this subject have failed to support these views. Salivary gland tumours do recur but are not connected with the original needle tract, as was proved by histological dissection of the needle tract. Haematoma is the only complication that occasionally occurs. It is important to stress the importance of good FNA technique—a thin needle should be used (maximum diameter 21 G) and negative pressure on the syringe and needle should be released before exiting the lesion.

Cytological appearances

Rather then try to classify lesions along the lines of histological classification, which is often difficult due to the variety of tumours and also appearances within individual tumours, cytological appearances can be classified into cystic, inflammatory, epithelial and hypocellular. There is sometimes overlap between different conditions showing similar appearances (particularly cystic). These present potential pitfalls, of which the cytopathologist needs to be aware and, if necessary, include differential diagnosis as part of the final report. The clinician will thus plan further management and decide about the need for surgery on clinical grounds, knowing that only the final histology will give the full answer. These present only a minority of cases and therefore should not distract from the fact that most salivary gland lesions can be confidently diagnosed as benign or malignant on cytological material.

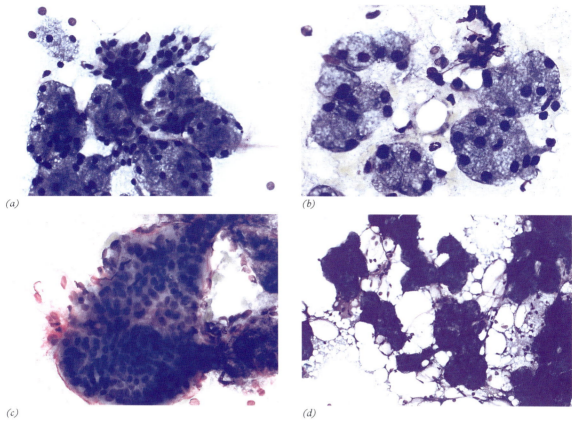

(a)

(b)

(c)

(d)

Fig. 11.1 Normal salivary gland acini

(a) MGG ×420 (b) ×1260 (c) ×1260 (d) ×840 (e) ×1260

FNA of the head and neck swellings sometimes contains normal salivary gland acini. These appear in rounded three-dimensional clusters of regular acinar cells. They have eccentric nuclei and abundant, well-outlined foamy cytoplasm. Ductal cells are rarely seen in normal glands. In patients with chronic sialadenitis or a history of irradiation to the neck, ductal epithelium may be hyperplastic (c) or show squamous metaplasia. In some cases there is a fatty infiltration of salivary gland with ductal and acinar atrophy (sialosis; d, e).

Sialosis is asymptomatic, non-inflammatory, non-neoplastic salivary gland enlargement usually affecting bilateral parotid glands. It is associated with hepatic cirrhosis, malnutrition, chronic alcoholism, diabetes mellitus, thyroid insufficiency and other diseases. There is a diminished salivary gland secretion due to degenerative changes in ducts and acini. Acini may be enlarged, and ducts atrophied with fatty replacement of the whole gland. There is no inflammatory cell infiltrate, an important negative finding to exclude inflammatory conditions and lymphoma (see Fig. 11.6).

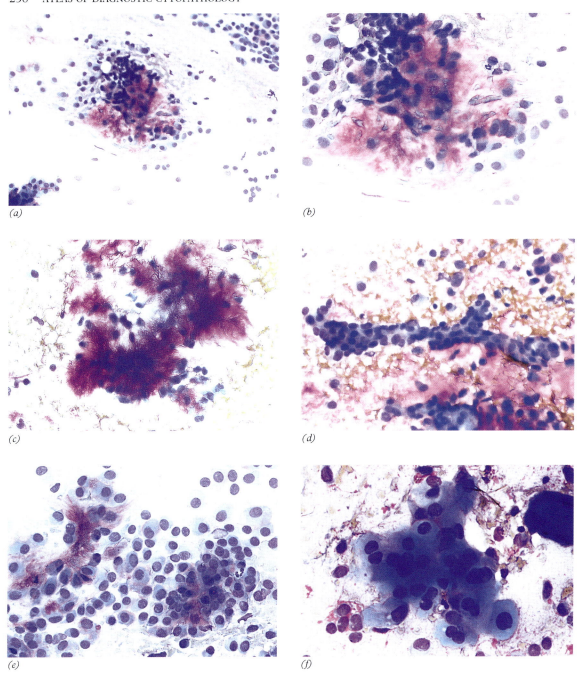

(a)

(b)

(c)

(d)

(e)

(f)

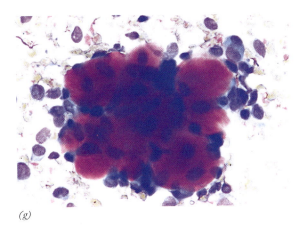

(g)

Fig. 11.2 Pleomorphic adenoma *(illustrations opposite and here)*

(a) MGG ×420 (b) ×1260 (c) ×840 (d) ×840 (e) ×1260 (f) ×2100 (g) ×2100

This is the most commonly diagnosed neoplasm of the salivary gland. Diagnosis is partly made on low power (a, b), where there is a characteristic mixture of epithelium and abundant chondromyxoid stroma in various proportions. Chondromyxoid stroma has characteristic fibrillary appearance and stains deep pink with May–Grünwald–Giemsa (MGG; c). Epithelium is either dissociated or in clusters, sometimes forming ducts (d). Myoepithelial cells in the background have a plasmacytoid appearance (e). Epithelium can undergo squamous metaplasia (f) and has to be distinguished from mucoepidermoid carcinoma. Chondromyxoid stroma sometimes forms amorphous globules surrounded by epithelium and can mimic adenoid (g).

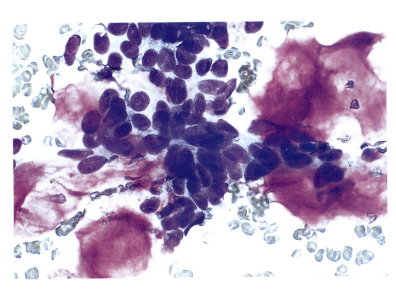

Fig. 11.3 Monomorphic adenoma

MGG ×1740 (courtesy of Dr A Rubin)

This tumour is of similar cytological appearance as pleomorphic adenoma, although it may appear to be more cellular. The typical fibrillary background material is a key to the diagnosis.

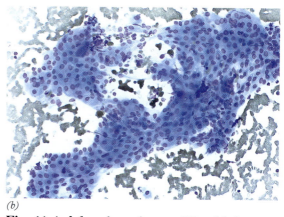

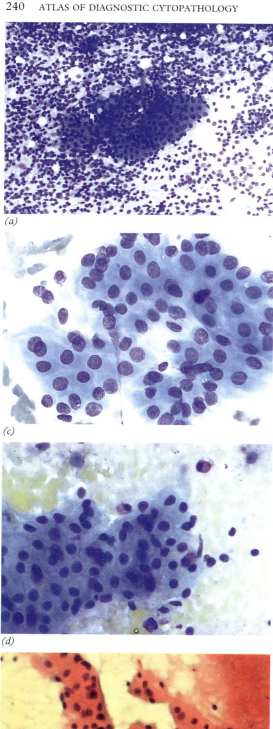

Fig. 11.4 Adenolymphoma (Warthin's tumour)

MGG (a) ×420 (b) ×840 (c) ×1260 (d) ×1260 (e) Papanicolaou ×840

Warthin's tumour is the second commonest tumour involving the major salivary glands. It often has a large cystic component reflected in numerous macrophages, admixed with background debris and lymphoid cells, including follicle centre cells as well as the epithelial component (a). The epithelium is oncocytic, presenting in flat sheets of cuboidal, well-outlined cells with dense (non-vacuolated) slate grey (MGG) or bright eosinophilic (Papanicolaou) cytoplasm (b-e). These can be admixed with mast cells (d). Aspirates lacking either lymphoid or epithelial component can also be suspected of being Warthin's tumour, but for definitive diagnosis both lymphocytes and oncocytes must be present. Differential diagnosis includes mucoepidermoid carcinoma which is often cystic. The characteristic appearance of oncocytes in flat sheets with no overlapping of nuclei and no cytoplasmic vacuolation helps to distinguish the two.

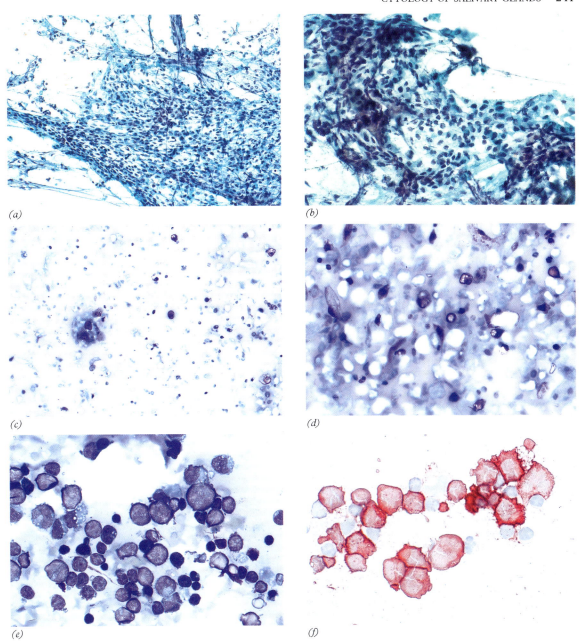

(a)   *(b)*   *(c)*   *(d)*   *(e)*   *(f)*

Fig. 11.5 Lymphoepithelial cyst

(a) Papanicolaou ×420 (b) ×840 (c) MGG ×420 (d) ×840 (e) MGG ×1260 (f) APAAP CD20 ×1260

Human immunodeficiency virus (HIV)-positive patients can present with parotid swelling which on FNA yields cystic fluid. The cytological appearances can be difficult to interpret. They contain either predominantly squamoid-type epithelium with very few lymphoid cells (a, b) or much debris; or cystic fluid in which only outlines of epithelial cells are seen and a few lymphoid cells are present (c). Both these appearances may mimic branchial cleft cyst,

squamous metaplasia in sialadenitis or even squamous cell carcinoma. The clinical history and precise anatomical site are important. Another appearance of lymphoepithelial cyst is that of predominantly lymphoid cells including many centroblasts, admixed with a few macrophages and very few or no epithelial cells. These appearances can be mistaken for lymphoma (d–f).

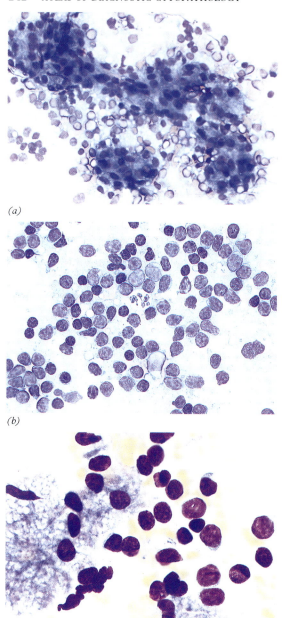

(a)

(b)

(c)

Fig. 11.6 Salivary gland lymphoma

(a) MGG ×840 (b) ×1260 (c) ×2100

Lymphoid infiltrates can accompany various lesions of the salivary gland. It is therefore important to establish morphological criteria and confirm monoclonal immunophenotype in order to diagnose salivary gland lymphomas and in particular to distinguish them from benign lymphoepithelial lesion. Lymphoma of mucosa-associated lymphoid tissue (MALT) is a special type of low-grade B-cell non-Hodgkin's lymphoma occurring in the salivary gland. It has an indolent clinical course and therapy is usually surgical removal of the gland. Cytological features are those of a monotonous population of centrocyte-like cells in close proximity and infiltrating the salivary gland cells (a–c). Not all low-grade lymphomas involving the salivary gland are of MALT type. High-grade non-Hodgkin's lymphomas should be distinguished from a poorly differentiated carcinoma preoperatively because management of the two is different.

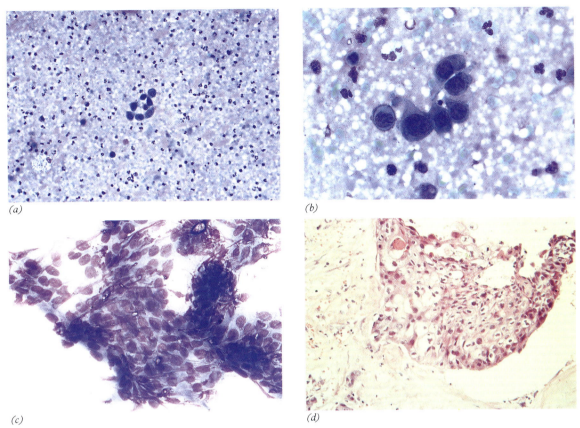

(a)   *(b)*

(c)   *(d)*

Fig. 11.7 Sialadenitis

(a) MGG ×420 (b) ×1260 (c) MGG ×840 (d) H&E ×420

Acute sialadenitis (a, b) contains numerous neutrophils with admixture of metaplastic salivary gland duct cells. This can occasionally present problems in differential diagnosis from branchial cleft cyst and squamous cell carcinoma, particularly when the lesion is clinically mimicking tumour. Chronic sialadenitis (b) often yields a sparsely cellular smear because of the fibrosis replacing most of the gland tissue. This is particularly true in cases following radiation of the neck. Aspirates often contain only a few cohesive and well-defined clusters of metaplastic salivary gland duct epithelium which can be mistaken for metastatic tumour in patients with a history of squamous cell carcinoma (c, d).

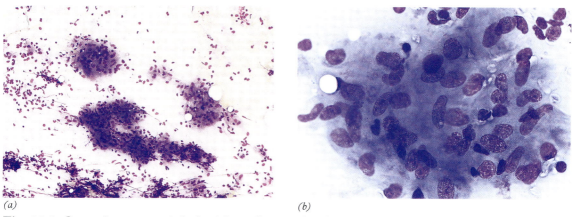

(a)   *(b)*

Fig. 11.8 Granulomatous sialadenitis: salivary gland sarcoid

(a) MGG ×420 (b) ×2100

Granulomatous inflammation without necrosis in the salivary gland is mainly associated with sarcoid which in some instances is the presenting symptom of the disease. Patients often have bilateral swelling of the parotid. Aspirates yield numerous epithelioid (b) and multinucleate giant cells with no necrosis (a, b). Very little residual

salivary gland epithelium, mainly ductal, is seen. When there is necrosis, tuberculosis and cat-scratch disease should be considered in the differential diagnosis. Cat-scratch disease can present as a rapid-growing preauricular swelling which clinically mimics tumour (see Fig. 10.2c, d).

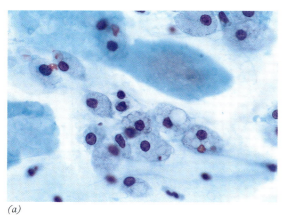 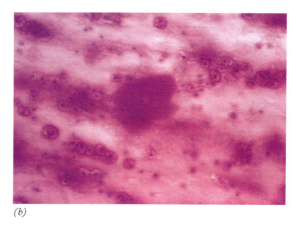

(a)   *(b)*

Fig. 11.9 Mucocoele

(a) Papanicolaou ×1260 (b) PAS-diastase ×1260

A salivary gland retention cyst can present as a unilateral or bilateral swelling. Aspirates characteristically yield tenacious transparent material resembling saliva. Smears contain

numerous macrophages amongst the thick background mucoid material. No inflammatory cells and no epithelium are seen.

Fig. 11.10 Mucoepidermoid carcinoma

MGG ×1740

FNA yields epithelial-rich aspirate, often admixed with cystic fluid, particularly the low-grade subtype where mucus-secreting cells are admixed with intermediate and squamous cells. The three cytological features shown to be most predictive of mucoepidermoid carcinoma are intermediate cells, squamous cells and overlapping epithelial groups. Intermediate cells have oval bland nuclei, small indistinct nucleoli and a negligible amount of cytoplasm. They are seen in most mucoepidermoid carcinomas, particularly in the low-grade lesions. The differential diagnosis of mucoepidermoid carcinoma includes pleomorphic adenoma undergoing squamous metaplasia. Immunoperoxidase staining shows pleomorphic adenomas to be glial fibrillary acid protein-positive whereas mucoepidermoid carcinomas are not. Demonstration of intracellular and extracellular mucin with mucicarmine is helpful in confirming the diagnosis.

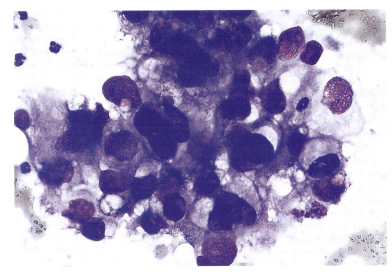

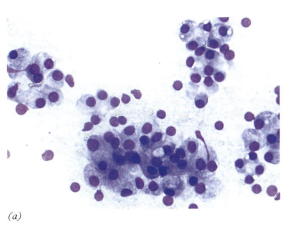

(a)

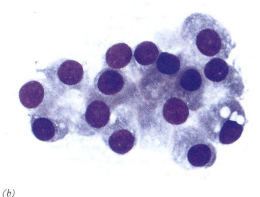

(b)

Fig. 11.11 Acinic cell carcinoma

(a) MGG ×840 (b) ×2100

Aspirate shows a monomorphic population of loose and cohesive cells with basally placed nuclei and oval well-outlined cytoplasm. This may be finely vacuolated, granular or slate-grey, resembling oncocytes. Psammoma bodies may be seen, although these are not specific to acinic cell tumour (see Fig. 11.13a). Differentiating these lesions from normal salivary gland is usually easy. Normal salivary gland aspirates contain a few round clusters of acinar cells, sometimes ductal epithelium and fat. Acinic cell carcinoma yields cellular smears containing sheets and irregular clusters of cells.

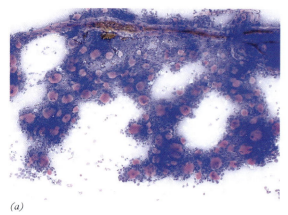

(a)

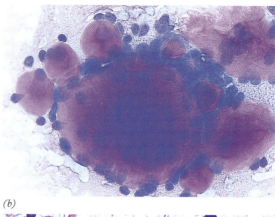

(b)

Fig. 11.12 Adenoid cystic carcinoma

(a) MGG ×420 (b) ×1260 (c) ×1260

Smears are characterized by cohesive, branching, multilayered fragments of epithelium. Diagnostic features are the homogeneous translucent cylinders known as mucoid globules surrounded by epithelial cells (a, b). These globules stain for basement membrane proteins on immunoperoxidase. They may be absent in a high-grade solid variant of adenoid cystic carcinoma. Conversely, they may be present in trabecular adenoma and pleomorphic adenoma. The key differences between these entities are the nuclear features: those of adenoid cystic carcinoma are coarser and usually have a nucleolus (c). Aspirates without mucoid globules could be mistaken for basal cell adenoma. Basal cell adenoma has a more haphazard cell arrangement compared to the relatively regular mosaic arrangement of adenoid cystic carcinoma but this feature is rarely sufficient to distinguish the two conditions. Basal cell adenoma cannot be diagnosed confidently from aspirates and, because of its rarity, it is always wise to consider other more common tumours. High-grade adenoid cystic carcinomas show nuclear atypia, making diagnosis of malignancy easy, although it may not be possible to type from the cytological preparation. Clinical information, e.g. nerve involvement, may help the surgeon reach management decisions.

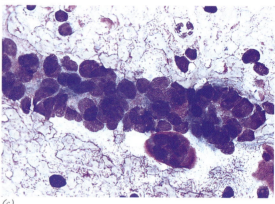

(c)

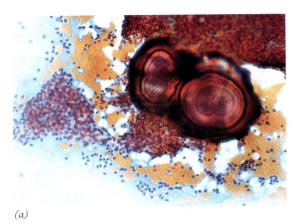

(a)

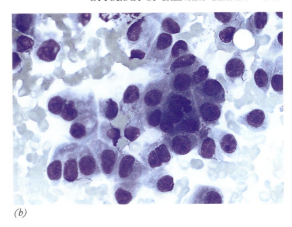

(b)

Fig. 11.13 Adenocarcinoma

(a) MGG ×420 (b) ×1260

Aspirates are cellular with cells showing features of malignancy (b). Psammoma bodies are sometimes seen (a). Adenocarcinoma is often indistinguishable from metastatic carcinoma. Epithelial myoepithelial carcinoma and terminal duct adenocarcinoma have been described in cytological preparations but their rarity rarely allows adequate typing

on FNA alone. Poorly differentiated carcinomas are often indistinguishable from high-grade lymphomas. Immunocytochemistry should be used to elucidate the findings. In some cases frozen section should be contemplated before the radical surgery involving the facial nerve is undertaken.

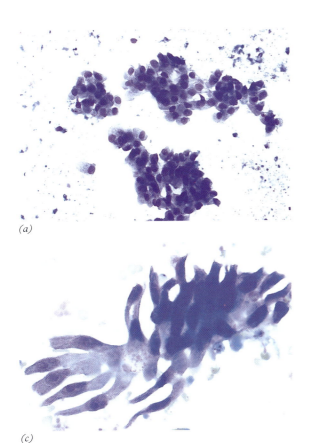

(a)

(c)

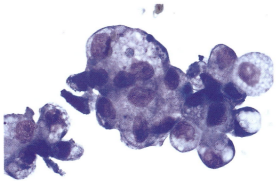

(b)

Fig. 11.14 Papillary adenocarcinoma

(a) MGG ×420 (b) ×1260 (c) ×1260

This is a rare well-differentiated salivary gland tumour which shows an instinctive cytological pattern of columnar cells in sheets and clusters (a) with cytoplasmic vacuolization (b) and cystic change.

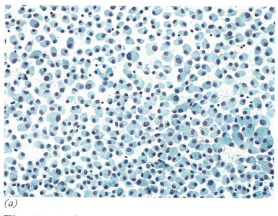
(a)

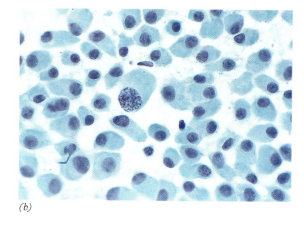
(b)

Fig. 11.15 Oncocytic carcinoma

(a) Papanicolaou ×840 (b) ×1260: FNA neck mass; history of oncocytic carcinoma

This is a rare tumour composed typically of sheets and single cells with characteristics of oncocytes (a, b). Cells have eccentric nuclei, prominent central nucleolus and abundant well-defined cytoplasm. This is finely granular, mauve (MGG) or blue-green (Papanicolaou). Nuclear pleomorphism is mild. Narrow intercellular spaces may be present, giving cells a squamoid appearance. The background is clean and contains no lymphocytes or necrotic material.

Correct cytological diagnosis may be difficult since oncocytes can be seen in other neoplastic and non-neoplastic conditions of the salivary gland. Cells display very little pleomorphism and the diagnosis of malignancy may be difficult.

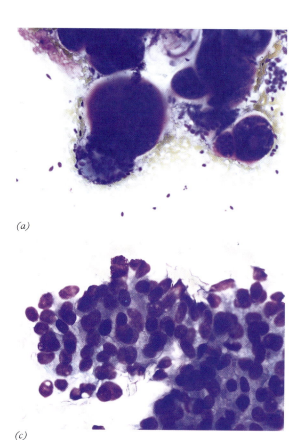
(a)

(c)

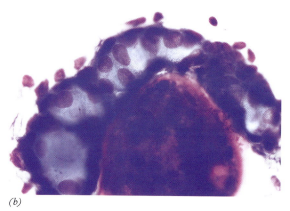
(b)

Fig. 11.16 Epithelial-myoepithelial carcinoma of the salivary gland

(a) MGG ×840 (b) ×1260 (c) ×1260

Epithelial-myoepithelial carcinoma is a rare tumour of the salivary gland of low grade malignancy. In its classic form it shows a biphasic pattern of inner layer of duct-like cells and outer layer of clear cells surrounded by basement membrane.

Cytological features include three-dimensional cellular aggregates surrounded by acellular hyaline material (a), clear cytoplasm of the peripheral cells (b) with the combination of the two cell types and hyaline matrix being the most characteristic. Some cells may exhibit pleomorphism (c). Differential diagnosis includes pleomorphic adenoma, adenoid cystic carcinoma, basal cell adenoma and other tumours with "clear cells": mucoepidermoid carcinoma, acinic cell carcinoma and metastatic renal or thyroid tumours.

Fig. 11.17
Rhabdomyosarcoma

Papanicolaou ×1160

Rhabdomyosarcoma yields a cellular aspirate composed of small, disaggregated spindle cells. These show positive staining for striated muscle, confirming the diagnosis.

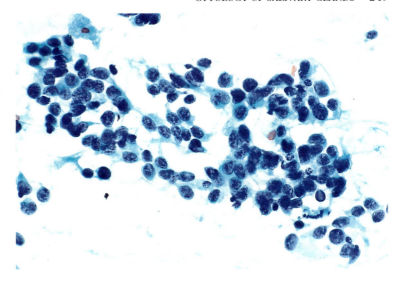

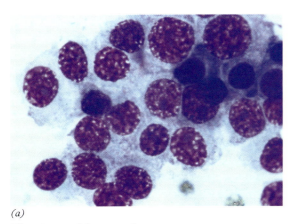

(a)

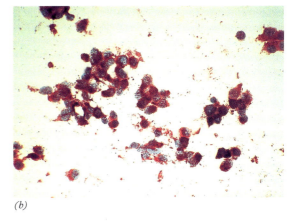

(b)

Fig. 11.18 Metastatic tumours

(a) MGG ×2100 (b) APAAP, PGP ×840

The salivary gland can be involved with spread of tumours from other parts of the body. The figures show neuroendocrine carcinoma demonstrating typical plasmacytoid cells in clusters (a). These stain positively with neural markers (b).

12. Skin and subcutaneous lesions

The role of cytology in the field of dermatological pathology is fairly limited. Fungal lesions may be identified by incubating a scraping of the affected skin or hairs detached from the lesion in 10% KOH until the epidermal elements are dissolved and hyphae become microscopically visible. Viral lesions are identified by their cytopathic effects in cells obtained from the base of a vesicle (Tzanck test). Round or oval parabasal cells with prominent eosinophilic nucleoli, seen in fluid aspirated from a bullous lesion are suggestive of pemphigus, a disorder characterized by dissolution of the intercellular bridges, or Acantholysis, in the lower epithelium. These cells, often referred to as Tzanck cells, may also be seen in bullous pemphigoid. Immunofluorescent demonstration of IgG antibodies to intercellular antigen at the precise site of Acantholysis is necessary to distinguish pemphigus, a serious condition, from the less significant pemphigoid. Keratoacanthoma is usually identifiable in a cytological preparation, but caution is indicated to avoid a false-positive diagnosis of squamous cell carcinoma. The many other benign lesions of the skin, whether topical or manifestations of systemic disorders, are outside the scope of cytopathology.

As regards the primary cancers of the skin, cytology is of particular value in the diagnosis of basal cell carcinoma. Melanotic melanoma is distinguished from benign pigmented lesions by its frankly malignant cellular features (see Figs 5.8, 10.7). Sensitivity for squamous cell carcinoma is lower as the cell yield from these tumours is often inadequate.

Diagnostic material may be obtained by direct scrape or by fine needle aspiration. The former is preferred for ulcerated lesions and the latter is used to sample sub-cutaneous nodules and soft tissue masses. Permanent preparation may be made by either the Papanicolaou or Romanowsky methods.

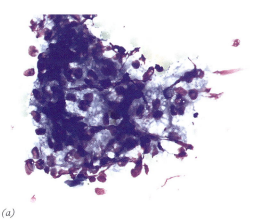 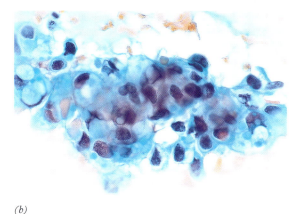

(a) *(b)*

Fig. 12.1 Sebaceous epithelial cells

(a) MMG ×1260: percutaneous FNA (b) Papanicolaou ×1260

Cells from the skin or its appendages may enter a needle during its passage through the skin. Squamous cells are easily recognized and unlikely to cause confusion. These micrographs illustrate epithelial cells from a sebaceous gland. These cells secrete oily sebum and their abundant cytoplasm is distended with lipid (a). This is removed by ethanol in a wet-fixed preparation leaving a clear cytoplasm (b).

Fig. 12.2 Basal cell carcinoma (BCC)

(a) Papanicolaou ×420 (b) ×1260 (c) MGG ×1260; skin scrape

The commonest primary cancer of the skin is a basal cell carcinoma, which, as its name implies, develops from the basal cells of the epidermis and its appendages. It occurs on areas exposed to sunlight or ultraviolet light, particularly the face in fair skinned subjects. The tumour is of low grade malignancy and infiltrates the subepithelial tissues but almost never metastasizes. It forms a nodular lesion which frequently ulcerates, hence it is popularly referred to as a rodent ulcer.

Diagnostic material may be obtained from a basal cell carcinoma either by needle aspiration of the nodule or by direct scrape of the base of the ulcer after the crust has been gently levered off with the back of a scalpel blade or a fine spatula. A permanent preparation may be stained by the Papanicolaou method (a, b) or MGG. An alternative rapid out-patient procedure is to suspend the cells in a drop or two of 1.0% aqueous methylene blue (b), (c), flatten them under a cover slip and examine the wet preparation with the microscope.

The characteristic cellular presentation consists of sheets of cohesive basal cells, the fragments of tissue appearing as microbiopsies (a). The cells have little or no apparent cytoplasm and consist largely of round or, more often, ovoid nuclei with finely granular chromatin (b, c). A somewhat greater amount of cytoplasm is evident in some cases and the cells may approximate in size to small parabasal cells and the tumour cells may show a basisquamoid morphology (c). Nucleoli are variable in number and size. Generally inconspicuous or absent in the smaller cells (a), they are usually evident in the cells with a greater volume of cytoplasm (c).

The neoplastic cells of BCC do not exhibit the usual criteria of malignancy and the diagnosis is based on the characteristic appearance of sheets of cohesive basal cells.

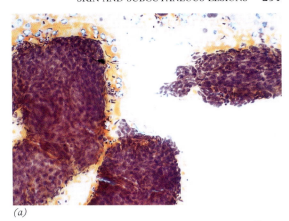

(a)

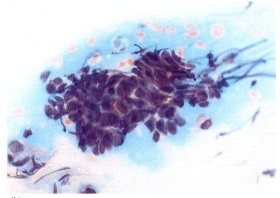

(b)

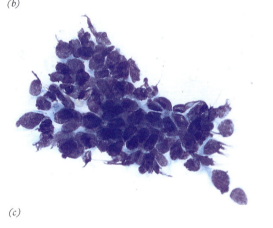

(c)

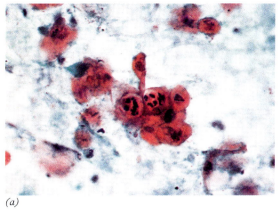

(a)

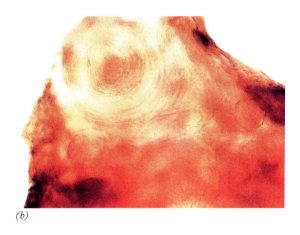

(b)

Fig. 12.3 Keratoacanthoma

Papanicolaou ×525: skin scrape (a) dyskeratotic cells (b) keratin

Keratoacanthoma, a disease of unknown aetiology, produces a nodular lesion with a central crater. The cells from the base of the crater are generally atypical in appearance (a). Although similar in size to the prickle cells, the intensely eosinophilic or orangeophilic cytoplasm indicates premature keratinization. Other features commonly associated with dyskeratosis, such as abnormality

of shape and pyknotic degeneration of the nucleus are also seen. The dyskeratotic atypical cells should not be overdiagnosed as squamous carcinoma cells. The presence of masses of keratin (b) which may be arranged in a concentric manner similar to that seen in squamous papilloma (see Fig. 1.20e), facilitates recognition of keratoacanthoma.

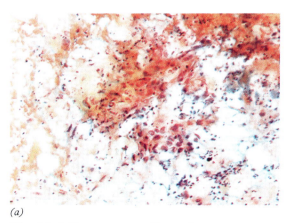

(a)

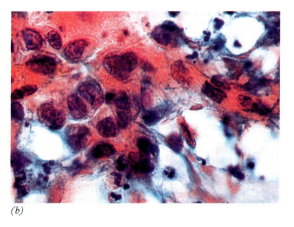

(b)

Fig. 12.4 Squamous cell carcinoma

Papanicolaou (a) ×133: skin scrape (b) ×525: same smear

Squamous cell carcinoma of the skin is much less common than basal cell carcinoma, but carries a graver prognosis as it spreads to the regional lymph nodes via the lymphaties. These tumours are generally well differentiated with abundant keratin formation. Because of this, they are difficult to scrape and the cell yield is often sparse and may be insufficient for a definitive diagnosis. Minor atypias of

and keratinization, which occur in benign skin lesions such as keratoacanthoma (Fig. 12.3a) are discounted in arriving at a diagnosis which is based on the presence of a sufficient number of cells (a) with unequivocal malignant characteristics (b) and morphological features of squamous origin (b).

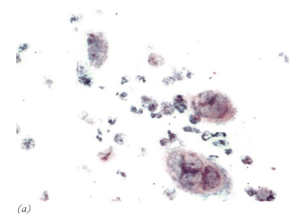

(a)

Fig. 12.5 Herpes zoster

Papanicolaou ×525: skin scrape

The cellular presentation of herpes zoster is identical with that of herpes simplex (see Figs 1.19, 3.29) and consists of menu- or multinculeated cells with moulded ground glass nuclei and margination of the nuclear chromatin. The vesicular lesions of Herpes zoster have a segmental distribution and appear on the skin along the course of the spinal or cranial nerve infected by the virus.

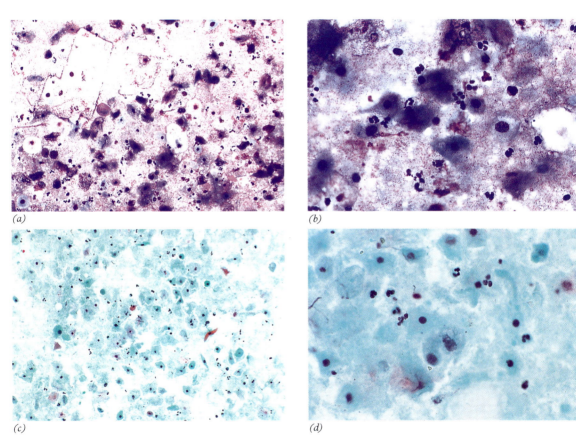

(a)　　　　　　　　　　　　　　　　*(b)*

(c)　　　　　　　　　　　　　　　　*(d)*

Fig. 12.6 Branchial cleft cyst

(a) MGG ×420 (b) ×1260 (c) Papanicolaou ×420 (d) ×1260

An anomaly of the branchial or visceral clefts which develop from the side of the embryonic pharynx may present in later life as a palpable or visible swelling at the angle of mandible.

The cyst is usually lined by squamous epithelium which is abundantly present in the cyst fluid. It is composed of both anucleate and mature squamous cells which can be keratinized (a, b). Cholesterol crystals may be seen (a). Lymphocytes from the cyst wall, seen on histology, are rarely present. More commonly, cyst fluid contains inflammatory cells (c, d). Differentiation from a well-differentiated squamous cell carcinoma may be difficult (b).

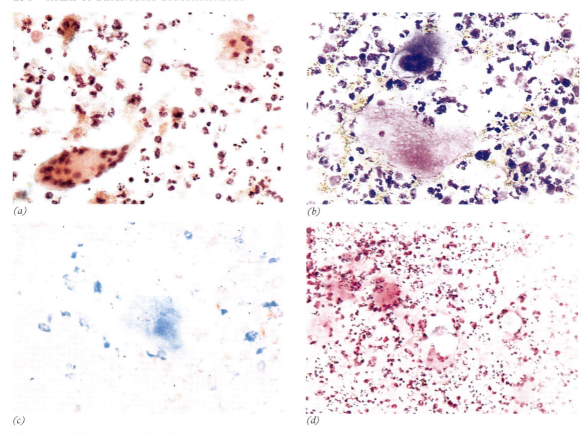

(a)   (b)   (c)   (d)

Fig. 12.7 Rheumatoid nodule

(a) Papanicolaou ×333: FNA; subcutaneous nodule on calf (b) MGG ×333: same specimen; another smear (c) Alcian blue ×133: same specimen; another smear (d) PAS ×133: same specimen; another smear

These micrographs illustrate the several components of a typical fully developed rheumatoid nodule (see also Fig. 4.18). The cells to note are the characteristic fish-shaped (a) and the round multinucleated giant epithelioid cells (a, b, d), the shift to the right and the pyknotic degeneration of the abundant neutrophils (a) and the moderate number of lymphocytes (b). The necrobiotic fibrinoid core of the nodule is represented in the May–Grünwald–Giemsa (MGG) smear by violet-coloured amorphous debris with a foamy honeycomb appearance (b). Being derived from collagen, it stains positively with Acian blue (c) and periodic acid-Schiff (PAS; d).

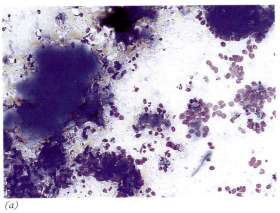

(a)

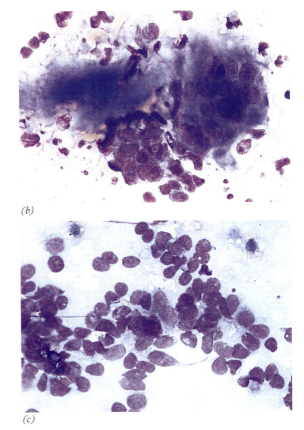

(b)

Fig. 12.8 Pilomatrixoma (calcifying epithelioma of Malherbe)

(a) MGG ×420 (b) ×1260 (c) ×1260

This case illustrates the variety of cells encountered in this benign skin appendage tumour. There are keratinized squamous cells, including 'ghosts' (a, b), multinucleate giant cells mainly associated with keratin (b), but there is also a population of small basal-type cells (c) which may form rosettes and acini. If the mixture of cells and reaction to it is not appreciated, one could possibly make an erroneous diagnosis of malignancy.

(c)

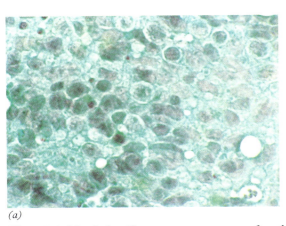

(a)

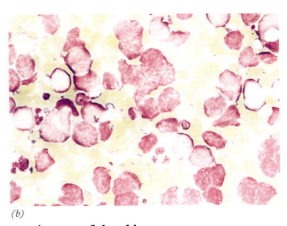

(b)

Fig. 12.9 Merkel cell tumour—neuroendocrine carcinoma of the skin

(a) Papanicolaou ×1260 (b) MGG ×1260 FNA skin nodule (courtesy of Dr Trutin-Ostovic)

This rapidly growing malignant tumour occurs most frequently in the face, neck and extremities of elderly people. Cytology of the tumour shows a monotonous cell population of bare nuclei with a tendency to form clusters, rosettes and a moulding effect. Cytoplasm is very sparse; chromatin is fine and granular and the nucleoli inconspicuous (a, b). Immunocytochemistry for epithelial and some neural markers is positive, differentiating this tumour from lymphoma. Differentiation from a metastasis of a small cell anaplastic carcinoma of the lung has to be made on the basis of clinical presentation and history because they may appear very similar cytologically.

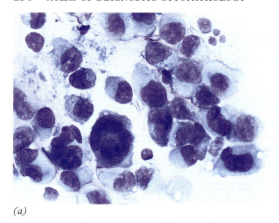

(a)

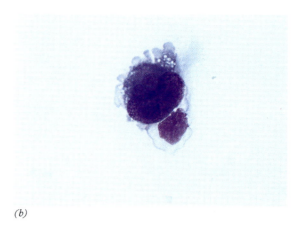

(b)

Fig. 12.10 Lymphomatoid papulosis

(a) MGG ×1260 (b) ×2100 imprint of the skin excision

This unusual lymphoid infiltrate of the skin is characterized by the large pleomorphic cells resembling Reed–Sternberg cells (a, b). The condition is benign. The differential diagnosis includes large cell anaplastic T-cell lymphoma.

13. Thyroid

INTRODUCTION

The thyroid is an endocrine organ showing a relatively limited span of cell morphology with considerable overlap between 'normal' functional changes and pathological conditions. Cell pleomorphism and other more traditional cytological features of malignancy may be associated with benign conditions whilst malignant tumours may appear cytologically bland. In this setting, features other than the morphology of follicular cells alone, e.g. cellularity, the presence of colloid or other background material, assume greater importance. Clinical information and understanding of the role of fine-needle aspiration cytology (FNAC) in the context of clinical management are of paramount importance.

The prime role of FNAC of the thyroid is reducing the rate of surgery for benign disease. The distribution of thyroid pathology depends on the geographic area. In a non-endemic area, such as the UK, approximately 15% of thyroid FNAC are neoplastic compared to 1–2% in endemic areas such as southern Germany. Therefore, most thyroid FNACs which will encountered are benign. Most of these can be diagnosed on the basis of clinical tests (ultrasound, isotope scan and hormone levels) and confirmed by FNAC. Despite the sophisticated clinical tests, we found that in 23% of patients who had undergone FNAC, this was the essential investigation for diagnosis. This is particularly true of thyroiditis and neoplasms. The sensitivity of the thyroid FNAC, as reported in the literature, is 94%, the specificity is 96% and the positive predictive value 93%. These values justify employing FNAC as the initial modality for investigating thyroid nodules and reaffirm its major role in determining where surgery is indicated and where it is not.

The method of performing thyroid FNAC is for the patient to be in the supine position, possibly with a pillow under the shoulders extending the cervical spine. The thyroid is palpated in the anatomical gutter formed by the trachea and sternocleidomastoid muscle. The patient is asked to swallow in order to establish the movement of the thyroid along with other neck structures. Having fixed the lesion between the fingers of one hand, pushing the muscle laterally at the same time, a fine needle (23–27 G) is directed vertically and slightly towards the midline, avoiding the carotid sheath and trachea or its perichondrium. Accidental puncture of the trachea produces loss of negative pressure and can yield mucus and respiratory epithelium, as well as the bone marrow if rings are aspirated. Apart from a slight cough, accidental puncture of trachea is harmless to the patient. Material expelled from the needle should be spread in a standard way, taking care that specimens with excess of fluid are handled appropriately—using either the special spreading technique of 'mopping' the fluid at the edge of the slide or cytospin preparations.

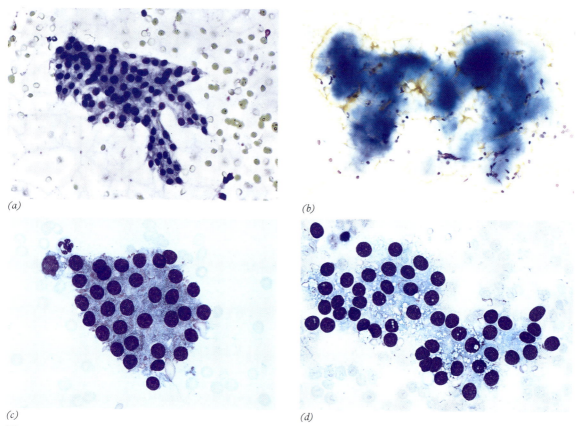

(a)

(b)

(c)

(d)

Fig. 13.1 Colloid goitre

(a) MGG ×420 (b) ×840 (c) ×1260 (d) ×1260

Aspirates from colloid goitre contain relatively few follicular cells and a thin layer of colloid in the background (a). Colloid may on occasions appear more viscous (b). Follicular cells are few: they are small and arranged in flat sheets. Nuclei are uniform; the cytoplasm is poorly outlined and often lost. Single cells in the background often appear as bare nuclei and have to be distinguished from lymphocytes (c). They can be arranged in microfollicles, although these are often very few and flat rather than three-dimensional. Cytoplasmic vacuolation and mild anisonucleosis may be seen (d).

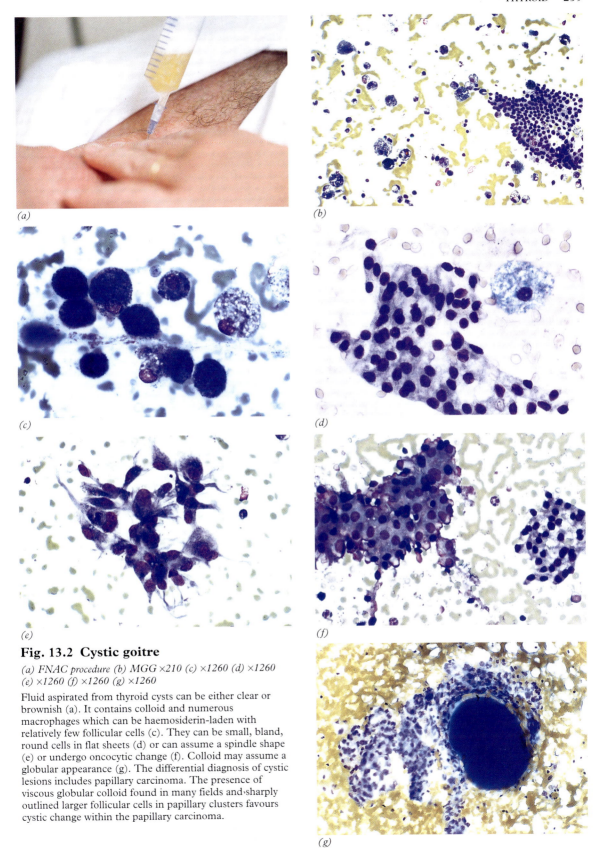

Fig. 13.2 Cystic goitre

(a) FNAC procedure (b) MGG ×210 (c) ×1260 (d) ×1260
(e) ×1260 (f) ×1260 (g) ×1260

Fluid aspirated from thyroid cysts can be either clear or brownish (a). It contains colloid and numerous macrophages which can be haemosiderin-laden with relatively few follicular cells (c). They can be small, bland, round cells in flat sheets (d) or can assume a spindle shape (e) or undergo oncocytic change (f). Colloid may assume a globular appearance (g). The differential diagnosis of cystic lesions includes papillary carcinoma. The presence of viscous globular colloid found in many fields and sharply outlined larger follicular cells in papillary clusters favours cystic change within the papillary carcinoma.

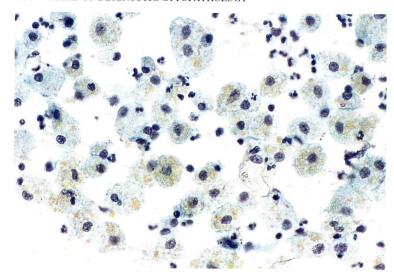

Fig. 13.3 Thyroglossal cyst

Papanicolaou ×1740

A thyroglossal cyst is usually a midline submental swelling which yields fluid. It contains numerous macrophages and may contain cholesterol crystals or inflammatory cells. It is invariably benign.

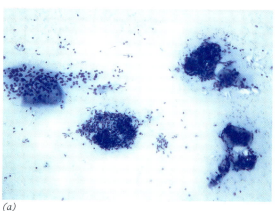

(a)

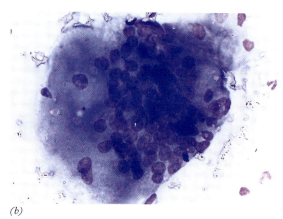

(b)

Fig. 13.4 Thyroiditis, subacute (de Quervain)

(a) MGG ×210 (b) ×1260 (c) ×1260

This condition rarely presents for FNAC since local symptoms, including pain, prompt initial treatment. Aspirates show very few follicular cells, multinucleate giant cells and epithelioid cells (c), suggesting a granulomatous process (a, b). These features are characteristic of the condition. Multinucleate giant cells can be found in chronic lymphocytic thyroiditis and also in papillary carcinoma (see Fig. 13.8g).

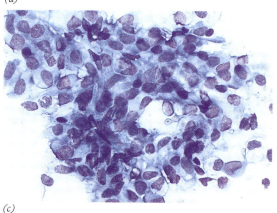

(c)

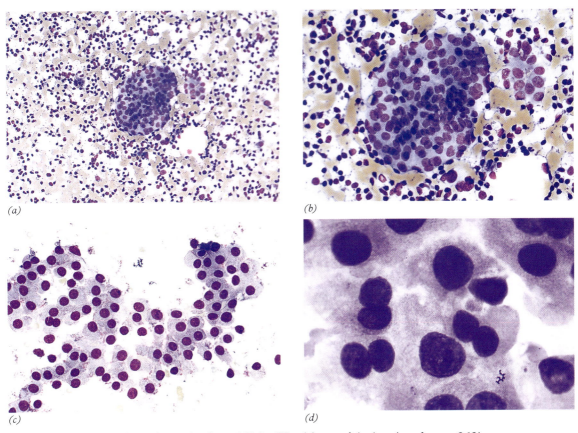

(a)

(b)

(c)

(d)

Fig. 13.5 Chronic lymphocytic thyroiditis (Hashimoto's) (continued on p. 262)

(a) MGG ×420 (b) ×1260 (c) ×1260 (d) ×1260 (e) ×1260 (f) ×840 (g) APAAP cytokeratin ×840

A low-power view of this condition reveals a background of lymphoid cells and an island of epithelium (a, b): the high-power view shows oncocytic epithelium (Hürthle cells, Askanazy cells; c). These are follicular cells which have slate-grey, dense, well-outlined cytoplasm with central nuclei (c). In addition to characteristic oncocytic epithelium there are forms which represent the transition between follicular and oncocytic epithelium. The nuclei of oncocytic epithelium can show marked anisonucleosis and pleomorphism, particularly in long-standing cases (d). In the absence of lymphoid background (if an oncocytic area was sampled) these can be mistaken for oncocytic neoplasm. A thorough search of the background for lymphoid cells and in particular follicle centre cells, including dendritic reticulum cells, centroblasts and plasma cells, is often the key to diagnosis (e). Epithelium can sometimes be hard to distinguish from follicle centre cells, in which case epithelial markers can be used (f, g). Oncocytic change is not specific to Hashimoto's thyroiditis. It can be seen in colloid goitre and in the Hürthle cell variant of papillary carcinoma.

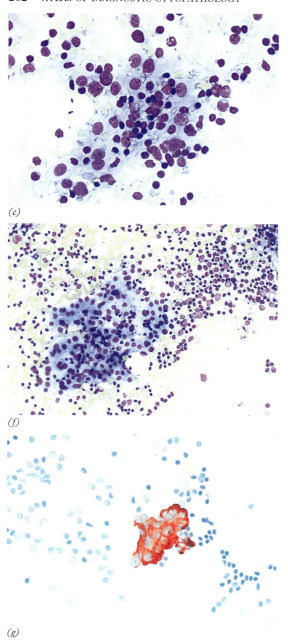

(e)

(f)

(g)

Fig. 13.5 Chronic lymphocytic thyroiditis (Hashimoto's) *(continued from p. 261)*

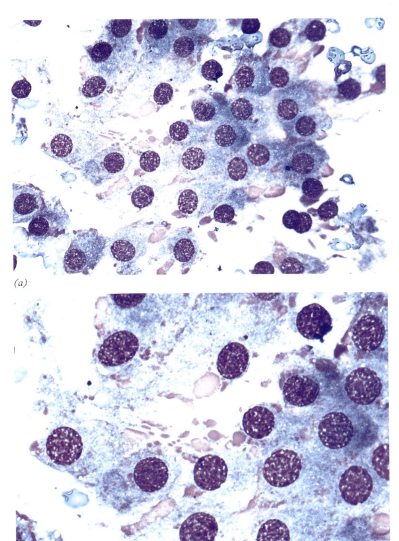

(a)

(b)

Fig. 13.6 Cellular "solid" nodules. Follicular hyperplasia

(a) MGG ×1160 (b) ×1740

In cases of thyroid hyperplasia (Grave's disease), patients are usually diagnosed on clinical investigation including hormonal assays. FNA is usually reserved for "hot" nodules within a goitre to distinguish hyperplasia from adenoma. Aspirates are rich in blood and show little, thin colloid. There is sometimes a marked anisonucleosis of follicular cells. They have abundant finely granular cytoplasm with numerous vacuoles which can be very small or as large as the nucleus (a). The vacuoles have homogenous thin content, which is stained pink in MGG, and tend to gather peripherally ("fire flares")(b). They suggest hyperfunction and are the result of pinocytosis of thyroglobulin from the small follicles. They are found in some but not all cases of hyperplasia. Similarly, they are not specific for primary hyperplasia and can be found in other conditions, e.g. Hashimoto's thyroiditis and neoplasia. Nuclei are the size of red cells and usually single. Nucleolus is single and may be prominent. Background colloid is thin and abundant, it may appear more solid in different shapes. Oxyphylic change and mild lymphocytic infiltrate may be present in thyroid hyperplasia reflecting the pathogenetic overlap between Hashimoto's thyroiditis and Grave's disease.

Aspirates from Grave's disease may show cytological atypia, particularly if the patient has undergone medical treatment or previous radioiodine ablative treatment (see Fig. 13.13). Dyshormonogenetic goitre can similarly give a picture of florid hyperplasia with papillary structures and atypia.

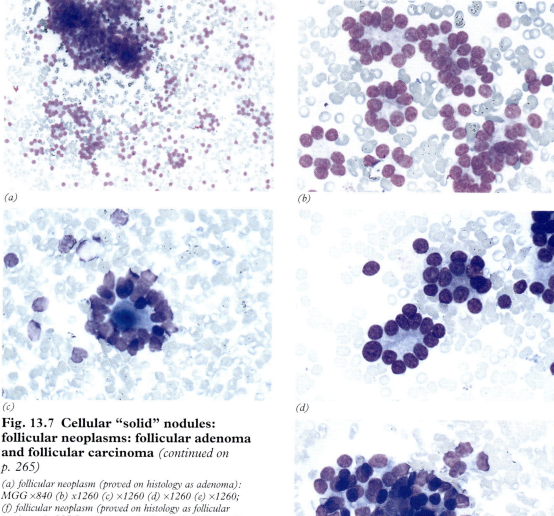

(a)

(b)

(c)

(d)

(e)

Fig. 13.7 Cellular "solid" nodules: follicular neoplasms: follicular adenoma and follicular carcinoma (continued on p. 265)

(a) follicular neoplasm (proved on histology as adenoma): MGG ×840 (b) x1260 (c) ×1260 (d) ×1260 (e) ×1260; (f) follicular neoplasm (proved on histology as follicular carcinoma): MCG ×1260 (g) ×1260 (h) ×840 (i) ×1260

Follicular neoplasms, i.e. follicular adenomas and follicular carcinomas, exhibit high cellularity with cells arranged in follicle-like structures. Together with the lack of colloid, this pattern can be recognised and cytological diagnosis of follicular neoplasia can be made. However, definitive diagnosis, i.e. whether follicular adenoma or carcinoma, should rest on histological examination, cytology having acted as a screening tool for nodules requiring surgical excision.

A characteristic cytological feature favouring neoplasia (both benign and malignant) over hyperplasia is the high cellularity with little, if any, colloid (a). Occasionally, due to haemorrhage, aspiration may yield a cystic, haemorrhagic fluid and may not be representative of the lesion. *Follicular adenoma* (a–e) yields cells arranged in monolayered sheets of equal sized, cohesive follicles with smooth surface ("complete" follicles) (a, b). Nuclei are even in size, round or slightly oval with regular chromatin distribution and barely visible nucleoli (c). In aspirates containing very little colloid and rich in monotonous cell population arranged in microfollicles, a tentative diagnosis of adenoma may be made. The possibility of follicular carcinoma cannot be ruled out on fine needle aspirates alone.

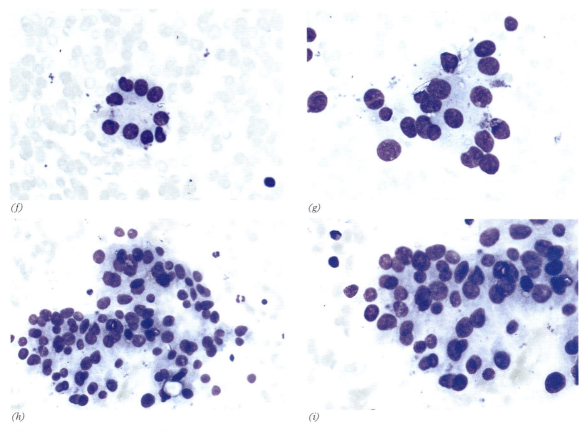

(f)   *(g)*

(h)   *(i)*

Fig. 13.7 Cellular "solid" nodules: follicular neoplasms: follicular adenoma and follicular carcinoma *(continued from p. 264)*

Follicular carcinoma, similar to adenoma, contains much blood and scant colloid with a number of epithelial cells (f–i). These may occur singly and in clusters and may be arranged in follicle like structures (f). Follicles with an amorphous background material in the centre are almost invariably neoplastic (c, e). Features favouring benign neoplasia are usually well outlined follicles (b, c, d, e) whilst loosely attached follicles are more often found in invasive carcinoma (f, g). Individual cells have poorly outlined cytoplasm, some of which may contain marginal vacuoles (g). Nuclei show moderate anisonucleosis and may vary in shape, they also appear larger than in adenomas and normal thyroid gland (g, h, i). Cell atypia may vary depending on the degree of tumour differentiation. However, atypia of poorly differentiated follicular carcinomas cannot be reliably distinguished from that occurring in atypical adenomas or adenomas with degenerative changes. The atypical features favouring malignancy are: high cellularity, crowding in cell groups, increased nuclear size, more than 75% of cells with nucleoli including three or more, irregular nuclear membrane and irregular chromatin distribution (h, i).

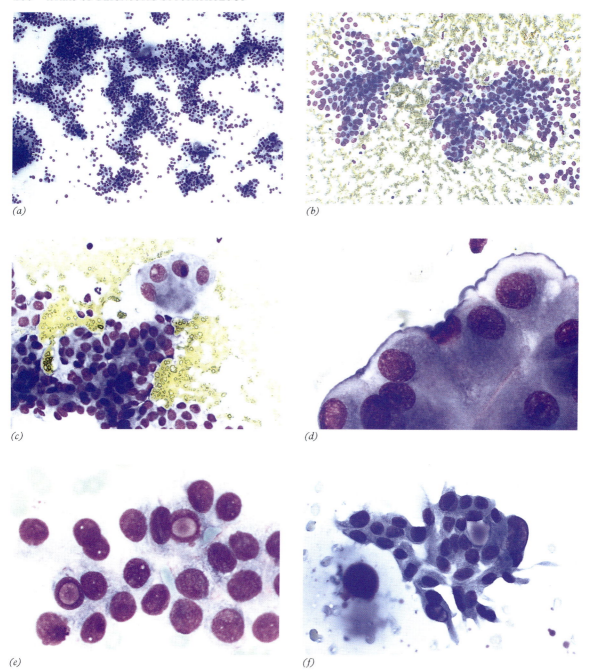

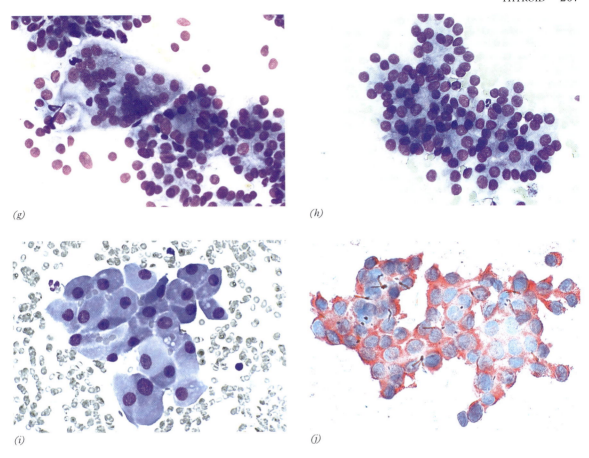

Fig. 13.8 Papillary carcinoma *(illustrations opposite and above)*

(a) MGG ×210 (b) ×840 (c) ×1260 (d) ×2100 (e) ×1260 (f) ×1260 (g) ×1260 (h) ×1260 (i) ×1260 (j) ×1260 APAAP antithyroglobulin

Aspirates are cellular-containing follicular cells in papillary aggregates and singly (a–c). Follicular cells may have visible nucleoli and sometimes well-outlined cytoplasm with 'scalloped' borders (d). Nuclei may show intranuclear cytoplasmic vacuolation ('orphan Annie') but this is neither a sensitive nor specific marker of papillary carcinoma (e). Psammoma bodies may be seen. They have to be distinguished from colloid, which can also be present (f). Multinucleate giant cells may be associated with epithelial clusters (g). Their nuclei are often indistinguishable from the epithelium. Cystic change can be present. Follicular and Hürthle cell variants of papillary carcinoma are recognized (h, i). Metastatic papillary carcinoma shows similar morphology and is characteristically found in the neck of relatively young patients as a presenting symptom of disease. Typical features and thyroglobulin antibody confirm the cell origin (j).

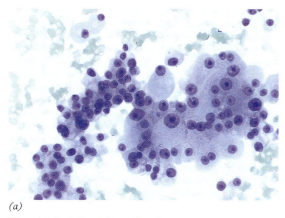

(a)

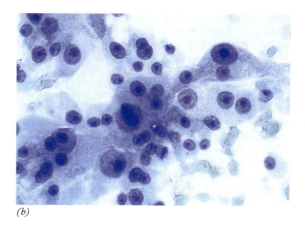

(b)

Fig. 13.9 Hürthle cell adenoma

(a) MGG ×840 (b) ×1260

Hürthle cell change can accompany various benign and neoplastic conditions of the thyroid: the finding of cellular smears with a single cell population of Hürthle cells is usually indicative of Hürthle cell neoplasm. Cells can show marked anisonucleosis and prominent nucleoli without being malignant (a, b). Histological examination for capsular or vascular invasion is the preferred method of distinguishing adenoma from carcinoma.

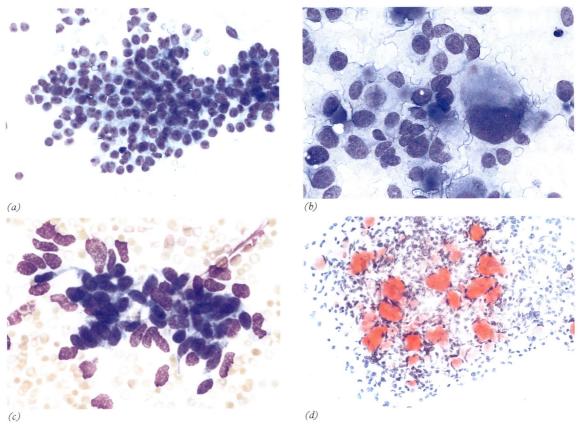

(a)　　　　(b)

(c)　　　　(d)

Fig. 13.10 Medullary carcinoma

(a) MGG ×840 (b) MGG ×1260 (c) MGG ×840 (d) Congo red ×210

FNAC from medullary carcinoma is either composed of monomorphic 'plasmacytoid' cells in loose aggregates or single cells with eccentric nuclei and basophilic cytoplasm. Eosinophils are frequently associated with cell groups (a). Alternatively, medullary carcinoma can present as a frankly malignant tumour with large cells, eccentric nuclei and prominent nucleoli (b). The spindle-cell variant of medullary carcinoma may appear sarcomatous (c). Background amyloid stains bluish green with May–Grünwald–Giemsa (MGG) and is present in dense patches. It mimics colloid, so special stains—Congo red and calcitonin—are indicated to confirm the true nature of this lesion (d).

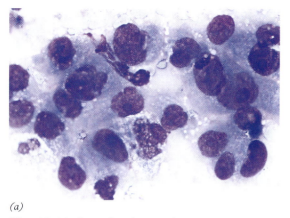

(a)

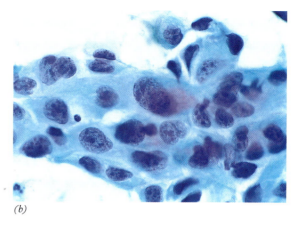

(b)

Fig. 13.11 Anaplastic carcinoma

(a) MGG ×1260 (b) Papanicolaou ×1260

Anaplastic carcinoma is a highly pleomorphic tumour with extreme anisonucleosis, prominent nucleoli and necrosis (a). This tumour has a very poor prognosis and is treated initially with radiotherapy rather then surgery. Histological variants have their parallel in cytology (e.g. squamous cell type) but the relevance of this subclassification is uncertain (b). Distinction from other tumours, including metastatic tumours and high-grade lymphomas, is important.

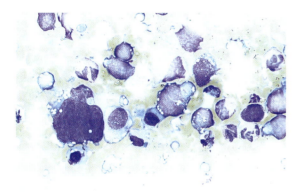

(a)

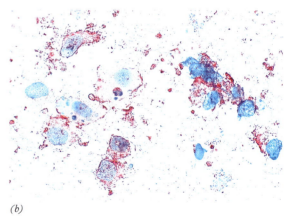

(b)

Fig. 13.12 Thyroid lymphoma

(a) ×1260 (b) APAAP for LCA

Thyroid lymphomas can present as a rapidly enlarging neck mass. They represent 0.04–0.2 % of thyroid FNAC and 1.2–6% of thyroid malignancies. Most are low-grade B-cell lymphomas. They may occur in patients with a history of lymphocytic thyroiditis or Hashimoto's. The two conditions should not be confused morphologically provided the sample is adequate. The presence of oncocytic epithelium and a mixture of follicle centre cells, including plasma cells in thyroiditis, as opposed to a monotonous population of lymphocytes expressing monoclonal phenotype should distinguish the two conditions.

Not infrequently, lymphomas are high-grade and not easily classified into any of the commoner cell categories (a). Immunocytochemistry to confirm the lymphoid nature of cells is important in the differential diagnosis with anaplastic carcinoma (b).

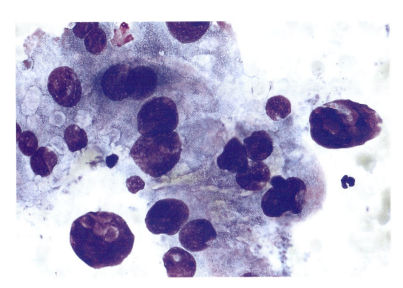

Fig. 13.13 Radioactive iodine effect

MGG ×1740

Patients with a history of radioiodine treatment to the thyroid may have highly pleomorphic cells in the FNAC. Large cells with bizarre hyperchromatic nuclei and a structureless chromatin pattern admixed with capillaries and fibroblasts may be mistaken for malignancy and even anaplastic carcinoma. The history and careful scrutiny of the entire specimen often reveal the benign nature of the lesion.

14. Bone and soft tissue

INTRODUCTION

Main indications for FNA of soft tissue tumours are: preoperative diagnosis of primary tumour, staging of a metastatic tumour and follow-up of recurrence. Whilst the use of FNA in determining metastases and recurrence is widely accepted, initial preoperative diagnosis is not. With good clinical/morphologic co-operation FNA can play a major role in the preoperative diagnosis.

Currently, soft tissue tumours are evaluated radiologically and clinically prior to surgical biopsy for histological diagnosis, followed by excision. Excision often depends on whether the tumour is benign or malignant, the site of the tumour (superficial, deep) and its relation to surrounding structures (nerves and vessels), rather than the histological subtype. The advantages of preoperative FNA are: the possibility of reducing the excision margin, the smaller risk of seeding sarcoma cells, that it does not require hospitalization, and that it allows planning of the management within 20 min of taking the sample.

The role of FNA diagnosis in preoperative management is to decide whether the lesion is a true soft tissue tumour or not and, if so, whether it is benign or malignant. Malignancy grades and histological subtypes are sometimes possible to assess although they are not absolutely necessary. Diagnostic categories best used are: (a) benign, (b) sarcoma, (c) malignant tumour other than sarcoma and (d) non diagnostic (either insufficient or inconclusive). Malignancy is assessed on the basis of cellular yield, necrosis, cellularity in tumour clusters, fascicles or fragments, chromatin, pleomorphism, nucleoli and mitoses.

FNA of soft tissues should be performed on the most accessible part of the tumour using a 22G needle. For deep lesions needles with stylet can be used and some centres (Lund, Sweden) recommend tattooing of the aspiration channel so that it can be surgically removed at operation, if a sarcoma. A combination of wet fixed and air dried smears gives best diagnostic information. May–Grünwald–Giemsa shows cartilage and myxoid background whilst Papanicolaou stained smears give good nuclear morphology. FNA material can be utilized for special techniques, e.g. electron microscopy, immunocytochemistry, chromosomal analysis and DNA ploidy studies. Chromosomal analysis gives best results in Ewing's sarcoma and primitive neuroectodermal tumours (PNET). Synovial sarcomas and alveolar rhabdomyosarcoma show cytogenetic abnormality in the majority of cases.

LIPOMATOUS TUMOURS

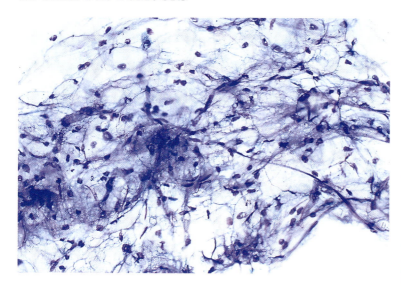

Fig. 14.1 Lipoma

MCG ×580

Lipoma is the most common soft tissue tumour. FNA smears usually contain fragments of monomorphic and univacuolated mature fat cells with small dark peripheral nuclei. *Intramuscular lipoma* may have fat intermixed with fragments of striated muscle which may show regenerative changes such as multinucleation. Angiolipoma is characterized by a delicate capillary network traversing the fat fragments. *Spindle cell and pleomorphic lipoma* occur in the back of the neck of elderly men. Spindle cell lipoma contains fibroblast-like cells and fascicles of spindle cells intermixed with fat. Pleomorphic lipoma is characterized by 'floret' cells; these have multiple, often irregular and hyperchromatic nuclei. *Hybernoma* has small fat cells with multivacuolated cytoplasm mixed with typical large fat cells.

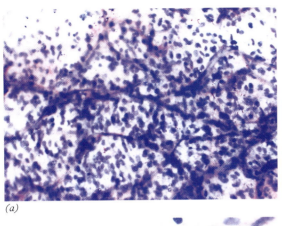

(a)

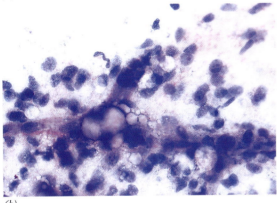

(b)

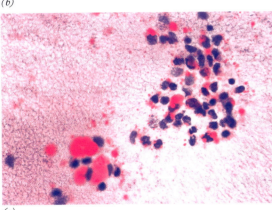

(c)

Fig. 14.2 Liposarcoma (myxoid)

(a) MGG ×840 (b) ×1260 (c) oil red O ×1260

Cytology of this relatively common sarcoma, which occurs predominantly as a deep-seated inter- or intramuscular tumour, has been described for myxoid, round cell and pleomorphic subtypes. Well-differentiated liposarcoma is difficult to distinguish from atypical lipoma.

Myxoid liposarcoma (a–c) yields typically gelatinous material which contains relatively cellular fragments composed of small round cells with noticeable vacuolation in some cells. The most prominent features of this tumour are myxoid background material, vascular meshwork ('chicken wire') of anastomosing capillaries (a) and occasional uni- or multivacuolated lipoblasts with scalloped nuclei (b). In cases of doubt as to the nature of cytoplasmic vacuoles, oil red O confirms their fatty content (c).

The pure round cell liposarcoma is very cellular, composed of atypical rounded tumour cells with vacuolated cytoplasm. The pleomorphic liposarcoma contains highly atypical, often multinucleated lipoblasts and can easily be recognized as a high grade sarcoma.

Well differentiated liposarcoma lacks sufficient diagnostic criteria on FNA and can be difficult to distinguish from atypical lipoma. Diagnostic pitfalls include hibernoma vs. well-differentiated liposarcoma, spindle cell and pleomorphic lipoma vs. well-differentiated liposarcoma and deep seated lipoma with degenerative changes and lipophages vs. myxoid liposarcoma. Intramuscular lipoma with its atrophic muscle fibres and multinucleate cells can be mistaken for malignancy. Nodular fasciitis, proliferative fasciitis and myositis ossificans can have myxoid component and may involve fat (see Fig. 14.16 on nodular fasciitis).

PERIPHERAL NERVE TUMOURS

Fig. 14.3 Benign nerve sheath tumour (neurilemmoma, schwannoma, peripheral nerve sheath tumour)

(a) MGG ×210 (b) ×1260 (c) ×840: FNA paravertebral tumour

Neurilemmoma is the most common peripheral nerve tumour. FNA yields different sized fragments of tumour tissue. The fragments are variably cellular composed of cohesive spindle-shaped cells with often indistinct cytoplasmic borders within fibrillary mesenchymal background material. Cells show orientation in various directions (similar to epithelioid cells; a). They have slender, oval pointed nuclei and elongated, tangled, wire-like cytoplasmic processes which may contain pigment (b, c). The overall uniformity indicates a benign soft-tissue tumour.

The differential diagnosis includes fibromatosis, fasciitis, leiomyoma, fibroblastic liposarcoma, fibroblastic malignant fibrous histiocytoma, monophasic synovial sarcoma, malignant schwannoma and melanoma.

Malignant peripheral nerve sheath tumour (MPNST) is not sufficiently characterized on FNA. It often appears as a pleomorphic sarcoma or atypical spindle cell neoplasm. Slender, atypical pointed nuclei may be a clue to the diagnosis.

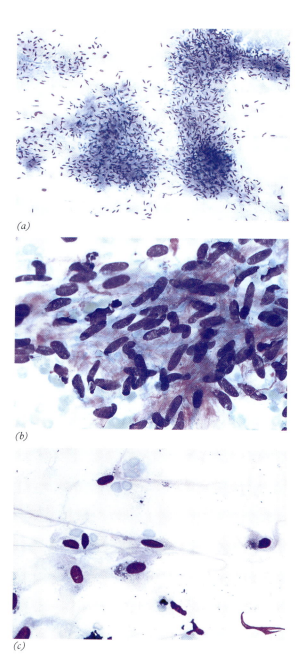

(a)

(b)

(c)

FIBROHISTIOCYTIC TUMOURS

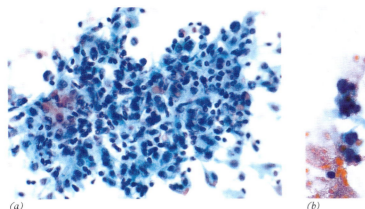

(a)

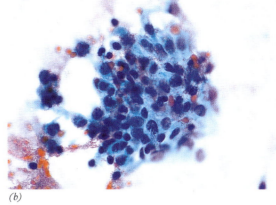

(b)

Fig. 14.4 Benign fibrous histiocytoma

(a) Papanicolaou ×840 (b) ×1260

Aspirates from this condition contain a mixture of fibroblasts, histiocytes, which may contain haemosiderin and inflammatory cells. Lesions are invariably superficial and well-defined as well as relatively small. Clinical information is important in making a diagnosis.

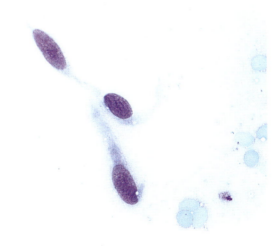

Fig. 14.5 Dermatofibroma

MGG ×1740

A dermatofibroma is a superficial lesion similar to fibrous histiocytoma. It contains sparse elongated fibroblasts with plump nuclei. The absence of inflammatory cells differentiates it from fibrous histiocytoma.

Fig. 14.6 Dermatofibrosarcoma protuberans

(a) MGG ×420 (b) ×1260 (c) ×1260: FNA breast lesion

Dermatofibrosarcoma protuberans is a tumour of borderline malignancy: a benign variant is dermatofibroma and malignant fibrous histiocytoma. It is usually a cutaneous nodule which grows slowly as either a plaque or a nodule and only in late stages protrudes above the skin surface. It is most commonly encountered on the trunk of adult males. Tumour infiltrates along the cutaneous connective tissue structures and commonly recurs if the initial surgery is incomplete.

Tumour cells are spindle and pleomorphic, occasionally resembling histiocytes. Unlike its benign and malignant counterparts, dermatofibrosarcoma protuberans rarely includes an admixture of inflammatory and Touton giant cells (c). Histologically it displays a characteristic storiform pattern which is unfortunately lost on cytological smears. Recurrent tumours tend to have myxoid change and prominent vascular network and may be mistaken for myxoid liposarcoma.

Cytology of dermatofibrosarcoma protuberans includes unexpectedly cellular smears from what clinically appear to be well-defined superficial lesions (a). Cells are usually represented by bare nuclei showing an irregular outline and are haphazardly arranged along fibrin streaks or associated with amorphous background material (b). Mitoses and overt pleomorphism are rare. Background stromal material and bare nuclei, vascular fragments as well as the absence of any cell organization suggest a mesenchymal lesion. Since histogenesis of this tumour is not yet entirely clear (? fibroblastic, ? schwannoma or histiocytic), special stains do not contribute much to the diagnosis. Tumour cells show weak positivity for vascular markers and may be mistaken for angiosarcomas. The cytology report should include a request for (wide) local excision biopsy and histology.

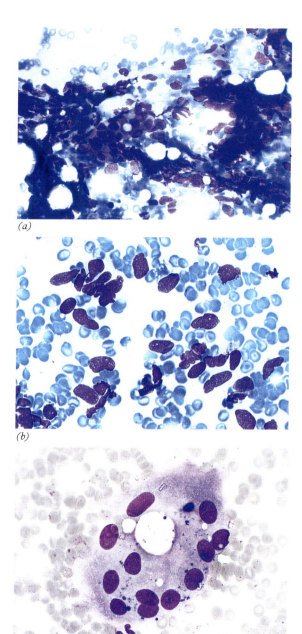

(a)

(b)

(c)

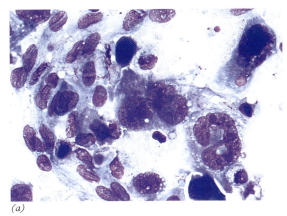

(a)

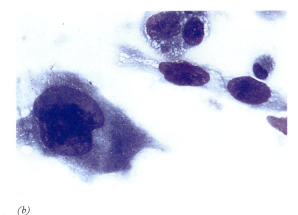

(b)

Fig. 14.7 Malignant fibrous histiocytoma

(a) MGG ×1260 (b) ×1260

Atypical, highly pleomorphic spindle cells admixed with similarly bizarre histiocyte-type cells found in malignant fibrous histiocytoma typically result in relatively cellular smears with most of the cells dispersed and admixed with blood, necrosis and inflammation. All the different histological subtypes appear cytologically as high-grade malignant tumours. Myxoid-type malignant fibrous histiocytomas may have a prominent myxoid background in which the cells are embedded. Spindle cells have fusiform nuclei and elongated, well-defined cytoplasm, whilst histiocyte-type cells are pleomorphic and often multinuclear with prominent nucleoli and vacuolated cytoplasm showing phagocytosis (a, b). Mitoses are frequent.

Differential diagnosis includes metastases of melanoma and anaplastic carcinoma. High-grade malignant peripheral nerve sheath tumour, leiomyosarcoma and pleomorphic liposarcoma may be difficult to distinguish from malignant fibrous histiocytoma.

Myxoid subtype occurs subcutaneously and contains myxoid background matrix and fragments of relatively large vessels within and outside tumour cell clusters. Differentiation from intramuscular myxoma may be difficult. *Intramuscular myxoma* is, in typical cases, a tumour with an abundant myxoid background material containing small clusters and dispersed cells which are fusiform with ovoid or elongated, uniform, benign nuclei and long, slender cytoplasmic processes. Plump cells with round nuclei representing regenerating muscle fibres may be seen.

SMOOTH MUSCLE TUMOURS

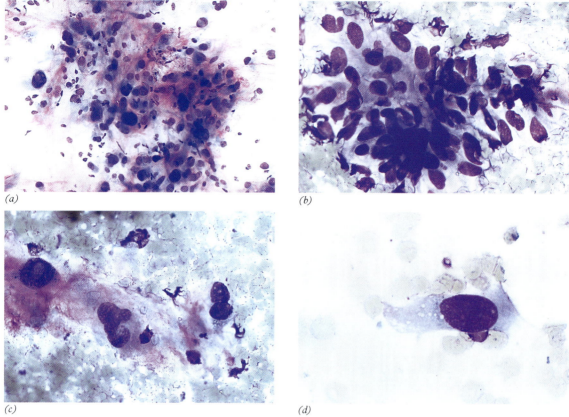

(a)   *(b)*

(c)   *(d)*

Fig. 14.8 Leiomyosarcoma

(a) MGG ×840 (b) ×1260 (c) ×1260 (d) ×1260

FNA of this malignant soft-tissue tumour yields variable cellularity with dominance of mesenchymal background material in which bundles and fascicles rather than single cells are seen (a). Cell pleomorphism varies from mild to bizarre multinucleate cells (b–d). Typical nuclei are oval, blunt, cigar-shaped with nuclear segmentation and intranuclear vacuole (b). Cytoplasmic vacuoles, corresponding to pinocytotic vacuoles, can be seen at the poles of the nuclei (d). Cytoplasm is usually blue to blue-grey in MGG

High grade leiomyosarcoma displays pleomorphism with multinucleated tumour cells and high grade MFH is an important differential diagnosis. Blunt ended, segmented although atypical nuclei and dense cytoplasm are, however, typical of pleomorphic leiomyosarcoma. Immunocytochemistry for muscle-specific markers may reveal the differentiation but further markers (myoglobin) may be necessary to exclude pleomorphic rhabdomyosarcoma.

Differential diagnosis on cytological smears includes ancient neurilemmoma (most common misdiagnosis), leiomyoma, malignant peripheral nerve sheath tumour, malignant fibrous histiocytoma and other high-grade malignant soft-tissue tumours.

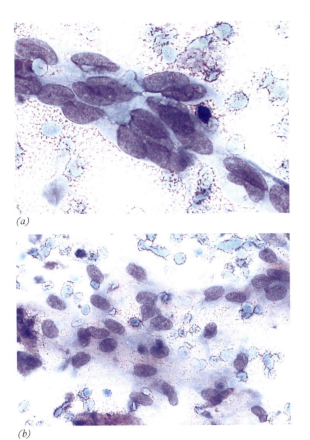

(a)

(b)

Fig. 14.9 Intestinal (epithelioid) leiomyoma

(a) MGG ×1260 (b) ×1260: imprint of gastric tumour

These most frequently occur in the stomach wall. Despite the ulceration of the overlying mucosa, cells can rarely be seen in gastric brushing. These have plump spindle-cell nuclei and poorly outlined cytoplasm (a). Background material is prominent (b).

MALIGNANT TUMOURS OF VASCULAR SPACES

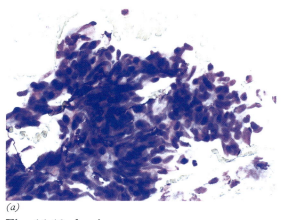

(a)

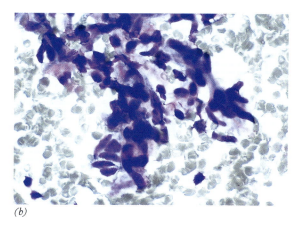

(b)

Fig. 14.10 Angiosarcoma

(a) MGG ×840 (b) ×1260: FNA breast (courtesy of Dr A Rubin)

Angiosarcomas are tumours rarely encountered in FNA smears. This is an example from the FNA breast of a young woman with breast mass. Cytology reveals cellular smears with spindle-shaped cells in clusters with pulled-out ill-defined edges. Individual cells are difficult to characterize due to admixture of mesenchymal background material. They show a haphazard arrangement and are sometimes forming vascular, tram-track structures, connecting aggregates of cells. These are features of high-grade angiosarcoma.

Differential diagnosis includes poorly differentiated carcinoma, dermatofibrosarcoma protuberans (vascular markers may be positive in both) and other soft-tissue tumours. Clinical history and site as well as immunocytochemistry are essential for diagnosis.

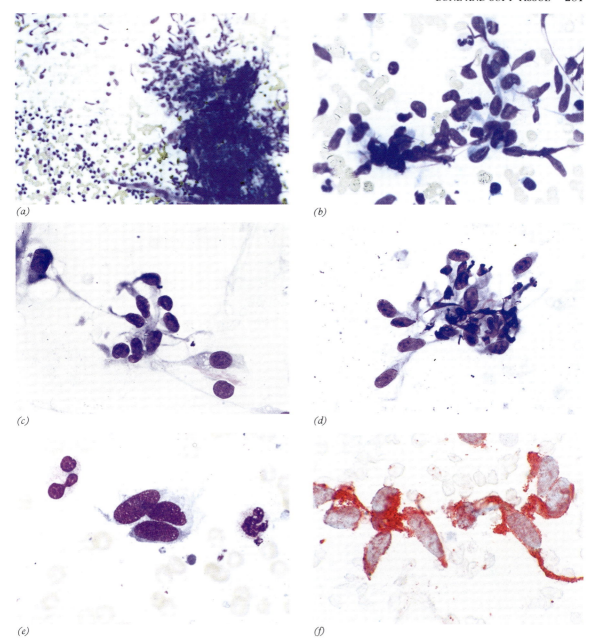

(a)

(b)

(c)

(d)

(e)

(f)

Fig. 14.11 Kaposi's sarcoma

FNA lymph node, HIV positive patient: (a) MGG ×400 (b–d) ×600 (e) ×1000 (f) APAAP: CD 34 ×1000

With the increased number of human immunodeficiency virus (HIV)-related pathology received in the laboratory, Kaposi's sarcoma has become a frequent consideration in the differential diagnosis of lymph node, lung and skin lesions.

Aspirates are usually blood-stained and hypocellular. They may contain tissue fragments of overlapping spindle cells (a) or loosely cohesive clusters of similar cells (b). Individual cells have plump oval nuclei with very little elongated cytoplasm containing vacuoles (c, d, e). Nucleoli may be prominent. Metachromatic stroma may be noted on MGG stain.

In the appropriate clinical setting and with the help of immunocytochemical markers for endothelium (f), diagnosis may be made on FNA material in most cases. Kaposi's sarcoma is an acquired immunodeficiency syndrome (AIDS)-defining diagnosis in HIV-positive patients.

PAEDIATRIC SMALL CELL TUMOURS

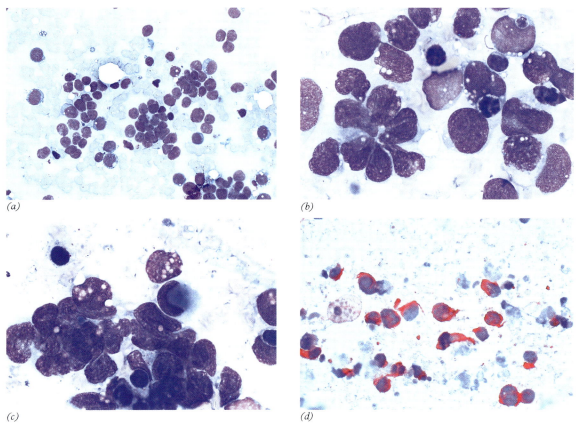

(a)   *(b)*

(c)   *(d)*

Fig. 14.12 Rhabdomyosarcoma

(a) MGG ×420 (b) ×1260 (c) ×1260 (d) APAAP antidesmin ×1260

Smears from rhabdomyosarcoma are cell-rich, composed of small round cells. Distinction between embryonal and alveolar type is difficult and often impossible because of the similar cytological features. Clinically, the distinction between rhabdomyosarcoma and other small blue cell tumours is more important—Ewing's/peripheral neuroectodermal tumour (PNET), lymphoblastic lymphoma/leukaemia and neuroblastoma.

Smears from rhabdomyosarcoma show single cells and aggregates (a). Cells have relatively large nuclei with fine reticular chromatin and a variable number of small irregular, inconspicuous nucleoli. Nuclear folds, lobulated appearance and grooves towards the scanty cytoplasm can be seen. This has prominent vacuolation (b). Occasional cells are spindle, strap or ribbon-like and may have deep blue (May–Grünwald–Giemsa: MGG) or eosinophilic (haematoxylin and eosin: H&E) dense staining cytoplasm at one pole, pushing the nucleus (c). This feature, together with the absence of prominent nucleoli, favours embryonal

rather than alveolar type. Similarly, embryonal type typically contains myxoid tissue fragments, whilst alveolar type contains small rounded cells with circular nuclei, sometimes arranged in acini (b). Distinction is best made on histology of the resection specimen.

Immunocytochemistry shows positivity for antidesmin antibody, which is diagnostic (d). Negative leukocyte common antigen (LCA) and MIC 2 antibodies exclude Burkitt's and Ewing/PNET tumours. This is important, since some PNET tumours can be desmin-positive and also some are MIC 2-negative. Cytoplasmic vacuolation can be seen in both rhabdomyosarcoma and Ewing/PNET as well as lymphomas. Periodic acid-Schiff (PAS) staining is therefore non-specific. The acinar arrangement (b) can mimic rosettes otherwise seen in Ewing's as well as classically in PNET and neuroblastomas. Chromosomal studies show typical translocation t(11;22) in Ewing's and PNET and t(2,13) in alveolar rhabdomyosarcomas.

Fig. 14.13 Ewing's sarcoma/peripheral neuroectodermal tumour (PNET)

(a) MGG ×1260 (b) MGG ×1260 (c) APAAP: MIC2

Ewing's sarcoma and PNET belong to the group of small round cell tumours of childhood and adolescence and share a number of similarities—age, sex, anatomical locations and phenotypic characteristics are cytologically indistinguishable. Both tumours have the same chromosomal abberations [t(11: 22)] and del (22). Both express the MIC 2 gene which can be detected by specific antibody. For all the above reasons Ewing's sarcoma/PNET are considered one entity.

Smears from Ewing's sarcoma/PNET are usually very cellular: cells are arranged in aggregates and singly (a, b). Rosette formation may be prominent (c). Cells are round and polygonal, some with scanty vacuolated, well-defined, granular cytoplasm (which is particularly prominent when cells are suspended in fluids), and others with bare nuclei showing moulding and much smearing artefact. Chromatin is finely granular; nucleoli are inconspicuous.

Immunocytochemistry shows positive staining for MIC 2 antibody, which is diagnostic (c). Desmin is negative (exceptionally some cells may be positive); LCA and epithelial markers are negative; vimentin is positive. PAS staining shows coarse granules in the cytoplasm and overlying the nucleus.

Differential diagnosis includes other small round cell tumours of childhood such as: neuroblastoma, retinoblastoma, medulloblastoma, blastemic nephroblastoma, rhabdomyosarcoma, small cell osteosarcoma and lymphoblastic lymphoma. MIC 2 antibody is diagnostic, although it has been shown to stain other cells, for example of lymphoid lineage, ependymal and endocrine cell and therefore also tumours, such as insulinoma and ependymoma.

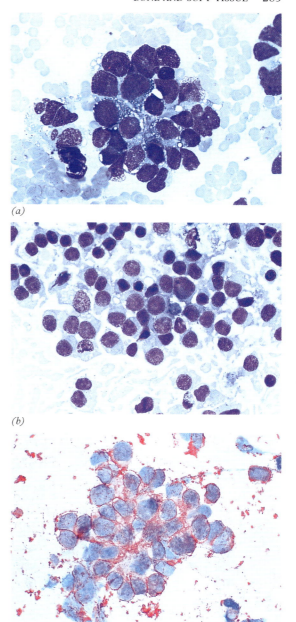

(a)

(b)

(c)

SPINDLE CELL SARCOMAS

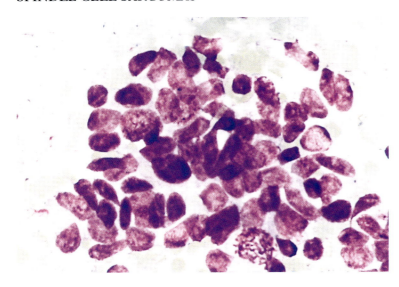

Fig. 14.14 Synovial sarcoma

MGG ×1160: FNA lesion on the dorsal part of the hand (courtesy of Dr Trutin Ostovic)

Soft tissue tumours with predominant spindle cell component are most difficult to diagnose. Synovial sarcoma, along with desmoid, deep seated leiomyoma, fibrosarcoma and haemangiopericytoma, belongs to this group of tumours which are, as yet, not sufficiently characterized on FNA.

Synovial sarcoma frequently shows irregular fragments of tightly packed small ovoid or rounded cells with blunt nuclei. Biphasic tumour pattern is uncommon; cytological appearance of biphasic synovial sarcomas does not always exhibit two distinct cell populations, stromal and epithelial. Biphasic tumours are cell-rich and composed of a mixture of large, ramifying, tightly packed cell clusters and dispersed cells. At the periphery of the clusters the cells can be arranged in acinar-like structures. Cells are usually small to medium-sized with an oval or round blunt nucleus. Cytoplasm is moderate in amount and can be unipolar or bipolar. The nuclear structure is finely granular with small nucleoli. Mast cells are common in both types of synovial sarcoma. Mitoses are common. Cells show positivity for cytokeratins and vimentin and are negative for carcinoembryonic antigen. Monophasic synovial sarcoma contains spindle-shaped cells only and is difficult to distinguish from other high-grade sarcomas, namely malignant schwannoma and haemangiopericytoma.

The differential diagnosis of biphasic synovial sarcoma includes malignant fibrous histiocytoma, epitheliod mesothelioma, glandular schwannoma, Wilms tumour and skin adnexal tumours. Monophasic sarcoma can mimic fibrosarcoma, malignant fibrous histiocytoma, schwannomas, desmoplastic melanoma and desmoplastic carcinoma.

MISCELLANEOUS SOFT TISSUE LESIONS

Fig. 14.15 Pigmented villonodular synovitis (PVNS)

(a) MGG ×210 (b) ×1260 (c) ×1260: synovial fluid

Cellular material from this synovial fluid contained papillary fragments of tissue (a). Cells forming these papillae were ill-defined and haphazardly arranged (b). Some resembled histiocytes and others synovial cells (c). Very few inflammatory cells were noted. The lesion was diagnosed clinically and confirmed cytologically, mainly on the basis of papillary pattern and the blandness of the cells.

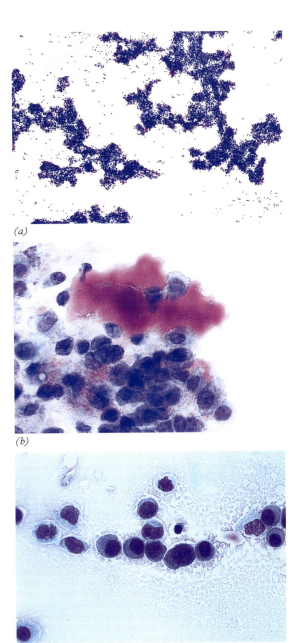

(a)

(b)

(c)

PSEUDOSARCOMATOUS LESIONS

Nodular fasciitis, proliferative myositis and myositis ossificans are often clinically misdiagnosed as sarcoma. Co-operation of clinical data, radiological findings and cytological features usually allows for accurate preoperative diagnosis. All three conditions have plump proliferative fibroblast-like cells, some with ganglion-like appearance. Nodular fasciitis has a myxoid background whilst myositis ossificans has osteoblast-like cells. Proliferative myositis has large rounded cytoplasm-rich cells with a double peripheral nuclei.

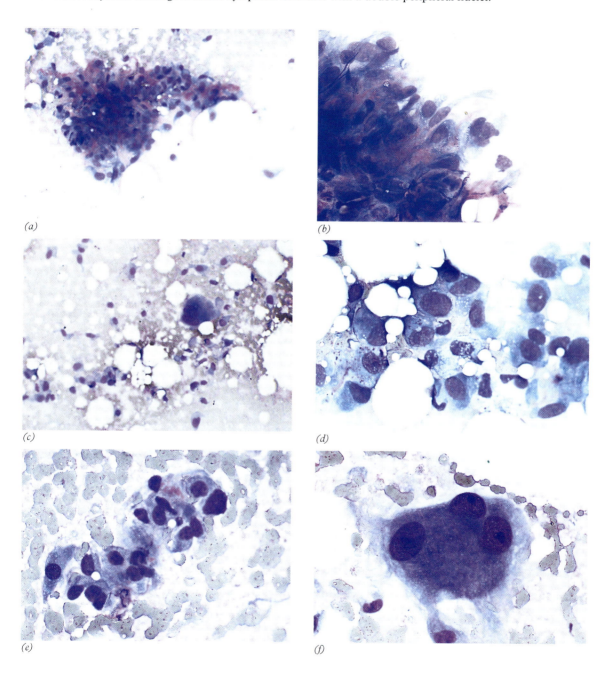

(a)

(b)

(c)

(d)

(e)

(f)

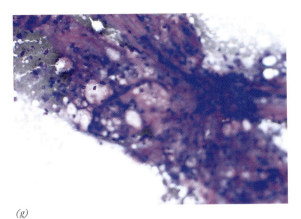

(g)

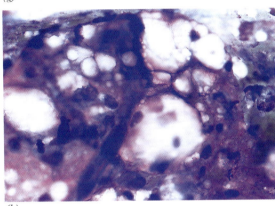

(h)

Fig. 14.16 **Nodular fasciitis** *(illustrations opposite and here)*

FNA subcutaneous lesion, MGG: (a) ×840 (b) ×1260 (c) ×420 (d) ×1260 (e) ×840 (f) ×1260 (g) ×840 (h) ×1260

Aspirates from this subcutaneous lesion in the forearm of a 45-year-old surgeon yielded tenacious material. Smears are cellular with the majority of cells embedded in the myxoid matrix with some fibrillary collagen (a, b). There are also many cells haphazardly dispersed in the background (c). These vary from plump to slender spindle-shaped cells. Some have very large oval nuclei with prominent, sometimes irregular nucleoli and relatively abundant cytoplasm containing fine vacuoles (d). Some cells have distinct basophilic cytoplasm. Occasional large ganglion-type cells are noted, both singly and within large clusters where they may mislead into an overall impression of cell pleomorphism (c, f). Cells are sometimes forming whorls and sheaves along collagen bundles. Adipose tissue cells and fat droplets may form part of the lesion and have prominent vascular pattern (g, h). This may be mistaken for myxoid liposarcoma. The site, clinical history (recent onset, superficial lesion, history of trauma, tenderness) should point to this benign self-limiting condition which can be cured by excision.

BONE

Normal cells

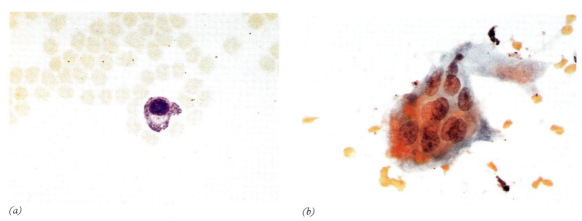

(a)   *(b)*

Fig. 14.17 Osteoblast: osteoclast

(a) MGG ×525: lumbar vertebra; osteoblast (b) Papanicolaou ×525: lumbar vertebra; osteoclast

Two types of bone cells concerned with maintaining the integrity of the skeletal system by continuous dynamic remodelling of bone may be met with in a needle aspiration of bone. Each has a different function which is reflected in its morphology.

The osteoblast, derived from a precursor cell probably of the stromal cell system, synthesizes and secretes osteoid, the non-mineralized extracellular matrix of bone. It is a mononuclear cell of moderate size and has a basophilic cytoplasm which stains less intensely in its central portion due to the presence of a large paranuclear Golgi apparatus. This gives the osteoblast a superficial resemblance to another actively secretory cell, the plasma cell. The latter is smaller in size and has a clock-face nucleus.

The osteoclast is responsible for the resorption of osteoid, and its precursor, like the precursors of other phagocytic cells, is probably of haematopoietic origin. The osteoclast is a large cell, and may contain one or many nuclei, in which form it resembles a giant multinucleated histiocyte. Its cell outline is often indistinct or irregular and, with the Papanicolaou stain, its cytoplasm is generally amphophilic. The nuclei are oval or round, and each contains an eosinophilic nucleolus.

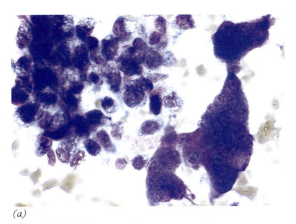

(a)

Fig. 14.18 Giant cell tumour of bone

MGG (a) ×600 (b) ×600 (c) ×600

This lesion has its peak occurrence in the second and third decade and is more common in women. Most frequently it affects the epiphyses of long bones and particularly either knee joint.

Aspirates are cellular with spindle mononuclear cells, singly and in large clusters (a). Cells have oval, regular nuclei and one or two nucleoli. They have well-outlined cytoplasm which may contain vacuoles and granules and has extensions making for variable cell shape (b). Binucleate, trinucleate and characteristic multinucleate cells seen in this tumour appear to be direct transitions from mononuclear forms (c). The multinucleate cells may contain up to 100 nuclei and have abundant cytoplasm resembling osteoclast giant cells.

Differential diagnosis of giant cell tumour is: (a) benign lesions: aneurysmal bone cyst, metaphyseal fibrous defect (non-ossifying fibroma), chondromyxoid fibroma, chondroblastoma, osteoblastoma, osteitis fibrosa cystica and brown tumour of hypeparathyroidism; (b) malignant lesions: osteosarcoma. In practice, aneurysmal bone cyst and osteosarcoma are the most common differential diagnoses of giant cell tumour.

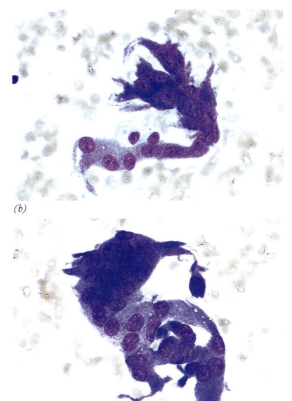

(b)

(c)

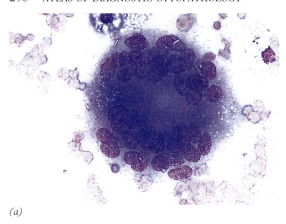

(a)

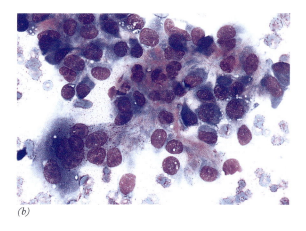

(b)

Fig. 14.19 Aneurysmal bone cyst

(a) MGG ×1260 (b) ×1260

An aneurysmal bone cyst is a solitary intraskeletal cystic lesion occurring most frequently in females in the first two decades of life. The most common sites are metaphyses of long bones and vertebrae. Aspirates characteristically contain much blood and haemosiderin-laden macrophages as evidence of old haemorrhage (a). In addition, multinucleate osteoclast-like giant cells and fibroblast-like spindle cells, similar to giant cell tumour of bone, are seen (b).

Differential diagnosis of bone lesions that may contain giant cells includes: reparative granuloma of jaw, metaphyseal fibrous defect (non-ossifying fibroma), chondromyxoid fibroma, chondroblastoma, osteoblastoma, osteitis fibrosa cystica (brown tumour of hyperparathyroidism) and telangiectatic osteosarcoma.

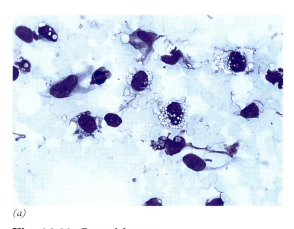

(a)

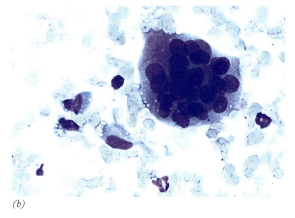

(b)

Fig. 14.20 Osteoblastoma

(a) MGG ×1260 (b) ×1260

Osteoblastoma is a rare tumour which may yield numerous giant cells on aspiration. It also contains osteoblasts which are different from mononuclear cells of a giant cell tumour. Osteoblasts are round cells with eccentrically placed nuclei and vacuolated cytoplasm (a). The intertrabecular matrix contains giant cells (b).

The behaviour of these tumours is different, with a benign to aggressive range. The differential diagnosis includes aneurysmal bone cyst, giant cell tumour, histiocytic fibrous histiocytoma and osteosarcoma.

CARTILAGINOUS TUMOURS
Chondromyxoid lesions

A subgroup of soft tissue lesions may yield a large amount of chondromyxoid stroma (CMS) as part of the aspirate. The most common malignant neoplasm containing CMS is extraskeletal chondrosarcoma followed by myxoid liposarcoma and malignant fibrous histiocytoma. Benign entities include ganglion cyst, myxoma and neurofibroma.

Fig. 14.21 Chondrosarcoma

FNA soft tissue mass: (a) ×400 (b) ×600 (c) ×600

Chondrosarcoma is a tumour of adult age (40–60), the most common sites being pelvis, scapula and upper end of the humerus. The most remarkable feature on the aspirate is the presence of fibromyxoid background material staining deep purple on MGG (a). Well-differentiated chondrosarcoma have prominent matrix and relatively few cells. Uninuclear or binuclear cells may be seen enclosed within this matrix, sometimes in clear lacunae, sometimes poorly discernible due to the density of the background material preventing the penetration of the MGG stain. Toluidine blue may be used to demonstrate nuclei better (b). Wet fixed smears stained with Papanicolaou or H&E show better nuclear detail but may not show appreciable background material. Fragments of capillaries may be seen (c).

Well-differentiated chondrosarcoma cannot reliably be distinguished from a chondroma, in particular a cellular chondroma (periosteal chondroma and chondroma of small peripheral bones). Clinical presentation and radiological appearances should be carefully considered before making a cytological diagnosis.

Poorly differentiated (high grade) chondrosarcomas are more cellular and show binucleation and nuclear atypia. A potential pitfall in diagnosing a poorly differentiated chondrosarcoma, particularly if the smears are stained by H&E or Papanicolaou, is metastatic carcinoma because of cellularity and weak staining of characteristic matrix. Another differential diagnosis is between a chondrosarcoma and chondroblastic osteosarcoma.

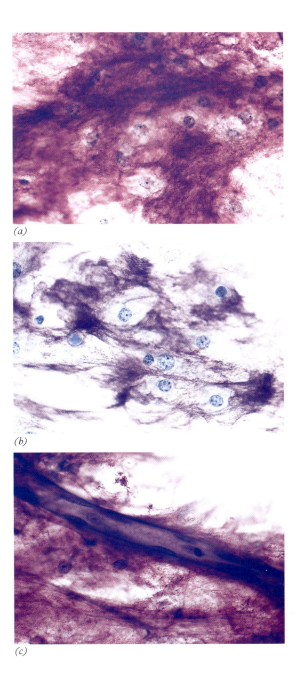

(a)

(b)

(c)

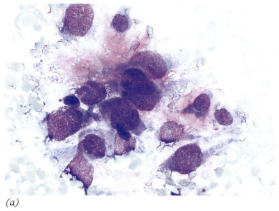

(a)

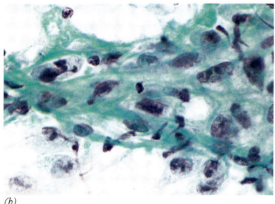

(b)

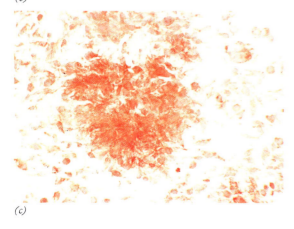

(c)

Fig. 14.22 Osteosarcoma

(a) MGG ×1260 (b) ×525 (c) alkaline phosphatase ×840

This rare but important primary cancer of bone is derived from osteoblasts or possibly osteoprogenitor cells. It affects mainly young subjects, the usual sites being the lower end of the femur or the upper end of the tibia. In the older patient, it is usually a complication of a predisposing disorder such as Paget's disease of the bone or fibrous dysplasia. The case illustrated is of a 56-year-old male with long-standing polyostotic fibrous dysplasia and a recent pathological fracture of the neck of the femur. Large fragments of softish tissue were obtained in a needle aspirate of the fracture site (a). At higher magnification (b) the tissue is seen to consist of pleomorphic cells with ill-defined cell borders, and high nuclear-cytoplasmic ratios. The plump nuclei are markedly variable in shape and size and contain one or several prominent macronucleoli. The preponderance of fusiform or sausage-shaped malignant nuclei and the absence of epithelial-type cell borders is consistent with a diagnosis of sarcoma. The type of sarcoma—whether, for example, an osteosarcoma or a fibrosarcoma—is identified by its characteristic extracellular matrix. Osteoid may be noted on routinely stained preparations (a) and confirmed by alkaline phosphatase stain (c).

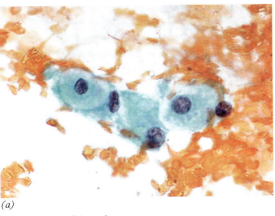
(a)

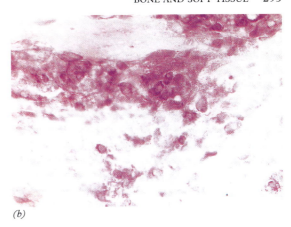
(b)

Fig. 14.23 Chordoma

(a) Papanicolaou ×525: lumbosacrum (b) PAS ×133: same specimen; another smear

A chordoma is a locally invasive, jelly-like tumour which develops from the notochord, essentially an embryonic structure which persists in the adult in the central pulp of the intervertebral discs. Microscopically, the tumour has a characteristic appearance, being composed of large, clear, epithelium-like cells. The nuclei, usually one per cell, occasionally multiple, are small and bland and contain one or two pinpoint nucleoli (a). The abundant cytoplasm contains many intracytoplasmic granules of glycogen and the cells are embedded in a mucoid substance which is also PAS-positive (b). A chordoma may develop from any part of the vertebral canal: the lumbosacrum and the base of the cranium are the commonest sites.

Immunocytochemistry shows that chordoma cells are positive for vimentin as well as keratin, thus distinguishing chordoma from other primary bone lesions.

METASTATIC TUMOURS

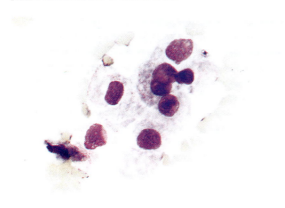
(a)

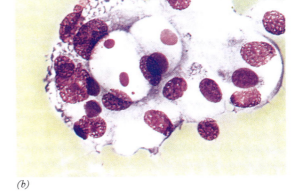
(b)

Fig. 14.24 Metastatic renal cell carcinoma

Papanicolaou ×525: (a) lumbar vertebrum (b) renal aspirate; same case

Bone is a common site of blood-borne metastases and metastatic disease which is much more common than primary cancer is the most frequent indication for FNA cytology. The diagnosis of secondary carcinoma based on recognition of neoplastic epithelial cells is relatively simple. Comparison with the cells of the primary lesion is helpful. The large, circumscribed epithelial cells with abundant clear cytoplasm, relatively small nuclei and prominent nucleoli in (a) are comparable with the cells from a primary carcinoma of kidney (b).

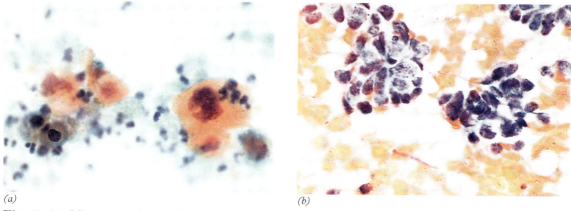

(a) *(b)*

Fig. 14.25 Metastatic bronchogenic carcinoma

Papanicolaou ×525: lumbar vertebra (a) squamous cell carcinoma (b) small cell carcinoma

Bronchogenic carcinoma is one of the commonest sources of metastatic deposits in the skeleton. Micrograph (a) illustrates well-differentiated, large, variable, orangeophilic malignant squamous cells obtained from a vertebra of a male with lung carcinoma.

The cells in (b) are small and virtually filled with nuclei which mould one another and have a 'salt-and-pepper' chromatin. The appearance is so typical of a small cell carcinoma that a bronchogenic origin may be easily deduced from the secondary tumour.

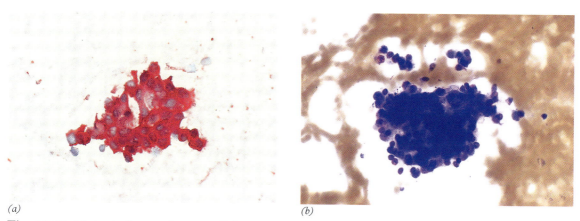

(a) *(b)*

Fig. 14.26 Metastatic carcinoma of the prostate

(a) MGG ×420 (b) APAAP PSAP ×420: bone marrow aspirate

Carcinoma of the prostate may present with bone marrow metastases. Cells are usually small and in tight aggregates (a) with no specific features. The primary origin of the tumour can be confirmed by applying prostate-specific antibodies to the cells (b). In this case, it was a so far unknown primary, so that cytological examination had a major clinical relevance.

HAEMATOPOIESIS

Fig. 14.27 Haematopoietic cells

MGG: lumbar vertebrum (a) ×183
(b) ×720: same smear; another field
(c) ×720: another specimen

Haematopoietic tissue present in the intertrabecular spaces of bone consists of both red and white blood cells in various stages of maturation, and of the platelet-forming megakaryocytes (a). Whilst it is not necessary for the cytopathologist to be able to identify each red and white cell precursor, familiarity with the overall appearance of haematopoietic tissue is required if a misdiagnosis of a small-celled malignancy is to be avoided. The megakaryocyte, with its coarsely reticulate, giant polyploid nucleus (b), needs to be distinguished from a bizarre carcinoma or sarcoma cell. The nucleus of the megakaryocyte is occasionally seen stripped of its cytoplasm (c), and in this form mimics a group of oat cells. Distinguishing features are the indentation and lobulation of the megakaryocyte nucleus rather than moulding of adjacent separate nuclei, its coarsely reticulate chromatin and the absence of any cytoplasm round it.

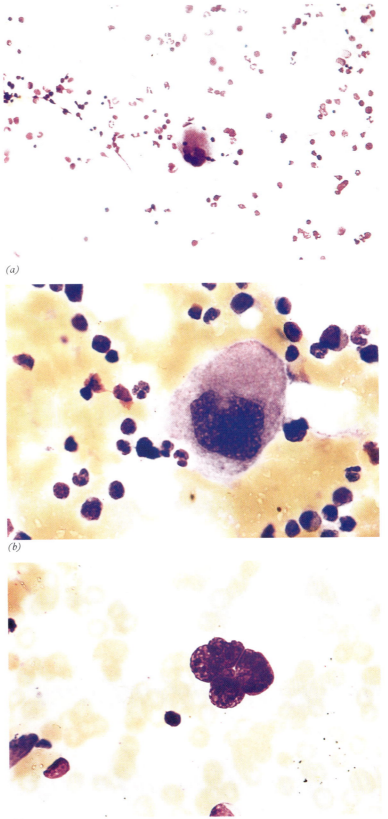

(a)

(b)

(c)

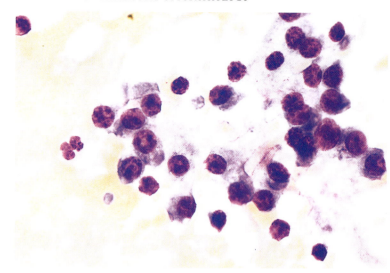

Fig. 14.28 Plasmacytoma

MGG ×720: sacrum

Plasmacytoma, a neoplasm of plasma cells in the marrow, is a localized form of multiple myelomatosis. Unlike the latter, a plasmacytoma is not generally associated with anaemia and hypercalcaemia and gammopathies are either absent or occur in a milder form. The tumour may be single or multiple and produces lytic lesions in bone. Focal collections of neoplastic plasma cells are seen in aspirates of these lesions. The cells may be similar in morphology to normal plasma cells, or they may be larger and less mature, as in the example illustrated.

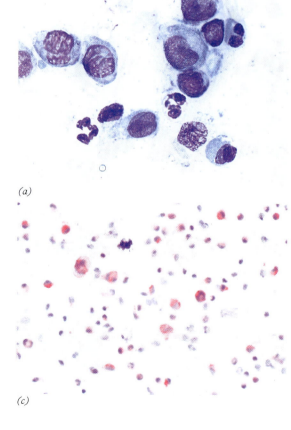

(a)

(c)

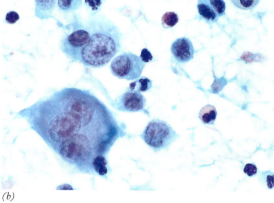

(b)

Fig. 14.29 Langerhans cell histiocytosis/eosinophilic granuloma

(a) MGG ×1260 (b) ×1260 (c) APAAP S100 ×1260: FNA rib lesion

The lesion affects any bone, with a predilection for skull, mandible, ribs, femur, vertebrae and humerus. FNA on low power appears to contain an inflammatory background. On close scrutiny, predominance of eosinophils, occasional giant cells and many typical Langerhans-type histiocytes are noted (a, b). These have characteristic grooved, folded, eccentric nuclei and non-phagocytic, well-outlined cytoplasm reminiscent of epithelioid cells. Cytoplasmic granules may be seen. Charcot–Leyden crystals, a product of eosinophils, may be noted. Immunocytochemistry for S100 protein (c) and electron microscopy detection of Birbeck granules is diagnostic.

15. Cellular changes due to treatment

A variety of therapeutic agents, the most important of which are the anticancer agents, alter the morphology of cells. There is often a loss of the distinctive cytoplasmic features that help in the identification of the cell type. Benign cells may be so altered by ionizing radiation that distinction from malignant cells becomes exacting. Neoplastic cells may show features of complete necrosis, partial degeneration which raises the question of possible or probable viability or may remain virtually unaffected. The success or failure of treatment may be assessed to some degree by the number and the morphological features of tumour cells in a posttreatment specimen. Some of the commoner treatment-induced changes in cell morphology and smear pattern are considered in this chapter.

Fig. 15.1 Radiation effects: polychromasia

Papanicolaou (a) ×183: vaginal smear
(b) ×720: same smear

A Papanicolaou smear of a woman with good response to recent radiotherapy has a dramatic appearance. This is due to marked changes in the tinctorial properties, shape and size of the benign cells.

Benign cells in a vaginal smear taken 6 weeks after completion of a course of caesium for invasive squamous carcinoma of the cervix are illustrated in this and the next three figures.

The immediate impact is of the polychromasia of the cytoplasm and the vividness of the colours (a). The peripheral portion of the cells is essentially basophilic and the central part acidophilic (a, b). The basophilia ranges from bright blue to yellowish green and a corresponding range of shades from salmon pink to apricot is displayed by the acidophilic part of the cells. The nuclei are small and the majority are condensed and hyperchromic.

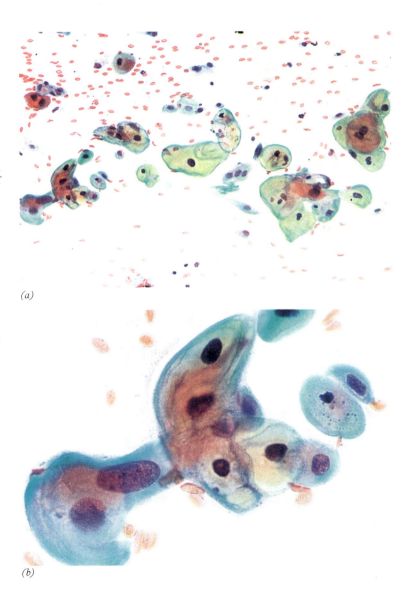

(a)

(b)

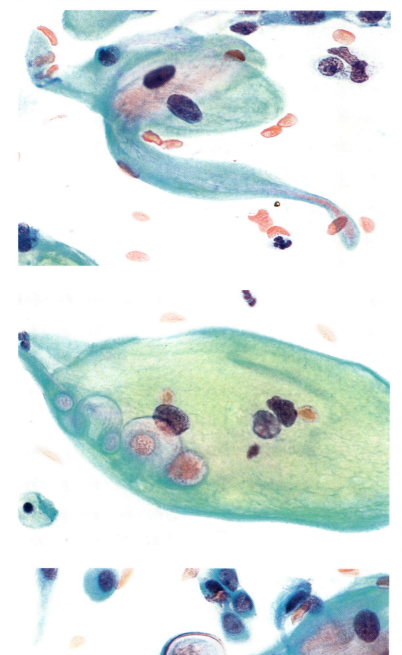

Fig. 15.2 Radiation effects: abnormal shapes

Papanicolaou ×720: same smear as in Figure 15.1

The two cells in this field have tail-like extensions of the cytoplasm which terminate in club-shaped expansions; the cells are similar in appearance to caudate cells frequently met with in well-differentiated squamous cell carcinoma. A suggestion of a Herxheimer spiral is seen in the lower cytoplasmic process. Compare these cells with normal squamous cells (Figs 1.1–1.3) and note their larger size and the substantial increase in the volume of their cytoplasm. The nuclei of irradiated benign cells remain normal in size or enlarge to a lesser extent than the cytoplasm; the nuclear-cytoplasmic ratio is reduced.

Fig. 15.3 Radiation effects: macrocytosis

Papanicolaou ×720: same smear as in Figure 15.1

The increase in the volume of the cytoplasm may be so gross that the cell cannot be assigned to any of the layers of normal stratified squamous epithelium. The giant cell in this micrograph has the ovoid shape of a navicular cell but it extends beyond one high-power field and is several times the size of any normal squamous cell. It also shows two other features commonly met with in irradiated cells—multinucleation and intracytoplasmic vacuoles. The vacuoles may form a fine honeycomb (right) or they may be circumscribed with central zones of condensation or inclusions (lower left).

Fig. 15.4 Radiation effects: vacuolization

Papanicolaou ×720: same smear as in Figure 15.1

A sharply outlined vacuole, especially one with central condensation, may mimic a large intracellular mucin globule. It is seen here in a parabasal squamous cell which has acquired a resemblance to a glandular cell.

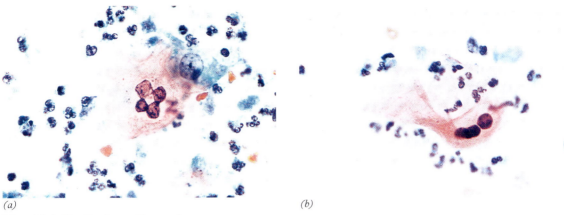

(a)   (b)

Fig. 15.5 Radiation effects: long-term

Papanicolaou ×525: vaginal smear (a) pseudoeosinophilia; multinucleation (b) vacuolization of cytoplasm

As a general rule, the changes induced in benign cells by ionizing radiation gradually fade and disappear within 3–6 months of treatment. In a small proportion of cases, they last longer and in a few individuals, persist for life: marked irradiation effects have been seen by the author in follow-up smears for 10 years or more.

This micrograph illustrates changes seen 12 months after caesium therapy. Polychromasia and macrocytosis are no longer present, but multinucleation (a) and binucleation and some abnormality of shape remain. The size and shape of the cells, the pseudoeosinophilia, loss of definition of cell outline and vacuolization of the cytoplasm (b) are consistent with non-specific inflammatory changes in a mature squamous epithelium: in an older or castrated woman with an atrophic epithelium, it is more often associated with previous radiotherapy.

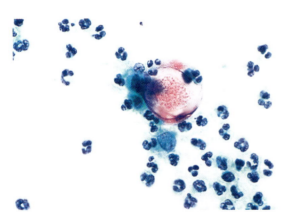

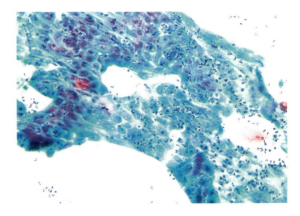

Fig. 15.6 Radiation effects: long-term

Papanicolaou ×525: vaginal smear

The vacuolated parabasal cell with the appearance of a mucin-secreting columnar cell, shown in this micrograph, was seen in a vaginal smear $2\frac{1}{2}$ years after caesium treatment for a cervical squamous carcinoma.

Fig. 15.7 Radiation effects: increased exfoliation

Papanicolaou ×133: vaginal smear

The cellularity of a postradiotherapy smear varies. There is generally an increase of exfoliation during and for some months after the course of treatment. Thereafter the cell yield diminishes and in the majority of cases, the smear reverts to an atrophic pattern and may indeed become quite sparse. In exceptional cases, massive exfoliation may persist for longer periods. This micrograph shows a representative field in a follow-up smear 12 months after treatment. A microbiopsy of hypertrophic immature metaplastic squamous cells is seen together with an occasional mature squamous cell.

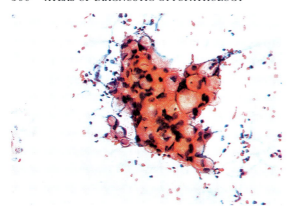

Fig. 15.8 Radiation effects: apparent alteration of cell type

Papanicolaou ×133: vaginal smear

A combination of continued irradiation change and excessive exfoliation may produce a problematical appearance. The vacuolated parabasal cells in a sheet illustrated in this micrograph are suggestive of signet-ring cell carcinoma. They were seen in a vaginal smear over a year after total hysterectomy and radiotherapy for a squamous cell carcinoma. This case illustrates the importance to the cytopathologist of relevant clinical data which should include details of the therapeutic protocols and information about the cell type of the original tumour.

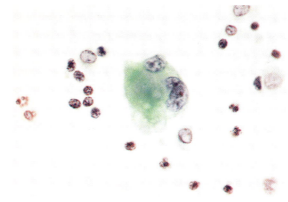

Fig. 15.9 Radiation effects in metastatic malignant cell

Papanicolaou ×525: ascitic fluid

Treatment-induced changes of morphology are also seen in malignant cells which are the target of cancer therapy. Persistence or recurrence of disease is indicated by the presence of intact cells, the nuclei of which retain malignant characteristics. The cell illustrated in this micrograph was one of several present in the ascitic fluid of a woman previously treated for cervical squamous carcinoma by radiotherapy. The finely stippled, irregularly distributed chromatin, characteristic of malignancy, is indicative of metastatic squamous carcinoma despite the peripheral alignment of the nuclei more commonly seen in cells which originate in glandular tissue.

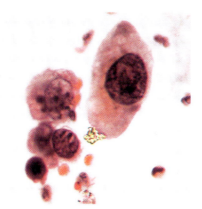

Fig. 15.10 Radiation-resistant carcinoma cells

Papanicolaou ×525: urine

This micrograph illustrates cells which continued to exfoliate after a course of radiotherapy for a carcinoma of the bladder. The coarse granularity of the nuclear chromatin, the high nuclear-cytoplasmic ratio and the anisocytosis are indicative of persistent tumour. The large size of the cell to the right probably reflects minimal radiation change but the majority of the tumour cells appear to be unaffected.

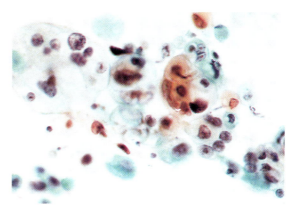

Fig. 15.11 Degenerative changes in irradiated carcinoma cells

Papanicolaou ×525: sputum

The probable viability of severely altered cancer cells seen soon after completion of treatment is difficult to assess. The abnormal cells seen here are derived from a squamous carcinoma of lung treated by deep X-irradiation (DXR). Degenerative changes are seen in the cytoplasm which is swollen in some cells and in the nuclei, several of which are fragmented. Note the three prominent nucleoli near the centre of the field. Large nucleoli may occur in both benign and malignant irradiated cells and are not helpful in the assessment of malignancy in a posttreatment specimen. Continued exfoliation of cells of the type illustrated would be suggestive of persistent tumour.

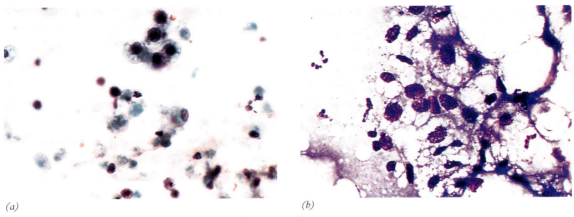

(a)   *(b)*

Fig. 15.12 Necrosis of irradiated carcinoma cells

(a) Papanicolaou ×525: FNA; breast (b) MGG ×525: same specimen; another smear

The patient whose cells are illustrated in this micrograph had been treated for carcinoma of the breast by DXR. There are no viable well-preserved tumour cells in this posttreatment specimen which shows necrotic change. In (a), this consists of pyknotic degeneration in the few recognizable cells and cytoplasmic remnants of disintegrated cells. The cells in (b) are foamy and histiocytic in appearance and the nuclei condensed or crenated.

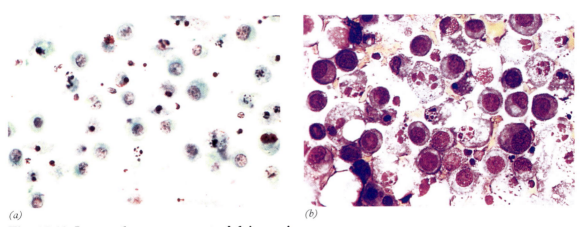

(a)   *(b)*

Fig. 15.13 Incomplete response to Adriamycin

(a) Papanicolaou ×525: pleural fluid (b) MGG ×525: same specimen; another smear

Both well-preserved and necrotic tumour cells are seen in the pleural fluid of a woman treated for disseminated carcinoma of the breast with Adriamycin. The viable tumour cells have basophilic cytoplasm and stippled nuclei (a). A high nuclear-cytoplasmic ratio is evident in the air-dried smear (b). The necrotic tumour cells show either karyopyknosis or karyorrhexis. In addition, there are several tiny fragments of cytoplasm with pinpoint chromatin inclusions such as are seen in apoptosis (see Fig. 1.13).

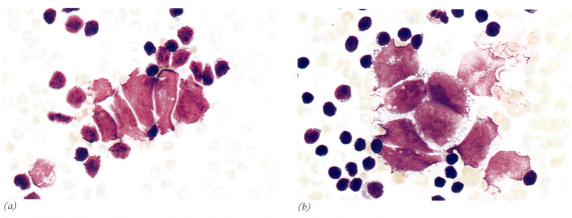

(a)   *(b)*

Fig. 15.14 Chemotherapy-induced change in small cell carcinoma

MGG ×525: pleural fluid (a) pretreatment specimen (b) posttreatment specimen

One effect of combined chemotherapy administered for small cell carcinoma of the lung illustrated above in Figure 3.60 is the emergence of a refractory large cell carcinoma. Another effect which is occasionally met with is a substantial increase in the size of cells with the characteristic morphology of oat cells. Compare the appearance of the tumour cells (a) before and (b) after treatment and note the increase in the volume and vacuolation of the cytoplasm of the posttreatment cells which may mimic non-Hodgkin's lymphoma. The three morphological features of oat cells stained by the May–Grünwald–Giemsa (MGG) method, namely violet coloration, a smudged appearance of the nuclei and fine internuclear clefts, are seen in both specimens.

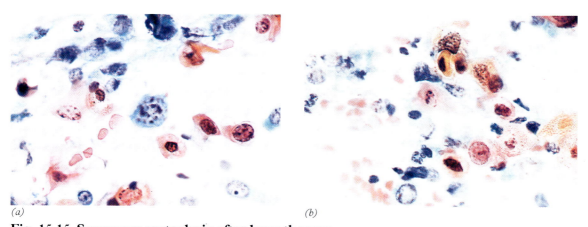

(a)   *(b)*

Fig. 15.15 Squamous metaplasia after laser therapy

Papanicolaou ×525: bronchial brush (a) abnormal shapes (b) dyskeratosis

Two representative fields from a bronchial brush smear obtained after laser treatment for a bronchogenic squamous cell carcinoma are illustrated in these micrographs. The size and shape of the cells seen are similar to that of atypical but benign metaplastic squamous cells with degenerate nuclei (compare with Figs 3.36–3.40).

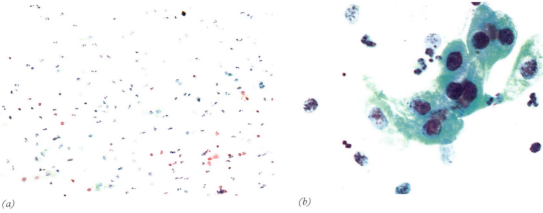

(a)   (b)

Fig. 15.16 Effect of hormones

Papanicolaou ×133: cervical smear; mature squamous cells (b) ×525: same smear; squamous metaplasia

The smear illustrated in these micrographs demonstrates the effect of female sex hormones on the atrophic epithelium of a 55-year-old postmenopausal woman receiving hormone replacement therapy. Maturation of the epithelium is indicated by the abundance of oestrogenized eosinophilic superficial cells and their precursors, the cyanophilic intermediate squamous cells (a). Further evidence of hormone-induced change is provided by metaplastic squamous cells (b) not normally seen in a postmenopausal smear.

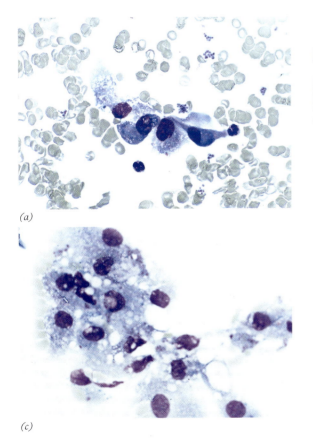

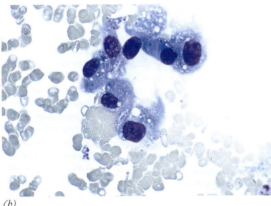

(a)   (b)

(c)

Fig. 15.17 Post surgery/radiotherapy changes: FNA of scar area after surgery and radiotherapy for breast carcinoma, ? recurrence

(a) MGG ×1260 (b) ×1260 (c) ×1260

FNA from indurated area in and around surgical scars is usually performed in order to establish the absence of local recurrence of malignant disease. This case illustrates radiation induced fibroblasts and macrophages with their plump nuclei (a, b). The large amount of cytoplasm present and the relatively sparse cellularity of these aspirates, as well as the absence of pleomorphism, favours benign granulation tissue type reaction.

Index

Abscess
  breast subareolar 55
  liver **199**
Acantholysis 250
Achlorohydria 174
Acinar cell pancreatic carcinoma 185
Acinic cell salivary gland carcinoma **245**
Actinomyces spp. **16,** 17
Actinomycetoma 16
Adenocarcinoma **124**
  breast **125, 145, 146, 152,** 170
  bronchogenic carcinoma **118–121,
    124, 144**
  colon **150, 182**
  liver **206**
  malignant effusions 143, **145, 146,
    149, 150, 151, 152**
  oesophagus **176**
  pancreas **125, 145**
  pancreatic duct **184**
  prostate **219**
  stomach **149, 151, 180–181**
Adenocarcinoma-in-situ (AIS), cervix
  30
Adenoid cystic carcinoma
  breast 67
  respiratory tract **123**
  salivary gland **246**
Adenoma
  pancreas 188
  salivary gland
    monomorphic **239**
    pleomorphic **238–239**
  thyroid
    follicular **264**
    Hürthle cell **268**
Adenosquamous pancreatic carcinoma
  185
Adriamycin incomplete response **301**
Alcoholism
  liver disease-associated ascites 137
  sialosis 237
Allergic bronchopulmonary
  aspergillosis 95
Allergic rhinitis 84
Alpha feto-protein 203
Alveolar epithelial lining 86
Alveolar macrophages 84, **88**
  anthracotic **88**
  cohesive **88**
  fat-laden (lipophages) **89**
  iron-laden (siderophages) **89**
  multinucleated **88**
Alveolar proteinosis **107**
Alveolar rhabdomyosarcoma 272, 282
Amelanotic melanoma, breast
  metastases **82**

Amiodarone, pulmonary toxicity **104**
Anaplastic carcinoma
  large cell of lung **122**
  small cell
    cervix **32**
    lymph node metastases from lung
      233
    thyroid **270**
Aneurysmal bone cyst **290**
Angiolipoma 272
Angiosarcoma **280**
  breast **81**
Anthracotic alveolar macrophages **88**
Antidesmin antibody 282
Apocrine breast carcinoma **77**
Apoptosis, cervical squamous
  epithelium **13**
APUD cells, respiratory epithelium 86,
  113
Arbovirus meningitis 166
Asbestos bodies **92**
Asbestos exposure 163
Ascites fluid 130, 133, 136, 161, 300
  alcoholic liver disease 137
  gallbladder papillary
    cystadenocarcinoma 147
  gastric adenocarcinoma 149, 151
  malignant squamous cells 156
  myeloid metaplasia 139
  ovarian cystadenocarcinoma 145, 147
  ovarian cystadenoma 153
  pancreatic adenocarcinoma 145, 148
  plasmablastic plasmacytoma 159
  serous cystadenoma 153
  Sézary syndrome 159
  transitional cell carcinoma 157
Askanazy cells 261
Aspergilloma 95
Aspergillus flavus 95
Aspergillus fumigatus **95**
Aspergillus niger 95
Aspergillus spp. 95, **96**
Aspergillus terreus 95
Aspirated tablets **103**
Asthma 102
  eosinophilic pleural effusion 138
  mucus 89
  pulmonary eosinophilia 91
Atrophic cervical smear 5, 10
  borderline nuclear changes 20
Atrophic vaginitis **12,** 13

Bacterial meningitis 166
Basal cell adenoma of salivary gland
  246

Basal cell carcinoma (rodent ulcer) 250,
  251
Benign breast lesions **56**
Benign cystic mastopathy *see* Benign
  breast lesions
Benign mammary dysplasia *see* Benign
  breast lesions
Bile 184, 194, 196
Bile duct
  cholangiocytes **197**
  epithelium **194**
  mucinous cystadenoma/
    cystadenocarcinoma **197**
  papillary carcinoma **184**
Bile duct brushings 194, 195
Bile pigment **198**
Bilharziasis *see* Schistosomiasis
Biliary tract **194–197**
Bladder
  reconstruction, intestinal mucosa **212**
  squamous cell carcinoma **211**
  secondary **212**
Bladder washings 207, 210
Blastomyces 93
Bone **288–296**
  haematopoietic tissue 295
Bone cells **288**
Bone tumour
  giant cell **289**
  metastatic **293–294**
  osteosarcoma **292**
  osteoblastoma **290**
Branchial cleft cyst **253**
Breast **52–82**
  benign conditions **53–67**
  collagenous spherulosis 67
  fine needle aspiration **52–53**
  malignant disease **68–82**
  phyllodes tumour **66**
Breast angiosarcoma **81**
Breast calcification 67
Breast carcinoid **80**
Breast carcinoma
  adenoid cystic 67
  adriamycin incomplete response **301**
  apocrine **77**
  with carcinoid features **80**
  ductal **69,** 78
    with Paget's disease of nipple **78**
    with squamous metaplasia **79**
  ductal *in-situ* **70**
  intracystic **70**
  lobular **71, 72**
    in-situ 71, 72
  male breast **79**
  medullary **74**
  metastases

Breast carcinoma *continued*
  cerebrospinal fluid (CSF) 170
  lung 125
  malignant effusions 145, 146, 152
  mucinous 75
  nuclear grading 68, 69
  oestrogen receptor status 80
  papillary 76
  post-radiation cells 301
  post-treatment scar area recurrence
    303
  primary 68
  triple assessment 68
  tubular 73
Breast cyst 57
  apocrine metaplasia 59
  papillary 58
  simple 58
Breast duct carcinoma 69, 78
  with Paget's disease of nipple 78
  with squamous metaplasia 79
Breast duct ectasia 56, 57
Breast duct epithelium 53
Breast fat necrosis 54
Breast fibroadenoma 62–63
  juvenile 64
  lactating breast 65
  in pregnancy 65
Breast fibroadenosis 60
Breast fibrofatty tissue 53
Breast mesenchymal lesions 81
Breast metastatic tumours 80, 82
Breast papilloma 66
Bronchial adenocarcinoma 102, 110
Bronchial brushings 83, 87, 88, 108,
    116, 118, 122, 123, 302
  bronchial lining cells 102, 103
Bronchial carcinoid 115–117
Bronchial epithelium 86
  mucosal hyperplasia 102–103
  regenerative changes 103
Bronchial obstruction 90
Bronchial washings 83, 84, 90, 98, 108,
    110, 112
  bronchial lining cells 102, 103
Bronchiectasis 102
Bronchiole epithelial lining 86
  cuboidal cells 87
Bronchitis, chronic 91, 102
  mucus 89
Bronchoalveolar carcinoma 118, 121
Bronchoalveolar lavage 83, 87, 104, 107,
    121
  flora/fauna 94, 95, 98, 99
Bronchoalveolar lymphocytes 87
Bronchogenic carcinoma 92, 108–123,
    129
  adenocarcinoma 118–121
  bone metastases 294
  large cell anaplastic carcinoma 122
  small cell carcinoma 113–115
    anaplastic carcinoma lymph node
      metastases 233
    chemotherapy-induced change 302
    malignant effusions 154, 155
  squamous cell carcinoma 108–112
    cerebrospinal fluid (CSF)
      metastases 170

laser therapy effects 302
serous effusions 157
Bronchopulmonary trap specimens 83,
    84
Bronchoscopy 108
Bullous pemphigoid 250
Burkitt's lymphoma 161, 231

Caecocystoplasty 212
Caecum carcinoma 182
Calcification, breast 67
Calcifying epithelioma of Malherbe
    (pilomatrixoma) 255
Calcospherite *see* Psammoma body
Candida albicans 94, 96
  cervical smear 15
Candida glabrata 94
Candida guilliermondi 94
Candida krusei 94
Candida parapsilosis 94
Candida spp.
  oesophagus/stomach 174
  respiratory tract 94, 96
Candida tropicalis 94
Carcinoid tumour
  breast 80
  bronchus 115–117
    atypical 115
  liver 201–202
Carcinomatous meningitis 170
Cartilaginous tumours 291
Cat-scratch disease, granulomatous
    lymphadenitis 227
CD30 229
CD45 159
Centroblastic lymphoma 160, 231
Centroblastic-centrocytic lymphoma
    160, 231
Centrocytic lymphoma 160, 231
Cerebrospinal fluid (CSF) 165–172
  benign conditions 165–167
  mycotic infections 167
  neoplasms 168–172
    metastatic carcinoma 170–171
Cervical adenocarcinoma-in-situ (AIS)
    30
Cervical ectopy/erosion 6
Cervical endometriosis 36
Cervical erosion of newborn 6
Cervical intraepithelial glandular
    neoplasia (CIGN) 30, 32
  benign conditions mimicking 33
  see also Endocervical
      adenocarcinoma
Cervical intraepithelial neoplasia 21,
    22–27
  false negatives/false positives 23
  mild dyskaryosis (CIN 1; low grade
      SIL) 21
  moderate dyskaryosis (CIN 2; high-
      grade SIL) 22
  severe dyskaryosis (CIN 3; high-
      grade SIL) 23
    endocervical gland involvement 27
    keratinizing dysplasia 26
    large cell non-keratinizing type 24

pale dyskeratosis 25
small cell non-keratinizing type 27
squamous intraepithelial lesions
    (SIL) 21
Cervical microglandular hyperplasia 34
Cervical polyp 10
Cervical small-cell anaplastic carcinoma
    32
Cervical smear 1–41
  apoptosis 13
  atrophic 5, 10, 20
  atrophic vaginitis 12, 13
  borderline nuclear abnormality 10,
      19, 20
  cervical intraepithelial neoplasia 21,
      22–27
  Döderlein's bacilli 3
  endocervical columnar cells 4
  endocervicitis 12
  endometrial adenocarcinoma 37, 38,
      39
  fallopian tube adenocarcinoma 37
  follicular cervicitis 13
  herpes simplex virus (HSV)-
      associated cell changes 18
  human papilloma virus-associated
      cell changes 19
  inflammatory 10, 11
  intrauterine contraceptive device
      (IUCD)-related changes 8, 10,
      17
  menstrual 8, 9
  navicular cells 3
  ovarian carcinoma 37, 40, 41
  pathogens 14–16, 18–19
  postcoital 9, 10, 13
  pregnancy 10
  reserve cells 6
  squamous cells 2
    hormone replacement therapy
        effect 303
  squamous metaplasia 6, 7, 20
Cervical squamous cell carcinoma
  invasive 29
  microinvasive 28
Cervicitis
  follicular 13
  Trichomonas vaginalis 14
Cervix uteri 1
  endocervical columnar cells 4
  endocervicitis 12
  squamous epithelium 2, 3, 4
  transformation zone 6
    epithelial repair 10, 11
Charcot-Leyden crystals 91, 138, 296
Chemotherapy-induced change 301,
    302
Chocolate cyst 45
Cholangiocarcinoma 195
  extrahepatic 196
  intrahepatic 205
Cholangiocytes 197
Chondroma 291
Chondromyxoid lesions 291
Chondromyxoid stroma 291
Chondrosarcoma 291
Chordoma 293
Chromosomal aberrations 272, 282, 283

Ciliated columnar cells
  bronchial mucosal hyperplasia 102, 103
  respiratory epithelium **86, 87**
Cimetidine 60
Cirrhosis 136, **199**, 203, 237
  transudates 130
Clara cell 86, 118
Coal miner's lung 92
Coccidioides 93
Collagenous spherulosis, breast **67**
Colloid goitre **258**
Colon **182–183**
Colonic adenocarcinoma 173, **182**
  malignant effusions **150**
Colonic brushings 182, 183
Colonic polyp with dysplasia **183**
Cone biopsy
  cervical endometriosis 36
  tubal metaplasia 35
Congestive cardiac failure 130, 132
Corpora amylacea
  bronchopulmonary passages **90**
  prostate secretions **218**
Corpus albicans 1
Corpus luteum 1
Corpus luteum cyst **44**
Coxsackie virus meningitis 166
Cryptococcal meningitis 97
Cryptococcoma 97
Cryptococcus neoformans
  cerebrospinal fluid (CSF) **167**
  respiratory tract samples **97**
Curschmann spiral **90**
Cutaneous T-cell lymphoma 226
Cystic acinar adenocarcinoma of
  pancreas 188
Cystic goitre **259**
Cystic MALT lymphoma of
  mediastinum 231
Cystic mammary dysplasia *see* Benign
  breast lesions
Cystic pancreatic lesions 188
Cytomegalovirus (CMV) **98**

de Quervain (subacute) thyroiditis **260**
Dermatofibroma **275**
Dermatofibrosarcoma protuberans **276**
  breast 81
Dermatopathic lymphadenopathy 226
Desmoid tumour **284**
Diabetes mellitus 237
Döderlein's bacilli **3**
Drug reactions, eosinophilic pleural
  effusion 138
Ductal breast carcinoma 69, 78
  with Paget's disease of nipple 78
  with squamous metaplasia 79
Ductal breast carcinoma *in-situ* 70
Duodenal cells **187**

Echinococcus granulosus (hydatid) **100**
ECHO virus meningitis 166
Embryonal rhabdomyosarcoma 282
Empyema

streptococcal **143**
  tuberculous **142**
Endocervical adenocarcinoma **31, 32**
  invasive 30
  microinvasive 30
Endocervical columnar cells **4**
Endocervicitis **12**
Endometrial adenocarcinoma 13, **37, 38,
  39**
Endometrial cells, menstrual smear **8**
Endometriosis
  cervix **36**
  pleura 142
Endometriotic ovarian cyst 45
Endoscopic retrograde brush cytology
  (ERBC) 184
Endoscopic retrograde
  cholangiopancreatography
  (ERCP) 173, 194
Eosinophilic granuloma **296**
Eosinophilic pleural effusion **138**
Eosinophilic pleurisy, idiopathic **138**
Eosinophils
  Charcot-Leyden crystals **91**, 138, 296
  respiratory tract specimens **91**
Ependymoma **168**
Epithelial pearl
  benign bronchial **85**
  squamous carcinoma of larynx 124
Epithelial-myoepithelial carcinoma of
  salivary gland **248**
Epithelioid leiomyoma **279**
Epstein-Barr virus meningitis 166
Ewing's tumour 272, 282, **283**
Exudates 130
  cancer patients 143

Fallopian tube 1, 130
Fallopian tube adenocarcinoma 37
Familial polyposis coli 183
Fat necrosis of breast **54**
Fat-laden alveolar macrophages
  (lipophages) 89
Female genital tract 1
Ferruginous bodies **92**
Feyrter cell 86, 113
Fibreoptic bronchoscopy specimens
  83–84
Fibroadenoma, breast **62–63**
  juvenile **64**
  lactation **65**
  in pregnancy **65**
Fibrocystic breast disease *see* Benign
  breast lesions
Fibrohistiocytic tumours **275–277**
Fibrolamellar carcinoma, liver **204**
Fibrosarcoma **284**
Fibrous dysplasia 292
Fibrous histiocytoma
  benign **275**
  malignant 277, 291
Fine needle aspiration
  breast 52–53, 303
    aspiration technique 52
    benign conditions 53–67
    clinical history 52

false positive cytology 62
  malignant disease 68–82
  preparation/staining 52
  reporting 52–53
kidney 210, 215–217
liver 197–206
lymph nodes 225, 226–232
  reporting 225
mediastinum 159
ovary 42–51
pancreas 184, 185, 186–193
prostate 218, 219, 220
respiratory tract samples 88, 92, 93,
    98, 102, 104–106
  bronchogenic carcinoma 108–110,
    115, 117, 119, 120
  lymphoproliferative disorders 126,
    127
  percutaneous fibreoptic
    bronchoscopy **83–84**
salivary gland 236–239
  needle tract seeding 236
scrotum 221
soft tissue tumours 269–287
  surgical removal of aspiration
    channel 272
subcutaneous lesions 250, 251, 254
testis 222
thymus 235
thyroid 257, 258–259
  procedure 257, 259
urinary system samples 207
Follicle-stimulating hormone (FSH) 1
Follicular cervicitis 13
Follicular cyst, ovary **42**
  stimulated ovulation **43**
Follicular thyroid adenoma **264**
Follicular thyroid carcinoma 265, 267
  papillary 267
Foreign body granuloma, breast 54
Franzen needle aspiration
  prostate 219
  rectal mucosa **219**
Fungal infection
  breast fat necrosis 54
  respiratory tract 93
  skin lesions 250

Gallbladder papillary
  cystadenocarcinoma **147**
Ganglion cyst 291
Gardnerella vaginalis 10, **15**
Gastric brushings 174, 176–182
Gastric carcinoma 173, 178
  adenocarcinoma **180–181**
  Candida/bacterial colonization 174
  malignant effusions **149**
  signet-ring carcinoma **179**
Gastric leiomyoma **182**, 279
Gastric lymphoma, primary **181**
Gastric mucosa **176**
  intestinal metaplasia **177**
  regenerating **177**
Gastric ulcer
  Candida/bacterial colonization 174
  Helicobacter pylori 174

Gastritis, chronic 177
  intestinal metaplasia 177
  pernicious anaemia 178
Genital tract
  female 1–41
  male 218–224
Germ cell tumours, lymph node
  metastases 234
Germinal inclusion cyst 45
Giant cell tumour
  bone 289
  pancreatic carcinoma 184–185
Giant cells, benign 184
Giant multinucleated alveolar
  macrophages 88
Giardia lamblia 173
Goblet cells
  bronchial mucosal hyperplasia 102,
    103
  respiratory epithelium 86, 87
    mucus 89
Goitre
  colloid 258
  cystic 259
Goodpasture's syndrome 89
Graafian follicles 1
Granuloma, liver 200
Granulomatous lymphadenitis 227–228
Granulomatous sialadenitis (salivary
  gland sarcoid) 244
Granulosa cell tumour 51
Granulosa cells 1
Graves' disease (thyroid hyperplasia)
  263
Gynaecomastia 60

Haemangiopericytoma 284
Haematopoiesis 295–296
Haematopoietic cells 295
Haemophilus influenzae meningitis 166
Haemosiderin 89
  aneurysmal bone cyst 290
  ferruginous bodies 92
  subarachnoid haemorrhage 165
  thyroid cysts 259
Hamartoma, lung 106
Hashimoto's (chronic lymphocytic)
  thyroiditis 261–262, 263, 270
Head and neck swellings 237
Heart failure cells 89
Heart failure, transudates 130, 132
Helicobacter pylori 174
Helminthic infection 91
Hepatic abscess 199
Hepatic carcinoid 201–202
Hepatic granuloma 200
Hepatic metastatic adenocarcinoma 206
Hepatic non-Hodgkin's lymphoma 206
Hepatitis, chronic active 133, 136
Hepatoblastoma 205
Hepatocellular carcinoma 203
  fibrolamellar 204
Hepatocytes 198
Herpes simplex virus (HSV)
  cervical smear changes 18
  penile lesion 218

respiratory tract specimens 98
Herpes zoster 253
  meningitis 166
Histiocytes
  cervical smear 8, 9
  in urine 213
Histoplasma 93
HIV infection/AIDS
  cerebrospinal fluid (CSF)
    Cryptococcus neoformans 167
    non-Hodgkin's lymphoma 169
  granulomatous lymphadenopathy 228
  immunoblastic lymphoma 161
  Kaposi's sarcoma 281
  parotid lymphoepithelial cyst 241
  Pneumocystis carinii 99
Hodgkin cells 229
Hodgkin's lymphoma 225, 229–230
  lung 126, 127
  serous effusions 158
Honeycomb lung (chronic interstitial
  fibrosis) 118
Hormone replacement therapy 303
HTLV I-associated T-cell lymphoma
  162, 231
Human papilloma virus, cervical smear
  19
  borderline abnormality 10, 20
Hürthle cell adenoma 268
Hürthle cells 261
Hürthle papillary thyroid carcinoma 267
Hybernoma 272
Hydatid cyst fluid 100
Hydrocoele 218, 221
Hypoalbuminaemia 130
Hypochlorohydria 174
Hypoproteinaemia 130

Ileal bladder 212
Immunoblastic lymphoma 161, 231
Immunocompromised host
  oesophageal Candida 174
  respiratory opportunistic infection
    93, 94, 95
Infectious mononucleosis 226
Inflammatory conditions
  cervical smear 10, 11
  lung 104–105
  serous effusions 136–143, 140–143
Inflammatory exudates 130
  acute 137
Interstitial airway disease 91
Interstitial fibrosis, chronic
  (honeycomb lung) 118
Intestinal (epithelioid) leiomyoma 279
Intestinal metaplasia
  dysplasia 178
  gastric mucosa 177, 178
Intestinal mucosa, reconstructed
  bladder 212
Intracystic breast carcinoma 70
Intrahepatic cholangiocarcinoma 205
Intramuscular lipoma 272
Intramuscular myxoma 277
Intrauterine contraceptive device
  (IUCD), cervical smear 8, 10, 17

Iron-laden macrophages
  alveolar macrophages (siderophages)
    89
  benign renal cyst fluid 215
Islet cell tumour 185, 193
Islet cells 187

Juvenile breast fibroadenoma 64

Kaposi's sarcoma 234, 281
Keratoacanthoma 250, 252
Kidney 215–217
Kulchitsky cell 86, 113
Kupffer cells 198

Lactation 61
  breast changes 56
  breast fibroadenoma 65
  breast lumps 61
Langerhans cell histiocytosis 232, 296
Large cell anaplastic carcinoma, lung
  122
Larynx, squamous carcinoma 124
Laser therapy effects 302
Left ventricular failure 132
Leiomyoma
  deep seated 284
  intestinal (epithelioid) 279
  stomach 182
Leiomyosarcoma 278
  stomach 182
Leucocyte common antigen (LCA) 282
Leukaemia, acute myeloid 162
Lipoid pneumonia 89
Lipoma 272
  atypical 273
Lipomatous tumours 272–273
Lipophages (fat-laden macrophages) 89
Liposarcoma 273
Liver 198–206
Lobular breast carcinoma 71, 72
Lobular breast carcinoma in-situ 71, 72
Lung hamartoma 106
Lung inflammatory conditions 104–105
Lung metastatic carcinoma 123–129
  adenocarcinoma 124
    breast 125
    pancreas 125
  malignant effusions 144
  renal cell carcinoma 125
Luteinizing hormone (LH) 1
Lymph node hyperplasia 225, 226
Lymph node metastases 233–234
Lymph nodes 225–234
  fine needle aspiration in diagnosis
    225
Lymphoblastic lymphoma 231
  Burkitt-like 161
Lymphocytes, CSF 166
Lymphocytic effusion 136
Lymphocytic thyroiditis, chronic
  (Hashimoto's) 261–262, 263, 270

Lymphoepithelial cyst, salivary gland **241**
Lymphoma
  HTLV I-associated T-cell lymphoma **162**, 231
  immunoblastic **161**
  kidney 217
  lymphoblastic Burkitt-like **161**
  lymphoplasmacytoid type 231
  serous effusions **159**, **160**
  see also Hodgkin's lymphoma; Non-Hodgkin's lymphoma
Lymphomatoid papulosis 256
Lymphoplasmacytoid lymphoma 231
Lymphoproliferative disorders
  lung **126–129**
  serous effusions **158–162**

Macrocytosis, radiation effect 298
Male breast 60
  carcinoma **79**
  gynaecomastia **60**
Male genital system **218–224**
Malignant effusions 130
  adenocarcinoma
    breast **145**, **146**, 152
    colon **150**
    lung **144**
    pancreas **145**
    stomach **149**, **151**
  carcinoma **143**
  malignant squamous cells **156**
    lung carcinoma **157**
  mesonephroid carcinoma of ovary **146**
  mucinous cystadenocarcinoma of ovary **145**
  papillary adenocarcinoma of pancreas **148**
  papillary cystadenocarcinoma of gallbladder **147**
  papillary cystadenocarcinoma of ovary **147**
  rhabdomyosarcoma **158**
  sarcoma **158**
  serous cystadenoma **153**
  small cell carcinoma of lung **154**, **155**
  transitional cell carcinoma **157**
Malignant peripheral nerve sheath tumour (MPNST) 274
Malnutrition
  sialosis 237
  transudates 130
MALT lymphoma
  cystic of mediastinum 231
  salivary gland **242**
  thymus **159**
Mammary carcinoid **80**
Maxillary sinus carcinoma 84
Mediastinum, cystic MALT lymphoma 231
Medullary breast carcinoma **74**
Medullary thyroid carcinoma **269**
Megakaryocytes 295
Melanoma
  amelanotic, breast metastases **82**

cerebrospinal fluid (CSF) **172**
lymph node metastases **234**
skin 250
Meningitis
  carcinomatous 170
  cerebrospinal fluid (CSF) **166**
Meningococcal meningitis 166
Menopause
  breast changes 56
  post-menopausal smear 5
    hormone replacement therapy effect **303**
Menstrual cycle 1, 2, 3
  breast changes 56
Menstrual smear **8**
  histiocytes **9**
Menstruation 8
Merkel cell tumour (neuroendocrine carcinoma of skin) 255
Mesenchymal lesions
  breast **81**
  lymph node metastases **234**
Mesonephroid carcinoma of ovary **146**
Mesothelial cells **131–136**
  active (reactive) forms **132**, **133**, **134**, **135**
  degenerate **135**
    signet ring forms **136**
  in malignant effusions **143**
  mitosis **135**
Mesothelioma 92, **163–164**
  benign 163
  malignant 163, **164**
Metastatic adenocarcinoma **206**
Metastatic breast tumours
  amelanotic melanoma **82**
  carcinoid **80**
Metastatic carcinoma
  cerebrospinal fluid (CSF) **170–171**
  kidney **217**
  lung **123–129**
Metastatic tumours
  bone **293–294**
  lymph node 225, **233–234**
  papillary thyroid carcinoma 267
  salivary gland **249**
  serous effusions **143–158**
    radiation effects **300**
MIC 2 antibody 282, 283
Microfilaria, hydrocoele fluid 221
Mucinous breast carcinoma **75**
Mucinous cystadenocarcinoma
  bile duct **197**
  ovary 50
    malignant effusions **145**
  pancreas 185, **188**, **191**
Mucinous cystadenoma
  bile duct **197**
  ovary 49
  pancreas 188
Mucocoele, salivary gland **244**
Mucoepidermoid carcinoma, salivary gland **245**
Mucus, obstructive airway disease **89**
  corpora amylacea 90
  Curschmann spiral **90**
Mucus-secreting goblet cells 86, **87**
Multiple myeloma, lung **129**

Mumps meningitis 166
Mycobacterium avium-intracellulare 228
Mycobacterium tuberculosis 93
Myeloid leukaemia, acute **162**
Myeloid metaplasia **139**
Myeloproliferative disorders, serous effusions **158–162**
Myositis ossificans 273, 286
Myxoid liposarcoma **273**, 291
Myxoid malignant fibrous histiocytoma 277
Myxoma 291
Myxovirus meningitis 166

Nasal secretions 84
Nasopharyngeal carcinoma, lymph node metastases **233**
Navicular cells **3**
Neck irradiation 237
Nephroblastoma (Wilms tumour) **217**
Nephrotic syndrome 130
Nerve sheath tumour, benign **274**
Neurilemmoma **274**
Neuroendocrine carcinoma of skin (Merkel cell tumour) 255
Neurofibroma 291
Nipple discharge 56, 57
Nocardia 93
Nodular fasciitis 273, **286–287**
Non-Hodgkin's lymphoma 225, **231**
  cerebrospinal fluid (CSF) **169**
  Kiel classification 231
  lung **128**
  metastatic 82, **206**
  salivary gland **242**
  stomach **181**
  thyroid **270**

Obstructive airway disease 89, 90
  mucus **89**
    corpora amylacea **90**
    Curschmann spiral **90**
Oesophageal adenocarcinoma **176**
Oesophageal brushings 174, 175, 176
Oesophageal carcinoma 173
Oesophageal squamous cell carcinoma **175**
Oesophagogastrointestinal tract **173–183**
  endoscopic sampling methods 173
  pathogens 173–174
Oesophagus **174–176**
Oestrogen 1, 6, 20, 60, 303
Oestrogen receptor status, breast carcinoma **80**
Onchocerca 221
Oncocytic carcinoma, salivary gland **248**
Opportunistic respiratory tract infection 93
Oral mucosa in respiratory tract specimens 84, 85
Oral steroid contraceptives 6, 15
Osteoblast **288**, 290

Osteoblastoma **290**
Osteoclast **288**
Osteosarcoma **292**
Ovarian carcinoma 37, 40, 47
    fine needle aspiration 47
    peritoneal washings 47
    psammoma bodies 40, 41
Ovarian cycle **1**
Ovarian cyst
    corpus luteum **44**
    endometriotic **45**
    fimbrial **46**
    follicular **42**
        stimulated ovulation **43**
    germinal inclusion **45**
    neoplastic **47**
    postovulatory luteinized **44**
Ovarian follicles 1
Ovarian granulosa cell tumour **51**
Ovarian mesonephroid carcinoma **146**
Ovarian metastases, malignant effusions **145, 146, 147**
Ovarian mucinous cystadenocarcinoma **50, 145**
Ovarian mucinous cystadenoma **49**
Ovarian papillary cystadenocarcinoma **147**
Ovarian serous cystadenocarcinoma 41
Ovarian serous cystadenoma **47, 153**
    papillary **48**
Ovarian tumours **47**
Ovary 1, 42–51
Ovulation, stimulated 43

Paediatric small cell tumours **282–283**
Paget's disease of bone 292
Paget's disease of nipple **78**
Pancreas **184–185, 186–193**
    acinar cells **186**
    ductal cells **186**
    islet cells **187**
Pancreatic adenocarcinoma
    cystic acinar 188
    metastases to lung **125**
    pancreatic duct 184
    pancreatitis differentiation 189
Pancreatic adenoma 188
Pancreatic carcinoma **184–185, 190**
    acinar cell 185
    adenosquamous 185
    cystic 184
    giant cell 184–185
    mucinous cystadenocarcinoma 185, **191**
    papillary 184
        cystic 185
    reporting 184
Pancreatic duct epithelium **186**
Pancreatic endocrine neoplasms 185
Pancreatic islet cell tumour 185, **193**
Pancreatic juice 173, 184, 194
Pancreatic metastases, malignant effusions **145, 148**
Pancreatic mucinous cystadenocarcinoma 188, **191**
Pancreatic mucinous cystadenoma 188

Pancreatic papillary and solid neoplasm **192**
Pancreatic pseudocyst **188**
Pancreatic retention cyst 188
Pancreatitis **189**
Papillary neoplasms
    bile duct carcinoma 184
    breast carcinoma **76**
    breast cyst **58**
    gallbladder cystadenocarcinoma **147**
    ovarian cystadenocarcinoma **147**
    ovarian serous cystadenoma **48**
    pancreatic adenocarcinoma **148**
    pancreatic carcinoma 184, 188
        cystic 185
    thyroid carcinoma **266–267**
Pelvic inflammatory disease 16
Pemphigus 250
Penile herpes simplex lesion **218**
Penile scrape 218
Percutaneous transhepatic cholangiography 196
Pericardial fluid 144, 161, 162
Pericardium 130
Peripheral nerve sheath tumour **274**
Peripheral nerve tumours **274**
Peripheral neuroectodermal tumour (PNET) **282, 283**
Peritoneal dialysis transudates 130
    malignant lymphoma 160
Peritoneal malignant mesothelioma 163
Peritoneal washings, ovarian carcinoma 47
Peritoneum 130
Pernicious anaemia **178**
    signet-ring carcinoma **179**
Pharyngeal carcinoma 84
Phyllodes tumour **66**
Pigmented villonodular synovitis (PVNS) **285**
Pilomatrixoma (calcifying epithelioma of Malherbe) **255**
Pinealoma **168**
Plasmablastic plasmacytoma **159**
Plasmacytoma 231, **296**
Pleomorphic adenoma, salivary gland **238–239**
Pleomorphic lipoma 272
Pleura 130
Pleural effusion 142, 162
    adenocarcinoma of breast 145, 146
    adenocarcinoma of lung 144
    eosinophilic **138**
    malignant mesothelioma 163, 164
    mesonephroid carcinoma of ovary 146
    serous cystadenoma 153
    small cell carcinoma of lung 154, 155
Pleural endometriosis 142
Pleural fluid 130, 132, 133, 135, 301, 302
    Hodgkin's lymphoma **158**
    malignant lymphoma 160
    malignant squamous cells **156**
    rhabdomyosarcoma 158
    rheumatoid effusion **140–141**
Pneumococcal meningitis 166
Pneumoconioses 92, 118
Pneumocystis carinii 98, **99**

Pneumocytes 86, 118
Pneumonia 102
Polio meningitis 166
Pollen in urine **214**
Polychromasia **297**
Polymorphs, cerebrospinal fluid (CSF) 166
Polyoma virus infection 213
Polyp
    cervix 10
    colon **183**
Postcoital smear 10, 13
    histiocytes 9
Post-menopausal smear **5**
    hormone replacement therapy effect **303**
Postovulatory luteinized cyst **44**
Postpartum smear 5, 6
Pouch of Douglas fluid 131
Pregnancy 6
    breast changes 56
    breast fibroadenoma **65**
    cervical smear 3, 10, 15
Primitive neuroectodermal tumours (PNET) 272
Progesterone 1
Proliferative fasciitis 273
Proliferative myositis 286
Prostate 218
    corpora amylacea **218**
    Franzen needle aspiration 219
Prostate adenocarcinoma **219**
Prostate carcinoma **220**
    bone metastases **294**
Prostate cells **219**
Prostate fluid 219
Psammoma bodies
    ovarian carcinoma 40, 41
    papillary thyroid carcinoma 267
    respiratory tract specimens **91**
    salivary gland adenocarcinoma 247
Pseudo-Meig's syndrome 146
Pseudosarcomatous lesions **286–287**
Puberty 6, 56
Pulmonary alveolar microlithiasis 91
Pulmonary eosinophilia, primary 91
Pulmonary haemosiderosis, idiopathic 89
Pulmonary infarct 135
Pulmonary sarcoidosis 87, **104**

Radiation effects **297–301**
    abnormal cell shapes **298**
    apparent cell type alteration **300**
    carcinoma cells **300**
        degenerative changes **300**
        necrosis **301**
    increased exfoliation **299**
    long-term **299**
    macrocytosis **298**
    polychromasia **297**
    vacuolization **298**
Radiation-resistant carcinoma **300**
Radioactive iodine **271**
Rectal mucosa 219
Red cell precursors 295

Reed-Sternberg cells 126, 127, 158, 229
Renal cell carcinoma 211, **215**, **216**
  bone metastases **293**
  lung metastases **125**
Renal cyst, benign **215**
Renal metastatic squamous cell
    carcinoma **217**
Renal pelvic brushings 210
Renal tract stones 208, 211
Respiratory epithelium **86**
  bronchial epithelial cells **86**
  bronchial mucosal hyperplasia
      102–103
  bronchiolar cuboidal cells **87**
  bronchoalveolar lymphocytes **87**
  ciliated columnar cells **86**, **87**
  goblet cells 86, **87**
  squamous metaplasia **100–101**
    atypical **101**
Respiratory tract 83–129
  benign conditions 84–107
  calcospherite (psammoma body) **91**
  eosinophils **91**
  flora/fauna **93–100**
  handling of pathogens 84
  lymphoproliferative disorders
      126–129
  sample staining methods 84
  sampling techniques **83–84**
Retention cyst, salivary gland 244
Rhabdomyosarcoma 282
  alveolar 272, 282
  cerebrospinal fluid (CSF) **172**
  malignant effusions 158
  salivary gland 249
Rheumatoid disease 130
Rheumatoid effusion **140–141**
Rheumatoid nodule 254
  lung **105**
Rodent ulcer (basal cell carcinoma of
    skin) 250, **251**

Saliva 85
Salivary adenolymphoma (Warthin's
    tumour) **240**
Salivary adenoma
  basal cell 246
  monomorphic **239**
  pleomorphic **238–239**
Salivary duct cell metaplasia 243
Salivary gland **236–249**
  cytological appearances 236
  mucocoele **244**
  normal acini 237
Salivary gland carcinoma **245–249**
  acinic cell 245
  adenocarcinoma 247
  adenoid cystic 246
  epithelial-myoepithelial 248
  mucoepidermoid 245
  oncocytic 248
  papillary 247
Salivary gland lymphoma 242
Salivary gland metastatic tumours 249
Salivary gland rhabdomyosarcoma 249
Salivary lymphoepithelial cyst 241

Sarcoidosis 184
  lung 87, **104**
  salivary gland (granulomatous
      sialadenitis) 244
Sarcoma 272
  malignant effusions 158
Scar cancers 118
  breast carcinoma **303**
Schistosoma haematobium **214**
Schistosoma japonicum 214
Schistosoma mansoni 214
Schistosomiasis 207, 211, **214**
Schwannoma 274
Scrotum 221
Sebaceous epithelial cells 250
Seminoma **223**, 224
  lymph node metastases 234
Serous cystadenocarcinoma of ovary 41
Serous cystadenoma **153**
  ovary 47, 153
Serous effusions **130–164**
  benign conditions 131–143
  centroblastic-centrocytic lymphoma
      160
  centrocytic lymphoma **160**
  exudates 130
  inflammatory disease **136–143**,
      140–143
  lymphoproliferative/
      myeloproliferative disorders
      158–162
  mesothelial cells **131–136**
  metastatic tumours **143–158**
  preparation methods 130–131
  transudates 130
Serous membrane 130
Sertoli cell tumour 222
Sézary syndrome **159**
Sialadenitis **243**
  chronic 237
  granulomatous (salivary gland
      sarcoid) 244
Sialosis 237
Siderophages (iron-laden alveolar
    macrophages) **89**, 215
Signet-ring carcinoma **179**
Silica dust exposure **92**
Simple breast cyst 58
Skin **250–256**
  sebaceous epithelial cells 250
  squamous cell carcinoma 250, **252**
Skin cancer
  basal cell carcinoma (rodent ulcer)
      250, **251**
  melanotic melanoma 250
Skin scrape 250, 251, 252, 253
Small cell anaplastic carcinoma of
    cervix 32
Small cell carcinoma of lung 88, **113–115**
  chemotherapy-induced change **302**
  malignant effusions **154**, **155**
  metastasis 82
    lymph node **233**
  origin 113
  subtypes 113
  treated **115**
Small round cell tumours of childhood
    283

Smooth muscle tumours **278–279**
Soft tissue tumours 269, **269–287**
  chromosomal aberrations 272, 282,
      283
  diagnostic categories 272
  fibrohistiocytic **275–277**
  lipomatous **272–273**
  malignant of vascular spaces **280–281**
  paediatric small cell tumours **282–283**
  peripheral nerve 274
  pseudosarcomatous lesions **286–287**
  smooth muscle **278–279**
  spindle cell sarcomas 284
Spermatocoele 218, **222**
Spermatozoa 218, 220, 222
Spindle cell lipoma 272
Spindle cell sarcoma **284**
Spironolactone 60
Sputum 83, 84, 87, 88, 89, 90, 91, 100,
    101
  bronchial lining cells 102
  flora/fauna 94, 95, 96, 98
  malignant cells 108, 110, 112, 113,
      114, 116, 118, 120, 124, 128
  mucus 89
Squamous cell carcinoma
  bladder 211
    secondary 212
  cells in serous effusions 156, 157
  larynx 124
  lung 108–112, 157
    cerebrospinal fluid (CSF)
        metastases 170
    laser therapy effects **302**
    poorly differentiated **110–111**
    well-differentiated **108–109**
  oesophagus 175
  renal metastases 217
  skin 250, 252
Squamous cells
  upper respiratory tract specimens 84,
      85
  vagina/ectocervix 2, 3, 4
    hormone replacement therapy
        effect 303
Squamous metaplasia
  breast carcinoma 79
  cervical smear 6, 7
    borderline nuclear abnormality 20
    hormone replacement therapy
        effect 303
  respiratory epithelium **100–101**
    atypical **101**
  salivary gland 237
Squamous pearl, benign **85**
Staphylococcal meningitis 166
Stomach **176–182**
Streptococcal empyema **143**
Streptococcal meningitis 166
Subarachnoid haemorrhage **165**
Subareolar breast abscess 55
Subcutaneous lesions **250–256**
Synovial cell sarcoma 272, **284**

T-cell acute lymphoblastic leukaemia
    161

T-cell lymphoma 231
  cutaneous 226
Teratoma
  lymph node metastases 234
  testis, undifferentiated malignant 224
Testicular tumours 218
Testis 222–224
  undifferentiated malignant teratomas
    224
Thymic carcinoma 235
Thymoma 235
Thymus
  fine needle aspiration cytology in
    diagnosis 225
  low-grade MALT lymphoma 159
Thyroglossal cyst 260
Thyroid 257–268
  colloid goitre 258
  cystic goitre 259
  fine needle aspiration cytology
    (FNAC) 257
  fine needle aspiration procedure 257,
    259
Thyroid adenoma
  follicular 264
  Hürthle cell 268
Thyroid carcinoma
  anaplastic 270
  follicular carcinoma 265, 267
  lymph node metastases 233
  medullary 269
  papillary 266–267
Thyroid cellular "solid" nodules 257,
  263
  follicular adenoma 264
  follicular carcinoma 265
Thyroid hyperplasia (Graves' disease)
  263
Thyroid insufficiency 237
Thyroid lymphoma 270
Thyroid radioactive iodine effect 271
Thyroiditis, subacute (de Quervain) 260
Toxoplasma lymphadenopathy 227, 228

Tracheal epithelial lining 86
Transbronchial biopsy 83
Transitional cell carcinoma 209, 210,
  211
  malignant effusions 157
  papillary 209
Transitional cells, urinary tract see
  Urothelial cells
Transudates 130
  cancer patients 143
Treatment-induced changes 297–303
  chemotherapy effects 301, 302
  hormone therapy 303
  radiation effects 297–301
Trichomonas vaginalis 14, 207
Tuberculosis 118, 184
  breast fat necrosis 54
  empyema 142
  granulomatous lymphadenitis 227
  lymphocytic effusion 136
Tuboendometrioid metaplasia (TEM)
  35
Tubular breast carcinoma 73
Tzanck cells 250
Tzanck test 250

Ulcerative colitis 183
Umbrella cells 207, 208
Upper respiratory tract
  benign squamous pearl 85
  oral mucosal squamous cells 84, 85
Ureteric brushings 208
Urethra, male, squamous cell neoplasia
  211
Urinary system 207–217
  sampling techniques 207
Urinary tract 207–214
  transitional cell carcinoma 209, 210,
    211
  papillary 209
  transitional cells 207, 208

umbrella cells 207, 208
Urine 207, 208, 209, 211–214, 216, 218,
  220, 300
  contaminating pollen 214
  histiocytes 213
Urothelial cells 207, 208
  reactive 208
  viral cytopathia 213
Urothelium
  transitional cells 207
    reactive cells 208
  umbrella cells 207, 208
Uterus 1

Vagina 1
  squamous epithelium 2
Vaginal smear, radiation effects 297,
  298, 299, 300
Vaginitis
  atrophic 12, 13
  Trichomonas vaginalis 14
Vascular space malignant tumours
  280–281
Villous adenoma
  biliary tract 195
  colon 183
Viral infection
  meningitis 166
  skin lesions 250
  urothelial cells 213
von Hippel-Lindau disease 188
Vulva 1
Vulvovaginitis 15

Warthin's tumour (salivary
  adenolymphoma) 240
Wegener's granulomatosis 91, 130, 184
White cell precursors 295
Wilms tumour (nephroblastoma) 217